FRONTIERS OF INFECTIOUS DISEASES
NEW STRATEGIES IN PARASITOLOGY

FRONTIERS OF INFECTIOUS DISEASES

NEW STRATEGIES
IN PARASITOLOGY
PROCEEDINGS OF AN INTERNATIONAL SYMPOSIUM
SPONSORED BY GLAXO RESEARCH,
BROCKET HALL, HERTFORDSHIRE
22–25 APRIL 1989

EDITED BY

KEITH P. W. J. McADAM

Wellcome Professor of Tropical Medicine
Department of Clinical Sciences
London School of Hygiene and
Tropical Medicine
London

ORGANIZING COMMITTEE

K. P. W. J. McADAM,	**P. K. PETERSON**,	**J. VERHOEF**,	**S. R. NORRBY**,	**H. C. NEU**,
London	Minneapolis	Utrecht	Lund	New York
United Kingdom	USA	Netherlands	Sweden	USA

CHURCHILL LIVINGSTONE
EDINBURGH LONDON MELBOURNE AND NEW YORK 1989

Distributed in the United States of America by Churchill Livingstone Inc., 1560 Broadway, New York, N.Y. 10036, and by associated companies, branches and representatives throughout the world.

First Edition 1989

ISBN 0-443-04257-8

British Library Cataloguing in Publication Data
New strategies in parasitology.
1. Man. Parasitic diseases
I. McAdam, K. P. W. J. II. Series
616.9′6
ISBN 0-443-04257-8

Library of Congress Cataloging-in-Publication Data
New Strategies in parasitology: proceedings of an international symposium, Brocket Hall, Hertfordshire, 22–25 April 1989 / edited by K.P.W.J. McAdam.
    p. cm. — (Frontiers of infectious diseases)
  ISBN 0-443-04257-8
  1. Medical parasitology—Congresses. I. McAdam, K. P. W. J. (Keith P. W. J.) II. Series.
  [DNLM: 1. Parasitic Diseases—congresses. WC 695 A244 1989]
QR251.A33 1989
616.9′6—dc20
DNLM/DLC
for Library of Congress 89-22105
                  CIP

Printed in Great Britain by Bell and Bain Ltd., Glasgow

Preface

This book provides the record of a meeting in the magnificent setting of Brocket Hall, Hertfordshire, England between 22 and 25 April, 1989. The meeting was the second in an ongoing series on Frontiers of Infectious Diseases, this year devoted to New Strategies in Parasitology. A group of 40 internationally recognized scientists and clinicians of different disciplines, approximately half from Europe and half from the United States, met for three days to discuss recent advances in their areas of research and to speculate about future directions in the subject of Parasitology. Even though there have only been two in the series so far, the first on New Antiviral Strategies and this second one on parasitology, the Brocket Hall meetings have clearly established themselves as a most desirable addition to the calendar of academic meetings on infectious diseases. The proceedings are scheduled to be published within six months of the meeting so that others can share the papers presented and summaries of the discussions by leading investigators in the field.

The meeting focused on parasites causing significant morbidity and mortality in man and domestic animals worldwide. Not only have the basic sciences of molecular genetics and immunology contributed to the understanding of parasitology, but working on parasitic diseases has contributed significantly to our better understanding of basic biological mechanisms. This meeting emphasized how findings at the cellular level have enhanced our understanding of the host–parasite interaction and helped to explain the diverse pathology and epidemiological patterns of parasitic disease. Ultimately, such studies will reveal the potential for rational parasite control strategies, development of vaccines and design of chemotherapeutic agents.

The complexity and sophistication of host–parasite interactions at the cellular level are exemplified by the African trypanosome. The ability to evade the host immune response by systematically changing their surface antigens (VSGs) is now a classic example of immune evasion by parasites. David Barry (Glasgow, UK) explained the genetic control mechanisms underlying the switching of VSGs by the trypanosome and Michael Ferguson (Dundee, UK) gave a detailed account of how the VSGs are anchored to the trypanosome membrane. The three-dimensional structure of the glycosylphosphatidylinositol (GPI) anchors has been defined by n.m.r. spectroscopy and such anchors are now known to be widely used by parasitic protozoa. Furthermore, the core regions of the GPI anchor appear to be highly conserved in eukaryote cells.

Several presentations at the meeting discussed vaccine development. Cestode vaccines have been developed for veterinary practice and the empirical approach has been highly successful within a short time frame, as described by Mike Rickard (Melbourne, Australia). On the other hand, a systematic logical approach is advocated for human parasites and this has inevitably yielded slow progress but great understanding of the mechanisms underlying host–parasite interactions. Robin Anders (Melbourne, Australia) revealed that intraspecies variation of merozoite surface antigens (MSAs) is expressed on the surface of infected erythrocytes. This antigenic variability may explain why acquisition of effective immunity to malaria is a protracted process in endemic areas where many different clonal populations of *Plasmodium falciparum*, expressing different MSAs, co-exist. Pierre Druilhe (Paris, France) emphasized the problems underlying the development of an effective malaria vaccine and highlighted the need for further characterization of antigens expressed during the hepatic stage of malaria parasite development, as potential immune targets for a vaccine. Georges Grau (Geneva, Switzerland) described the development of a valuable new mouse model for cerebral malaria, implicating tumour necrosis factor (TNF or cachectin) in the pathogenesis of this major lethal complication of malaria.

Richard Locksley (California, USA) described recent developments in the understanding of the immune system in relation to experimental leishmaniasis. Subsets of T-helper cells produce different patterns of cytokines so that the outcome of a parasitic infection is likely to depend on which of these two arms of the immune system is preferentially stimulated. Jacques Louis (Lausanne, Switzerland) continued this theme, presenting further evidence that antibodies to specific cytokines can be administered to infected animals as part of the therapeutic strategy for clearing infection with leishmaniasis.

Daniel Colley (Tennessee, USA) described regulation of T cell function in schistosome infection by antibodies produced as part of the polyclonal antibody response, commonly observed in patients suffering from parasitic diseases. This idiotype regulation of T cell function might be particularly important in regulating the response of children exposed to maternal idiotype or anti-idiotype antibodies during fetal development, which might modify the response of the child to later infection. Anthony Butterworth (Cambridge, UK) described his elegant field studies of schistosomiasis in Kenya where evidence for blocking antibodies has been found. Carlos Gitler (Rehovot, Israel) described the role of the plasma membrane in the parasite response to stress and illustrated this in relation to his studies on entamoeba histolytica. Unfortunately, Jonathan Rothbard's paper on the interaction of peptides with the major histocompatibility complex could not be presented but has been included in the proceedings.

The advent of the AIDS epidemic has given fresh relevance to parasitology and position papers presented current research on opportunistic parasitic infections. Several previously rare organisms have become everyday words including *Pneumocystis* and *Cryptosporidium*. Walter Hughes (Tennessee, USA) emphasized the extent of the problem due to *Pneumocystis carinii* pneumonia in AIDS patients: in terms of morbidity this infection is expected to exceed that due to all other infectious diseases in the USA by the early 1900s. Elmer Pfefferkorn (New Hampshire, USA) described the development of anticoccidial drugs that may be beneficial for the treatment of toxoplasmic encephalitis. Bill Current (S. Carolina, USA) reviewed his development of the in vitro culture system for *Cryptosporidium* and animal models for this opportunistic diarrhoeal pathogen.

Recent advances in immunology, molecular biology and pharmacology still need to be turned into effective products for the treatment and prevention of diseases that affect a large proportion of the population of the world. Strategies for the implementation of health care by targeting parasitic diseases were discussed by Ken Warren (New York, USA). The parasitic diseases affecting so much of mankind continue to require our urgent attention as scientists, physicians and health care decision makers and this meeting highlighted exciting developments in the science and clinical practice of parasitology.

I would like to thank the speakers and discussants for their excellent contributions and timely preparation of manuscripts. We acknowledge the generous support of Glaxo Research in promoting these annual meetings on Frontiers in Infectious Diseases. Without the enormously efficient organization of Carolyn Bennet and the support of Grahaem Brown and Richard Sykes at Glaxo Group Research these meetings would not be half as attractive as they have become. Finally, I would like to thank Helen Jackson of Glaxo who provided a useful summary of the meeting.

K.P.W.J.M.
1989

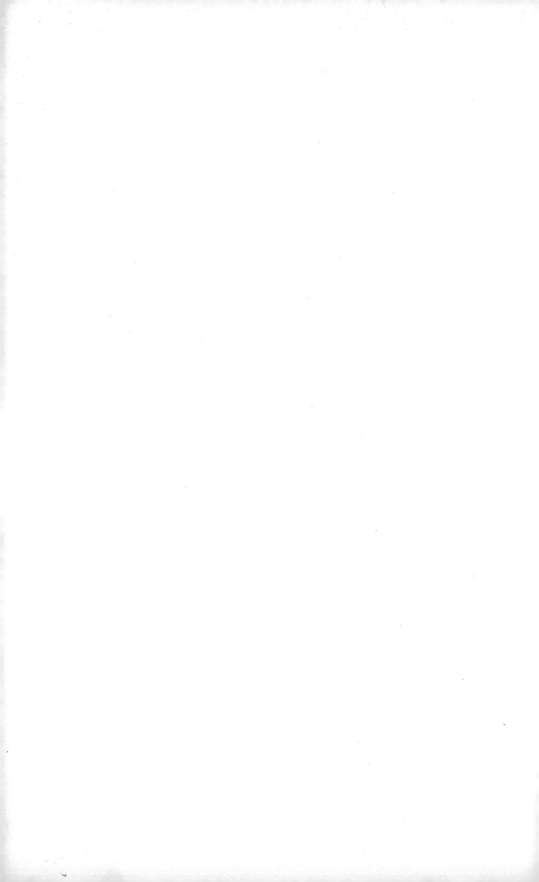

List of participants

ANDERS, Robin F, The Walter & Eliza Hall Institute of Medical Research, University of Melbourne, Australia

BARRY, J David, Institute of Genetics and Wellcome Unit of Molecular Parasitology, University of Glasgow, United Kingdom

BLACKWELL, Jennie M, Department of Medical Parasitology, London School of Hygiene and Tropical Medicine, United Kingdom

BRITTON, Sven, Department of Infectious Diseases, Karolinska Institute, Roslagstulls Hospital, Stockholm, Sweden

BUTTERWORTH, Anthony E, Department of Pathology, University of Cambridge, United Kingdom

CAPRON, André, Centre d'Immunologie et de Biologie Parasitaire, Institut Pasteur, Lille, France

CAPRON, Monique, Centre d'Immunologie et de Biologie Parasitaire, Institut Pasteur, Lille, France

COLLEY, Daniel G, Veterans Administration Medical Center and Vanderbilt University, Nashville, United States of America

CURRENT, William L, Infectious Disease and Fermentation Products Research, Lilly Research Laboratories, Indianapolis, United States of America

DAVID, John R, Department of Tropical Public Health, Harvard School of Public Health, Boston, United States of America

DOCKRELL, Hazel, Department of Clinical Sciences, London School of Hygiene and Tropical Medicine, United Kingdom

DRUILHE, Pierre, Department of Biomedical Parasitology, Institut Pasteur, Paris, France

FERGUSON, Michael A J, Department of Biochemistry, University of Dundee, United Kingdom

GITLER, Carlos, Department of Membrane Research and Unit of Parasitology, Weizmann Institute of Science, Rehovot, Israel

GRAU, Georges E, Department of Pathology, WHO-Immunology Research and Training Centre, University of Geneva, Switzerland

HART, Tony A, Department of Medical Microbiology, University of Liverpool, United Kingdom

HOLDER, Tony A, National Institute for Medical Research, Mill Hill, London, United Kingdom

HOMMEL, Marcel, Department of Tropical Medicine and Infectious Diseases, Liverpool School of Tropical Medicine, United Kingdom

HUDSON, Leslie, Biochemistry and Cellular Science Department, Glaxo Group Research Ltd, London, United Kingdom

HUGHES, Walter T, Department of Infectious Diseases, St Jude Children's Research Hospital, Memphis, United States of America

KEUSCH, Gerald T, Division of Geographic Medicine and Infectious Diseases, New England Medical Center, Boston, United States of America

KOVACS, Joseph A, Critical Care Medical Department, National Institutes of Health, Bethesda, United States of America

LANE, Richard, Department of Parasitology, London School of Hygiene and Tropical Medicine, United Kingdom

LOCKSLEY, Richard M, Department of Medicine, University of California, San Francisco, United States of America

LOUIS, Jacques A, Institute of Biochemistry, WHO-Immunology Research and Training Centre, University of Lausanne, Switzerland

McADAM, Keith P W J, Department of Clinical Sciences, London School of Hygiene and Tropical Medicine, United Kingdom

MAIZELS Rick, Department of Pure and Applied Biology, Imperial College of Science, London, United Kingdom

NEU, Harold C, Division of Infectious Diseases, Columbia University, New York, United States of America

NORRBY, S Ragnar, Department of Infectious Diseases, University of Lund, Sweden

OGILVIE, Bridget, Wellcome Trust, London, United Kingdom

PEREIRA, Miercio E A, Division of Geographic Medicine and Infectious Diseases, New England Medical Center, Boston, United States of America

PETERS, Wallace, Department of Medical Parasitology, London School of Hygiene and Tropical Medicine, United Kingdom

PETERSON, Phillip K, Department of Medicine, Hennepin County Medical Center, Minneapolis, United States of America

PFEFFERKORN, Elmer R, Department of Microbiology, Dartmouth Medical School, Hanover, United States of America

PIERCE, Raymond, Centre d'Immunologie et de Biologie Parasitaire, Institut Pasteur, Lille, France

RICKARD, Mike D, School of Veterinary Science, University of Melbourne, Australia

ROTHBARD, Jonathan B, ImmuLogic Pharmaceutical Corporation, San Francisco, United States of America

TAKLE, Garry B, Department of Molecular Biology, Wellcome Biotech, Beckenham, United Kingdom

TARGETT, Geoffrey A T, Department of Medical Parasitology, London School of Hygiene and Tropical Medicine, United Kingdom

Van der PLOEG, Leonardus H T, Department of Genetics and Development, Columbia University, New York, United States of America

VERHOEF, Jan, Department of Clinical Microbiology, University Hospital, Utrecht, The Netherlands

WARREN, Kenneth S, The Maxwell Foundation, Maxwell Communications Corporation, New York, United States of America

Contents

Plenary Lecture IV
Chairman: *Jan Verhoef*

Plenary Lecture I

Chairman: K. P. W. J. McAdam

1. A success in veterinary parasitology: cestode vaccines

M. D. Rickard

INTRODUCTION

The theme of this book emphasizes advances being made and problems faced in medical parasitology research. Parasites are a major problem in veterinary medicine, and many of the difficulties associated with drug resistance and in developing prophylactic vaccines are shared with medical parasitology. A huge amount of research is being devoted to developing recombinant DNA or synthetic peptide vaccines for important animal parasites, and information which can be usefully applied to studies on human parasites can be derived from such work. Substantial progress has recently been made in the area of anti-tick and anti-tick fever vaccines, but the most spectacular success thus far achieved has been in the field of vaccines against infection with the larval (metacestode) stages of tapeworm parasites. Several of these cestodes have direct relevance to human parasitology because they are important public health problems. This paper describes the development of a recombinant vaccine for a larval cestode parasite.

BACKGROUND

The most important cestodes with respect to their public health significance and economic importance belong to the family Taeniidae. The adult tapeworm parasites occur in the small intestine of their mammalian carnivorous or omnivorous final hosts (Fig. 1.1), and the mammalian intermediate host becomes infected by ingesting eggs from faecal contamination by the final host. The larval stages which develop in the tissues of their mammalian intermediate hosts can cause serious ill-health. Larval cestodes of public health and economic importance are illustrated in Figure 1.2. *Taenia solium* causes cysticercosis in man, and when the larval cysticercus stages are located in the central nervous system, this disease can be incapacitating or even fatal. *Echinococcus granulosus* larval cysts (hydatid) develop mostly in the liver and lungs of sheep and cattle but can also develop in man causing unilocular hydatid disease, which often necessitates multiple operations to effect a cure. *Echinococcus multilocularis* causes alveolar echinococcosis in man, and the parasite cysts proliferate in a tumour-like fashion in the liver with a

3

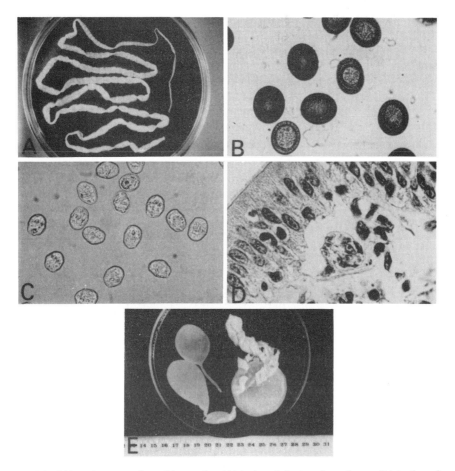

Figure 1.1 Life-cycle stages of taeniid cestodes. (A) is the adult stage from the small intestine of the final host. Eggs (B) released from segments passed in the faeces are ingested by the intermediate host and hatch releasing the oncosphere stage (C). The activated oncosphere penetrates the small intestine (D) and migrates via venules or lymphatics to its tissue location, where it develops into a mature infective larva (e.g. *T. hydatigena* (E)). The final host is infected by ingesting uncooked tissue containing the larval stage. The oncosphere (C) is a rich source of antigens which stimulate host-protective immunity in the intermediate host

usually lethal outcome. *Taenia saginata* occurs as an adult tapeworm in man, and the cysticercus stage in cattle causes substantial economic wastage. *T. ovis* and *T. hydatigena* in sheep are also of economic importance. Some species of the family Taeniidae which infect laboratory animals have been useful as experimental models for those infecting man and domesticated animals such as *T. taeniaeformis* in mice and *T. pisiformis* in rabbits. In addition, *E. granulosus* and *E. multilocularis* can infect some laboratory rodents.

Immunity in the mammalian intermediate hosts of taeniid cestodes plays a central role in regulating their natural transmission (Gemmell 1987). Almost complete immunity develops rapidly after infection, and although not life-long, persists if stimulated by occasional ingestion of eggs. This high level of immunity has made larval cestodes attractive candidates for the development of vaccines to

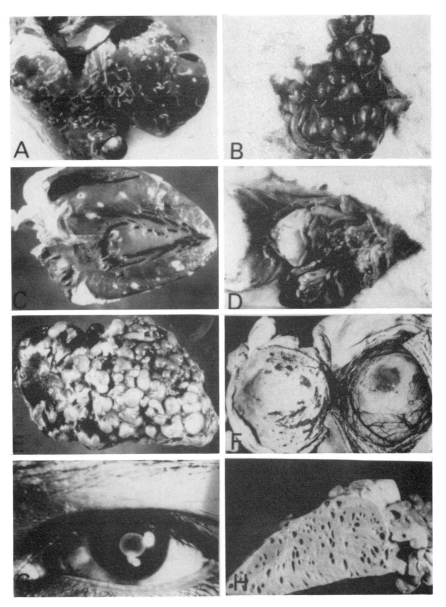

Figure 1.2 Important larval cestodes. Economically important species: (A) *T. hydatigena* migratory tracks in sheep liver, (C) *T. ovis* or *T. saginata* in sheep or cattle heart respectively, (E) *E. granulosus* cysts in sheep liver, (H) *T. solium* in pig muscle. Human infections: (F) *E. granulosus* cranial hydatid cyst (Begg et al 1957), (G) *T. solium* cysticercus in the eye (reproduced courtesy of A Flisser). Laboratory models: (B) *T. taeniaeformis* in mouse liver, (D) *T. pisiformis* in rabbit peritoneal cavity

assist in their control. Conventional methods for control of these parasites have been by prevention of infection and/or treatment of the definitive host, thereby reducing contamination of the environment with tapeworm eggs. As a result, many intermediate host animals are never exposed to infection early in life and so have never developed immunity. Chance contamination of the environment can result in massive infection, or 'cysticercosis storms', especially with the larger *Taenia* spp. which are prolific egg producers (Gemmell 1987). Under such circumstances, a vaccine to replace immunity acquired by natural infection of the intermediate host is necessary for effective control.

STUDIES ON VACCINATION AGAINST LARVAL CESTODES

Past studies on vaccination against larval cestodes have been extensively reviewed (Williams 1979, Rickard & Williams 1982) and effective vaccination has been described for *T. saginata* in cattle, *T. ovis* and *T. hydatigena* in sheep, *T. pisiformis* in rabbits and *T. taeniaeformis* in mice and rats. More recent publications have demonstrated vaccination against *E. granulosus* in sheep (Heath et al 1981, Osborn & Heath 1982), *T. multiceps* in sheep (Edwards & Herbert 1982, Verster & Tustin 1987) and *T. solium* in pigs (Molinari et al 1983). In general, antigens prepared from the oncosphere stage have been the most effective in stimulating immunity against challenge infection with eggs (Fig. 1.3), and it has been shown that:

1. Sheep and cattle can be vaccinated against infection acquired by grazing on contaminated pasture (*T. ovis*, *T. saginata*).

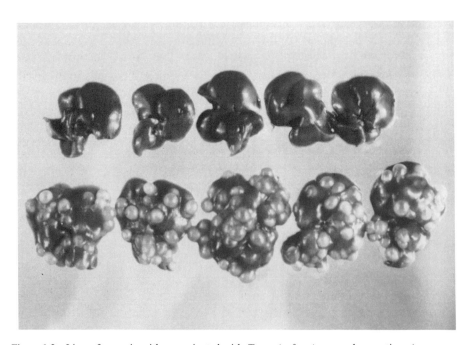

Figure 1.3 Livers from mice either vaccinated with *T. taeniaeformis* oncosphere antigen (upper row) or sham-vaccinated and killed 28 days after challenge infection with 250 *T. taeniaeformis* eggs each. The oncosphere antigen has stimulated almost absolute immunity against the challenge infection (Reproduced by courtesy of M W Lightowlers)

2. Vaccination of sheep and cattle in late pregnancy allows the passive transfer of immunity to their offspring via colostral antibody (*T. ovis* and *T. saginata*).
3. When Freunds' incomplete adjuvant is used, a single vaccination gives significant protection for 12 months (*T. ovis*).

These results suggest that vaccination against infection with these parasites should be feasible under normal farm management conditions, and this has been demonstrated with *T. saginata* infection in cattle (Rickard et al 1982). The major stumbling block in commercial development of anti-cestode vaccines has been in securing a cheap, plentiful supply of antigen. It is simply not feasible to rely upon supplies of adult worms from dogs and humans to provide oncosphere antigens for this purpose. Furthermore, the eggs of species such as *E. granulosus* and *T. solium* are dangerous to personnel required to handle them.

The advent of recombinant DNA technology provided a potential means for overcoming the problem of antigen supply. The host-protective activity of *T. taeniaeformis* oncosphere antigens includes protein components (Lightowlers et al 1984), suggesting that production of protective oncosphere antigens should be possible using recombinant DNA methods. Some preliminary studies have been carried out with *T. taeniaeformis* (Bowtell et al 1984, 1986) and *T. ovis* (Howell & Hargreaves 1988). Bowtell et al (1984, 1986) expressed a selection of clones from a λAmp3 *T. taeniaeformis* metacestode cDNA library as β-galactosidase (β-gal) fusion proteins. These fusion proteins were recognized by antisera to both metacestode- and oncosphere-stage antigens but stimulated no host-protective effect in vaccinated mice. Howell & Hargreaves (1988) prepared a cDNA library in the pEX series of plasmids using mRNA extracted from adult *T. ovis* tapeworms. Recombinants expressing antigenic determinants as β-gal fusion proteins were selected using antibodies in serum from sheep infected with *T. ovis*. Some fusion proteins were shown to correspond with native antigens (92.5–180 kD) present in adult and oncosphere stages of *T. ovis*, but trials on the host-protective nature of purified fusion proteins have not been reported.

It is important to ensure as far as possible that antibodies used to screen recombinant *E. coli* are known to be directed against putative host-protective antigenic epitopes. Monoclonal antibodies are attractive candidates for this purpose and Harrison & Parkhouse (1986) produced a mouse monoclonal antibody against *T. saginata* oncospheres which passively protected calves against infection. The monoclonal antibody was used to affinity-purify a host-protective antigen from oncospheres (Harrison et al 1986) but further experiments using this monoclonal antibody have not yet been reported. Lightowlers et al (1984) used sodium deoxycholate-polyacrylamide gel electrophoresis (DOC-PAGE) to identify a restricted subset of *T. taeniaeformis* oncosphere antigens (designated DOC FII) which stimulated significant protective immunity in mice. Attempts to further separate the four major antigens in DOC FII and identify a single host-protective component were unsuccessful (Lightowlers et al 1986). A cDNA expression library prepared in λgtll from *T. taeniaeformis* oncosphere mRNA was screened using a rabbit anti-DOC FII serum (Johnson & Cougle unpublished results). Several clones which were selected were expressed as β-gal fusion proteins for vaccination experiments in mice. None of these fusion proteins stimulated significant levels of host-protective immunity, even though fluorescent antibody studies using rabbit antibodies to the cloned antigens demonstrated antigenic specificities internally and on the surface of *T. taeniaeformis* oncospheres.

PRODUCTION OF A RECOMBINANT *T. ovis* VACCINE

In 1986 our laboratory undertook a collaborative project with Coopers Animal Health (NZ) Ltd and the New Zealand Ministry of Agriculture and Fisheries to produce a recombinant vaccine to prevent infection with *T. ovis* in sheep. The successful outcome of this research has been reported by Johnson et al (1989). In preliminary experiments (G B L Harrison & D D Heath unpublished results) Western blots of *T. ovis* oncosphere antigen reacted with sera from sheep immunized with immature *T. ovis* eggs (induces no protective immunity) and mature *T. ovis* eggs (induces strong protective immunity) showed strong recognition by antibodies in sera of immune sheep of antigens in the M_r range 47–52 kD. Sera from sheep previously infected with *T. ovis* oncospheres, and from lambs which had fed on their colostrum, as well as sera from sheep immunized with oncospheres solubilized in sodium dodecyl sulphate (SDS), also reacted strongly in Western blots with oncosphere antigens having the same relative mobilities.

The host-protective nature of the 47–52 kD antigens was examined more directly by solubilizing oncospheres in SDS, separating the antigens by poly-acrylamide gel electrophoresis (SDS-PAGE) and immunizing lambs with a region of the gel containing the 47–52 kD polypeptides (Johnson et al 1989). Immunized lambs were significantly protected (98%) against a challenge infection with *T. ovis* eggs. Furthermore, Western blots of oncosphere antigen which had been reacted with sera from the immunized lambs detected antibody reponses to the 47–52 kD antigens, as well as to other components within the gel cut-out region. Rabbit antibodies specific for the 47–52 kD region were prepared by affinity purification on nitrocellulose from a rabbit anti-*T. ovis* oncosphere serum and used as probes for identifying *T. ovis* cDNA clones in *E. coli* (Johnson et al 1989).

Hatched and activated oncospheres of *T. ovis* were used as the source of mRNA for constructing a cDNA library because it has been shown that they secrete potent host-protective antigens (see references in Rickard & Williams 1982). The *T. ovis* oncosphere cDNA library constructed in λgtll was screened with the affinity-purified antibodies, and two fusion proteins, β-gal-45W and β-gal-45S, purified from selected clones, were tested in vaccination trials in sheep (Johnson et al 1989). Host-protective immunity was not stimulated despite the fact that sheep immunized with the β-gal fusion proteins produced antibodies which reacted with native oncosphere antigens at 47–52 kD, corresponding to the region of the gel from which the original antibody probe had been affinity-purified.

It was possible that the β-gal fusion proteins failed to stimulate host-protective immunity due to unfavourable interaction between the β-gal or β-gal fusions and the host immune system, so that a different expression system was tested (Johnson et al 1989). A series of plasmid vectors has been recently developed which expresses antigens as fusion proteins with the enzyme glutathione S-transferase (GST) of *Schistosoma japonicum*. The vector chosen for these experiments was pSj10ΔBam7Stop7, a precursor of the pGEX-1 vector (Fig. 1.4) (Smith & Johnson 1988). The 45W and 45S cDNA were sub-cloned into this vector and expressed fusion proteins purified by affinity-purification using glutathione agarose (Figs 1.4, 1.5). The expressed fusion proteins GST-45W and GST-45S were tested in an immunization trial and the results showed that GST-45W stimulated significant (approximately 70%) host-protective immunity by comparison with the GST controls. Western blots of oncosphere antigen probed with sera from vaccinated sheep showed that antibodies to native antigens in the 47–52 kD region were produced by sheep inoculated with both fusion proteins. A further vaccination trial employed different adjuvants and doses of GST-45W (Johnson et al 1989). GST-45W at all dose levels in oil, FCA or saponin adjuvants induced significant levels of protective immunity, and a total dose of 50 μg of GST-45W in saponin gave 94% protection. The complete nucleotide sequence of 45W cDNA has been deduced (Johnson et al 1989) and encodes a sequence of 238 amino acids, giving a calculated molecular weight of 25 830 D.

The reason for the failure of *T. ovis* 45W to vaccinate sheep when injected as a C-terminal fusion with β-gal compared with the success of the C-terminal GST fusion is unknown. Some fusions with β-gal have been described as poor immunogens (Winter et al 1986) but in the experiments described by Johnson et al (1989) β-gal-45W generated antibodies to the native protein. It is not known which parts of the recombinant GST-45W polypeptide are immunogenic, and it is possible that protective epitopes of the *T. ovis* portion of the molecule are hidden when expressed as a C-terminal fusion with β-gal. Another possibility is that antigen solubility is important. Most C-terminal β-gal fusions are very insoluble, and in this instance the β-gal-45W was solubilized in SDS. The GST fusion was soluble in aqueous buffers, so that SDS treatment, which was shown to destroy its host-protective effect (Johnson et al 1989), was not necessary. Qualitative differences in the immune response of sheep to the two types of fusion protein cannot be discounted, although production of IgG_1 antibodies was stimulated by both β-gal and GST fusions (G B L Harrison unpublished results).

It is not known at this stage whether the *T. ovis* polypeptide encoded by 45W will stimulate protective immunity in the absence of the GST moiety. The parasite-encoded portion of the fusion protein differs substantially in molecular weight from the native parasite antigen. The remainder of the molecule may be made up of further polypeptide, carbohydrate, lipid, or a combination of these. Clones extending beyond the 5′ end of the 45W cDNA sequence have not been isolated (K L O'Hoy unpublished results), although the upstream regions do not appear to be necessary for effective vaccination. It is likely that the protective determinant(s) of GST-45W is conformational because dissociating conditions reduced its protective capacity (Johnson et al 1989).

The yield of fusion proteins with the pSj10ΔBam7Stop7 vector using standard bacterial cultures in 1-litre glass flasks was of the order of 2 mg. Several procedures are under investigation to increase the yield of antigen. A series of refinements of the vector is now available commercially and should give higher levels of expression than pSj10ΔBam7Stop7 which was a prototype of the pGEX vectors. In addition, two of the vectors, pGEX-2T and pGEX-3X, allow for enzymatic cleavage of the parasite-encoded polypeptide from the GST (Smith &

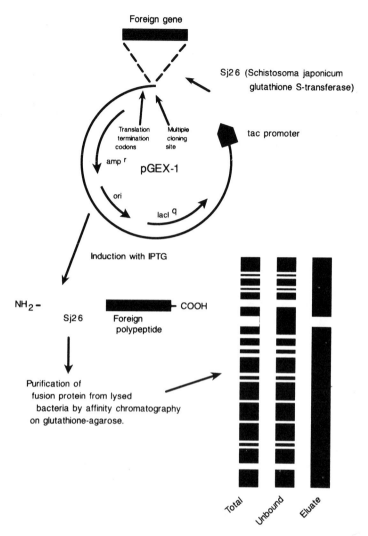

Figure 1.4 Illustration of pGEX-1 vector and purification of glutathione S-transferase–parasite antigen fusion protein (Reproduced by courtesy of D Smith and G F Mitchell)

Johnson 1988). The GST-45W fusion protein is soluble, but unstable (Fig. 1.5), and further modifications of the vector or the 45W cDNA are being explored to enable a more stable product to be expressed. Use of different adjuvants may also enhance the immunogenicity of GST-45W, and recently Craig & Zumbuehl (1988) reported encouraging results with *T. pisiformis* antigens incorporated into liposomes.

Studies on the nature of the native antigen and its location on, or in, the oncosphere should help to clarify the way in which the immune response affects the parasite. In this regard it would be most helpful to be able to clone a host-protective antigen of *T. taeniaeformis* oncospheres to use as an experimental model. A search of the *T. taeniaeformis* oncosphere cDNA library for 45W homo-

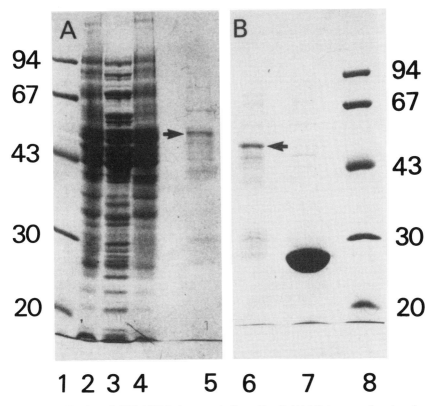

Figure 1.5 Purification of GST-45W fusion protein from *E. coli*. (A) Mini preparation; lane 1, molecular weight markers, lane 2, whole bacterial lysate solubilized in SDS and urea, lane 3, bacterial supernatant after sonication, lane 4, urea and SDS-solubilized bacterial pellet after sonication, lane 5, eluate from glutathione-agarose beads, purified GST-45W arrowed. (B) Large-scale preparation; lane 6, purified GST-45W, lane 7, purified GST from vector alone, lane 8, molecular weight markers

logues has been unsuccessful, and GST-45W does not confer host-protective immunity against *T. taeniaeformis* infection in mice (K L O'Hoy unpublished results). This supports data showing that *T. ovis* oncosphere antigen does not protect mice against *T. taeniaeformis* infection and vice versa (D D Heath unpublished results). A new approach is being undertaken in which antibodies collected by acid elution from the insoluble portion of a sonicate of *T. taeniaeformis* oncospheres (a potent host-protective material) have been used to screen a *T. taeniaeformis* oncosphere cDNA library in pGEX-1. Fusion proteins from several selected families of clones (some of which react with anti-DOC FII) are currently being tested in vaccination trials in mice (A Ito unpublished results).

RECOMBINANT VACCINES FOR OTHER SPECIES OF CESTODE

Many studies have demonstrated that oncosphere antigens of various taeniid cestode species can stimulate cross-protection (Rickard & Williams 1982). It is

11

possible, therefore, that antigens closely related to the *T. ovis* 45W native protein exist in other important species found in man and animals such as *E. granulosus, T. solium* and *T. saginata. T. ovis* 45W cDNA could be used to screen oncosphere cDNA libraries of these other species for homologous sequences, thereby providing a means for rapid development of vaccines against them.

STAGE-SPECIFIC IMMUNITY

Many early studies on cestode vaccines (see Rickard & Williams 1982) suggested that different developmental stages of larval cestodes stimulated qualitatively different immune responses. The most important models in this regard have been *T. taeniaeformis* in mice and *T. pisiformis* in rabbits where both the oncosphere and metacestode stages are known to contain host-protective antigens. Bogh et al (1988, in press) have carefully analysed stage-specific immunity in *T. taeniaeformis* infection in mice. Immunity stimulated by oncosphere antigens acts only against the earliest invasive stages, and has no effect on their subsequent survival if they evade the early immune response (Fig. 1.6 D). On the other hand, immunity stimulated using metacestode (28-day-old larvae) antigens does not prevent early invasion and development of the parasite (Fig. 1.6 B), but by 15–20 days post-infection most parasites are dying (Fig. 1.6 C), and all parasites are dead by

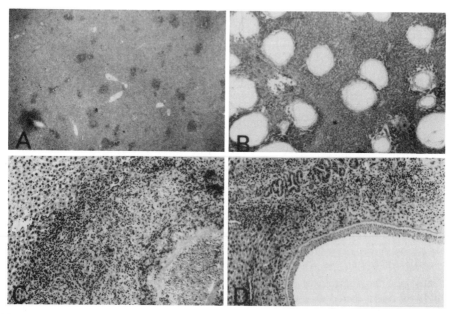

Figure 1.6 Liver sections from mice vaccinated with either oncosphere (TtO) or larval metacestode stage (TtM) antigens of *T. taeniaeformis* and challenged with *T. taeniaeformis* eggs. (A) TtO vaccinated, 6 days post-challenge there are no normal developing larvae visible. (B) TtM vaccinated, 6 days post-challenge there are many normal looking larvae. (C) TtM vaccinated, 20 days post-challenge all larvae are dead and surrounded by host inflammatory reaction. (D) TtO vaccinated, 20 days post-challenge the very few oncospheres which have survived the early immune response develop into normal larvae (Reproduced by courtesy of H O Bogh)

60 days post-infection. Bogh (unpublished results) has purified antibodies to a putative metacestode stage-specific antigen from Western blots of metacestode antigens, and has used these antibodies to screen a *T. taeniaeformis* 28-day-old larval-stage cDNA expression library (Bowtell et al 1984, 1986). GST fusion proteins of several clones have been prepared and are now being used in vaccination trials. It would be useful to have a cocktail vaccine of both recombinant oncosphere- and metacestode-stage antigens which not only prevented most oncospheres from establishing infection, but also killed those which survived early attack and commenced development in the host.

CONCLUSIONS

Several factors may have contributed to the success in isolating a host-protective recombinant *T. ovis* antigen.

1. The host–parasite system is naturally characterized by a high level of host-protective immunity.
2. Antibody clearly plays a major role in host-protective immunity (Rickard & Williams 1982), so that antibody probes provide a rational means for selecting potential host-protective recombinant clones.
3. The most appropriate stage of the parasite (the activated oncosphere) was selected as the source of mRNA for construction of the cDNA library.
4. Affinity purification of the antibody by Western blotting on to putative host-protective antigen gave probes with excellent signal-to-noise ratio. This was especially important as GST-45W gave a weak signal because the fusion protein is unstable and the clone would almost certainly not have been picked using whole anti-oncosphere serum as the probe (K S Johnson personal communication).
5. The use of the GST vector appears to have been crucial, and suggests that if one is confident of having identified a clone which should possess a host-protective epitope, it is important to experiment with different vector systems before discarding it.

REFERENCES

Begg N C, Begg A C, Robinson R G 1957 Primary hydatid disease of the brain–its diagnosis. NZ Med J 56: 84–98
Bogh H O, Rickard M D, Lightowlers M W 1988 Studies on stage-specific immunity against *Taenia taeniaeformis* metacestodes in mice. Parasite Immunol 10: 255–264
Bogh H O, Lightowlers M W, Sullivan N D, Mitchell G F , Rickard M D 1989 Stage specific immunity to *Taenia taeniaeformis* infection in mice: an histological study of the course of infection in mice vaccinated with either oncosphere or metacestode antigens. (Parasite Immunol (in press))
Bowtell D D L, Saint R B, Rickard M D, Mitchell G F 1984 Expression of *Taenia taeniaeformis* antigens in *Escherichia coli*. Mol Biochem Parasitol 13: 173–185
Bowtell D D L, Saint R B, Rickard M D, Mitchell G F 1986 Immunochemical analysis of *Taenia taeniaeformis* antigens expressed in *Escherichia coli*. Parasitology 93: 599–610
Craig P S, Zumbuehl O 1988 Immunization against experimental rabbit cysticercosis using liposome-associated antigen preparations. J Helminthol 62: 58–62

Edwards G T, Herbert I V 1982 Preliminary investigations into the immunization of lambs against infection with *Taenia multiceps* metacestodes. Vet Parasitol 9: 193–199

Gemmell M A 1987 A critical approach to the concepts of control and eradication of echinococcosis/hydatidosis and taeniasis/cysticercosis. Int J Parasitol 17: 465–472

Harrison L J S, Parkhouse R M E 1986 Passive protection against *Taenia saginata* infection in cattle by a mouse monoclonal antibody reactive with the surface of the invasive oncosphere. Parasite Immunol 8: 319–332

Harrison L J S, Joshua G W P, Parkhouse R M E 1986 Identification of protective antigens in *Taenia saginata* cysticercosis. Proceedings of VIth International Congress for Parasitology, Abstract 277

Heath D D, Parmeter S N, Osborn P J, Lawrence S B 1981 Resistance to *Echinococcus granulosus* infection in lambs. J Parasitol 67: 797–799

Howell M J, Hargreaves J J 1988 Cloning and expression of *Taenia ovis* antigens in *Escherichia coli*. Mol Biochem Parasitol 28: 21–30

Johnson K S, Harrison G B L, Lightowlers M W, O'Hoy K L, Cougle W G, Dempster R B, Lawrence S B, Vinton J G, Heath D D, Rickard M D 1989 Vaccination against ovine cysticercosis using a defined recombinant antigen. Nature 338: 585–587

Lightowlers M W, Mitchell G F, Bowtell D D L, Anders R F, Rickard M D 1984 Immunization against *Taenia taeniaeformis*: studies on the characterization of antigens from oncospheres. Int J Parasitol 14: 297–306

Lightowlers M W, Rickard M D, Mitchell G F 1986 Immunization against *Taenia taeniaeformis* in mice: identification of oncospheral antigens in polyacrylamide gels by Western blotting and enzyme immunoassay. Int J Parasitol 16: 297–306

Molinari J L, Meza R, Suarez B, Palacios S, Tato P 1983 *Taenia solium:* Immunity in hogs to the cysticercus. Exp Parasitol 55: 340–357

Osborn P J, Heath D D 1982 Immunization of lambs against *Echinococcus granulosus* using antigens obtained by incubation of oncospheres in vitro. Res Vet Sci 33: 132–133

Rickard M D, Williams J F 1982 Hydatidosis/cysticercosis: immune mechanisms and immunization against infection. Adv Parasitol 21: 229–296

Rickard M D, Brumley J L, Anderson G A 1982 A field trial to evaluate the use of antigens from *Taenia hydatigena* oncospheres to prevent infection with *T. saginata* in cattle grazing on sewage-irrigated pasture. Res Vet Sci 32: 189–193

Smith D B, Johnson K S 1988 Single step purification of polypeptides expressed in *Escherichia coli* as fusions with glutathione S-transferase. Gene 67: 31–40

Verster A, Tustin R C 1987 Immunization of sheep against the larval stage of *Taenia multiceps*. Onderstepoort J Vet Res 54: 103–105

Williams J F 1979 Recent advances in the immunology of cestode infections. J Parasitol 65: 337–349

Winter M D, Allen G, Bomford R H, Brown F 1986 Bacterially expressed antigenic peptide from foot-and-mouth disease virus capsid elicits variable immunologic responses in animals. J Immunol 136: 1835–1840

Discussion of paper presented by M. D. Rickard

Discussed by R. Maizels
Reported by K. P. W. J. McAdam

Maizels observed that veterinary vaccines were ahead of medical vaccines. There was considerable advantage in using the natural host rather than having to use a model in which to design human vaccines. In fact, the only currently available vaccine for a parasite is the veterinary vaccine for *Dictylocaulus*. Rickard's paper demonstrated the importance of knowing the parasite. Once the biotechnology became available, he knew where to go and the critical stages of the parasite on which to focus. The remarkable speed of progress in less than 2 years has been spectacular compared with the relatively slow progress with human parasite vaccines. It shows that a vaccine can be developed notwithstanding a certain amount of ignorance about the actual killing mechanisms.

With most of the helminths, parasites do not replicate or reproduce in the final host; 90% protection is adequate and indeed most investigators working on schistosome vaccines would be delighted with 90% protection. For most helminths, including nematodes, 90% protection is achievable and, in contrast to protozoa, different species of helminths can cross-protect as demonstrated by the *Taenia* species described by Rickard. The commercial vaccine against hookworm protects dogs against different species of hookworm so that is is unnecessary to make a new vaccine for every species.

In answer to questions about the protective antigen and its expression in the life cycle of *Taenia*, Rickard explained that the protective antigens were insoluble or particulate. If oncospheres were sonicated and centrifuged at 100 000g protection could be obtained with the pellet but not with the supernatant. Preliminary immunogold histology using monoclonals to the cloned antigen suggest that the protective antigen may be associated with glands in oncospheres which are prominent at the time they first enter the host and penetrate the intestinal wall. These glands contain secretory particles surrounded by membrane. Since the cestode vaccine had been expressed in the new pGEX expression vector system, based on the *Schistosoma japonicum* glutathione S-transferase, it was speculated that the vaccine might protect both against schistosomiasis and cestodes. However, preliminary data on protection with *S. mansoni* GST have perhaps not lived up to early expectations.

There were interesting discussions on the financial aspects of a successful vaccine. Each sheep was given 3 doses, 3 weeks apart and experiments with oncosphere antigens suggest that immunized ewes will protect their lambs for 8 weeks, although the lambs might have to be immunized to protect them for their next 3–5 months of life before going to slaughter. Oncosphere antigen has been shown to protect for 12 months. Mutton does not have a large economic margin of profit but, in New Zealand, market research has suggested that the vaccine will be economical, compared with the effort it takes to detect and reject meat infected with the parasite in the abattoir. It was suggested that it might be simpler to immunize the definitive host by finding a vaccine for dogs rather than sheep. However, Dr Rickard pointed out that evidence for an effective vaccine in dogs was not convincing. An infected dog with one worm might contaminate a whole pasture, since each terminal segment of the worm contains about 70 000 eggs. Evidently, in some parts of China where echinococcosis is a major problem, huge numbers of people are infected, 28% of the dogs are infected and 70–80% of the sheep are infected. Mathematical models have suggested that with the large *Taenia* species treatment of the definitive host alone will not control infection; immunity in the intermediate host has to be utilized.

Considerable discussion centred on the fusion protein which provided protection in sheep. The β-gal fusion peptide induced an antibody response but no protection whereas the pGEX fusion peptide protected. The GST fusions gave good IgG_1 responses in sheep to the oncosphere antigen. It was suggested that one of the reasons why the pGEX fusion peptide was more protective related to the method of isolation of the peptides; the pGEX peptide was purified by affinity chromatography whereas the β-gal peptide was isolated in SDS reducing buffer, thereby losing native conformation. In the future, antigens will be expressed in the more recently developed pGEX vectors containing enzyme cleavable sites.

The selection of 45W as the successful construct was particularly interesting since it represented a weak reactivity. The reason for this weak reactivity on Western blotting perhaps reflected the fact that antibodies were selected on the basis of reactivity with a denatured specificity. By selecting the weak specificity as well as the strong one, these studies have demonstrated that it pays to try a range of clones rather than going for the hottest spot on the Western blot which reflects antibodies against denatured antigens. Rickard pointed out that the 45S nucleotide sequence is totally contained within 45W with only one or two amino acid changes. Epitope mapping is in progress.

To date the best adjuvant has been saponin mixed with antigen, although other adjuvants are being investigated. Liposomal presentation had not been tried. The question was raised whether lambs passively protected by colostrum could be successfully vaccinated. Britton suggested that there would be no problem immunizing in the presence of colostral antibody for a non-live vaccine although Rickard reported that different experiments had provided variable results so far. The possibility of using *Salmonella typhi* vectors was questioned since this might provide immunity in the gut where infection is initiated. To date this has not been tried although Williams had successfully immunized rats and mice with orally administered cestode antigens.

The spectacular success of an empirical approach to the development of a cestode vaccine contrasted with the complicated and frustrating rational approaches being undertaken for human vaccines against protozoa such as malaria.

Section I:
Malaria

Chairman: G. A. T. Targett

2. Antigenic diversity of the asexual blood stages of *Plasmodium falciparum*

R. F. Anders   J. A. Smythe   N. G. Barzaga
K. P. Forsyth   H. J. Brown   P. E. Crewther
L. M. Thomas   R. L. Coppel   J. G. Culvenor
and G. V. Brown

INTRODUCTION

Diversity within different species of parasites is a major reason why parasites survive despite the ability of their hosts to mount immune responses which are effective in eliminating a particular infecting population. Recent studies on isolates of *Plasmodium falciparum* established in long-term culture as well as on field isolates have dramatically extended our understanding of the extent of diversity in this important human pathogen. Diversity in *P. falciparum* is seen in a variety of characteristics which include isoenzyme patterns, two-dimensional electrophoretic protein patterns, levels of drug resistance, morphology and karyotype in addition to antigenic diversity which will be discussed here. Significant antigenic diversity in malaria parasites of humans was demonstrated when individuals deliberately infected with malaria were found to be relatively more resistant to subsequent infection with the homologous strain than with a heterologous strain (see for example, Jeffrey 1966). The slow development of immunity in people living in areas where malaria is endemic is consistent with the hypothesis that immunity only develops after exposure to a large number of different parasite strains.

In recent years there has been great progress in characterizing antigens of the different life-cycle stages of *P. falciparum* and the molecular basis for much of the antigenic diversity among different parasite populations is now known. In this paper we will discuss some of the molecular aspects of diversity, in particular with respect to the protein antigens of asexual blood stages of *P. falciparum* and the antibody response to these antigens.

ANTIGEN TYPES

S-antigens
Antigenic differences among parasites causing infections in humans were first demonstrated in studies of soluble antigens detected in the serum of infected individuals or extracts of infected placental blood (Wilson et al 1969). Wilson and his colleagues classified these soluble antigens primarily by their heat stability. One group of antigens, termed S-antigens, which were stable to heating at 100°C, were

found to exhibit extensive antigenic diversity. The structural basis of diversity in S-antigens has recently been determined and these studies will be reviewed briefly.

The S-antigen of *P. falciparum* isolate FCQ27/PNG (FC27) was the first antigen of *P. falciparum* to be cloned and sequenced (Coppel et al 1983, Cowman et al 1985). A λgt11 cDNA clone which was selected by immunoreactivity with antimalarial antibodies affinity-purified from human serum was found to encode a segment of an isolate-specific heat-stable antigen that was released into the medium when FC27 was cultured in vitro (Coppel et al 1983). Sequencing of the insert in this clone revealed that the corresponding fragment of the protein was composed of a tandem array of 23 copies of an 11-amino-acid sequence. Subsequently, when the gene was sequenced this S-antigen was seen to be composed of a central block of on or about 100 copies of this 11-amino-acid sequence flanked by short non-repetitive sequences (Cowman et al 1985). Antisera raised in rabbits to a fusion protein composed of the 23 repeats of the FC27 11-amino-acid sequence and β-galactosidase reacted strongly with the antigen expressed in FC27 but not the S-antigen in a number of other isolates (Coppel et al 1983, Saint et al 1987). Furthermore, sera from individuals living in endemic areas, which contained antibodies to the FC27 S-antigen, reacted strongly with synthetic peptides or recombinant proteins containing only repeats, and the anti-S-antigen activity of these sera could be totally removed by adsorption with the repeat sequences. Thus the sequence repeats encode isolate-specific epitopes which are immunodominant.

The N-terminal sequence has the characteristics of a signal sequence with a hydrophobic domain of 16 residues commencing 4 residues from the N-terminus (Cowman et al 1985). Between the signal sequence and the start of the repeats 33 of 76 residues are charged. The C-terminal non-repetitive sequence is unremarkable and lacks any hydrophobic sequence. Thus the primary structural features of the S-antigen are those of a secreted, but not a membrane, protein consistent with the observations from immunoelectron microscopy that the S-antigen is transported into the parasitophorous vacuole (Fig. 2.1) before it is released into the serum at the time of schizont rupture. The full sequences for the S-antigens of 5 different isolates of *P. falciparum* have now been established and all have the same structural features with a central block of repeats, and an N-terminal non-repetitive region which includes a signal sequence and a highly charged region (Cowman et al 1985, Brown et al 1987, Saint et al 1987, Mattei et al 1988, Nicholls et al 1988). Despite the overall similarity in structure, there were dramatic sequence differences among the different S-antigens (Fig. 2.2). These differences were particularly evident in the repeats and not only were the sequences different, but the lengths of the repeat units and the number of repeats also varied. For example, the FC27 S-antigen has 100 copies of an 11-amino-acid repeat sequence whereas the NF7 and Wellcome S-antigens contain 43 and 80 copies of 8- and 12-amino-acid repeats, respectively. Although there are changes in the FC27 and Wellcome repeats at the nucleotide level, these are because alternative codons are used, the amino-acid sequences remaining unchanged.

In contrast, there are two different 8-amino-acid repeats in the NF7 S-antigen because of a substitution of leucine for arginine at 1 of the 8 positions in the repeat (Cowman et al 1985). NF7 differs from FC27 and Wellcome additionally in that there is a second sequence of 15 amino acids which occurs in tandem twice at the

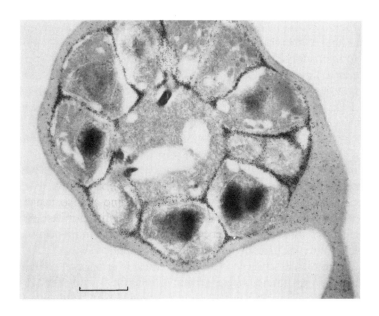

Figure 2.1 Post-embedding immunolabelling of the FC27 S-antigen using affinity-purified rabbit antibodies raised against the cloned antigen, and protein A-5-nm gold. The electron-micrograph of a schizont-infected erythrocyte shows dense labelling over the parasitophorous vacuole space surrounding the developing merozoites. Bar equals 0.5 μm

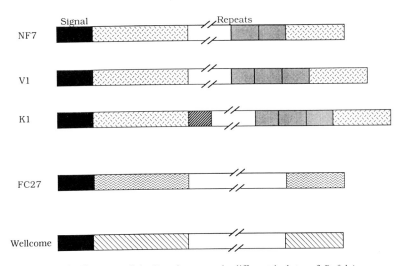

Figure 2.2 Schematic diagrams of the S-antigen gene in different isolates of *P. falciparum*

C-terminal end of the major block of repeats. This second repetitive sequence is also found in the K1 and V1 S-antigens which appear closely related to the NF7 antigen (Brown et al 1987, Saint et al 1987).

The major repeats in both the K1 and V1 S-antigens are encoded by sequences contained within the 45-base-pair (bp) sequence that encodes the 15-amino-acid minor repeat common to NF7, K1 and V1. The V1 repeat is encoded by a 33-bp sequence which is read in the same frame as the 45-bp sequence. In contrast, the 36-bp sequence encoding the 12-amino-acid sequence, which is the major repeat in the K1 S-antigen, contains within it 24 bp derived from the 45-bp sequence, translated in a different reading frame. These relationships are the most obvious but there is additional nucleotide sequence homology between the repeats in the Wellcome, FC27 and NF7 S-antigens which indicates a common evolutionary origin (Saint et al 1987, Mattei et al 1988, Nicholls et al 1988).

The flanking sequences of NF7, K1 and V1 are nearly identical but different from both FC27 and Wellcome. In turn, the flanking sequences of FC27 and Wellcome are considerably different from each other (Nicholls et al 1988). Hence there are at least 3 different types of allele based on the non-repetitive regions of the S-antigen and this represents a very different source of diversity from repeat variation. Palo Alto has the same repeat as Wellcome but because only a partial sequence is available the relationship between the flanking sequences of Palo Alto and the other isolates is unknown (Mattei et al 1988).

In the early studies S-antigens were detected with antibodies in the serum of selected individuals with long-term exposure to malaria (Wilson et al 1969, 1975a, Wilson 1980, Anders et al 1983, Winchell et al 1984a, 1984b, Howard et al 1986a). With the cloning and sequencing of several different S-antigens, monospecific antisera, raised against cloned S-antigens or synthetic peptides, and monoclonal antibodies are now available to detect circulating S-antigens (Forsyth et al 1988, 1989) or for the serotyping of parasites by, for example, indirect immunofluorescence microscopy (Schofield et al 1985). The world-wide distribution of S-antigens observed by Wilson and colleagues (Wilson 1970, Winchell et al 1984a) has been confirmed by Schofield et al (1985) for the FC27 serotype using a monoclonal antibody. We have used monospecific reagents for 5 different S-antigens to examine, by immunoblotting, the S-antigens in the plasma of 111 infected children from the Madang region of Papua New Guinea (Table 2.1). By far the most prevalent S-antigen detected was FC27 (16%), followed by K1 (4.5%), Palo Alto/Wellcome (2.7%) and V1 (0.9%). No NF7 S-antigens were detected. One plasma contained both an FC27 and a K1 S-antigen. As these 5 serotypes probably represent a small proportion of the total number of S-antigen serotypes, infections with mixed serotypes must occur commonly as indicated by the studies of Wilson et al (1975a).

In another study in the Madang region, Forsyth et al (1988) found that the NF7 serotype was absent over a 3-year period whereas the frequency of the K1 and FC27 S-antigen serotypes remained relatively constant. Forsyth et al (1988, 1989)

Table 2.1 S-antigens identified in plasma of infected individuals

Number examined	Number containing S-antigen											
	FC27		NF7		K1		V1		PA		FC27 + K1	
	(n)	(%)	(n)	(%)	(n)	(%)	(n)	(%)	(n)	(%)	(n)	(%)
111	18	16	0	0	5	4.5	1	0.9	3	2.7	1	0.9

These individuals were from the Madang region of Papua New Guinea (N G Barzaga & R F Anders unpublished results)

used the antibodies to the FC27 S-antigen to examine the prevalence of this serotype in different villages in the Madang region. Remarkable variation occurred in space and time in the prevalence of this S-antigen indicating that, despite the world-wide distribution of the FC27 serotype (Schofield et al 1985), transmission at the village level is periodic. In some villages the majority of FC27 S-antigens were found in the serum of individuals who were parasitaemic whereas in other villages a large number of individuals who had an antigenaemia were not parasitaemic. It is known that S-antigens may persist in the serum for some weeks after clearance of parasites from the blood (Wilson et al 1975b) but nevertheless this observation suggests that epidemics of a particular serotype within an endemic area may be relatively short-lived.

Because the sequence repeats in S-antigens are relatively short, synthetic peptides corresponding to the repeats can be prepared and used to measure antibody responses to individual S-antigens. Using peptides conjugated to bovine serum albumin with glutaraldehyde, we have measured anti-S-antigen antibody responses in sera from individuals in the Madang area (N G Barzaga and R F Anders unpublished results). The antibody specificity most frequently found was to the FC27 serotype, although antibodies to V1 and Palo Alto/Wellcome were also found frequently. The failure to find antibodies to the K1 S-antigen serotype (parasites of this serotype were found in the Madang region) may have been due to the use of a 12-amino-acid peptide which is a single repeat; longer peptides representing 2 or 3 repeats were used to detect the other S-antigen antibodies. Parasites of the NF7 S-antigen have been found in Papua New Guinea (Saint et al 1987) but, consistent with the failure to find S-antigens of this serotype in this more recent study, antibodies of this specificity were found in only 2 individuals.

Antibodies to S-antigens were found in 65 of the 140 sera examined and 24 of these had more than one specificity (Table 2.2). The great majority of adults over the age of 30 had antibodies to at least 1 S-antigen but antibodies were less commonly found in children and no child (1–10 years of age) had antibodies to more than 1 of the S-antigens. This, and the fact that all 7 individuals in the 1–10 years age group who had a detectable S-antigen antibody also had a parasitaemia, suggests that the antibodies in this age group were generated by the current infection. It seems probable that seropositivity in children may be relatively short-

Table 2.2 Age-specific prevalence of antibodies to S-antigens

Age group	Number examined	S-antigen antibodies		
		Antibody + ve	> 1 Serotype	Parasitaemic
1–10	44	7 (16%)	0	7
11–20	35	15 (43%)	5	9
21–30	22	10 (45%)	3	2
31–40	13	12 (92%)	7	2
> 40	26	21 (81%)	10	4

Antibodies were detected by ELISA. Because the V1 sequence is totally contained within the 15-mer, individuals with antibodies to both of these peptides are not included in the > 1 serotype group. These individuals were from the Madang region of Papua New Guinea but a different population from that studied in Table 2.1 (N G Barzaga & R F Anders unpublished results)

lived and that seropositivity in adults is a more stable reflection of previous infections with *P. falciparum*. Nevertheless, the seropositivity rate for antibodies to the FC27 S-antigen in adults was higher in villages where the FC27 S-antigen was detected (Forsyth et al 1989).

Thus, it appears that some adults with decades of exposure to *P. falciparum*, which must have included previous exposure to the FC27 serotype given its prevalence, convert from seronegative to seropositive with a new infection of this serotype. Village-to-village variation in antibody prevalence was not so marked as for antigenaemia but there were considerable differences (from 3% to 87%) particularly in the younger age group (Forsyth et al 1989). Generally, the higher seropositivity rates for FC27 antibodies in children were found in villages where the prevalence of FC27 antigenaemia was highest as would be expected if most antibody responses in children reflect relatively recent infections. However, there was a notable exception where 40% of the children had an FC27 S-antigenaemia but only 8% had antibodies to this S-antigen serotype. This village was exceptional also in that almost all children with an S-antigenaemia had a parasitaemia as well. Thus transmission of the FC27 serotype in this village may have commenced shortly before the time of the survey and antibody responses had not had time to develop (Forsyth et al 1989).

The original studies on S-antigens used sera which usually contained multiple antibody specificities (Wilson et al 1969, 1975a, Wilson 1980). In our Madang study, 17% of all individuals examined and 70% of those over 20 years of age had antibodies to more than 1 of the S-antigens tested for. Almost every possible combination of different antibody specificities was found (Table 2.3) but the combination of antibodies to the FC27 and V1 S-antigen serotypes was found most frequently and occurred more frequently than expected from the prevalence of the individual specificities ($\chi^2 = 11.1$, $p < 0.001$).

The role of S-antigens in inducing protective immune responses is unknown. Saul et al (1985) reported that a monoclonal antibody to the FC27 S-antigen

Table 2.3 Prevalence of different combinations of antibodies to S-antigens

S-antigen antibody						Number of individuals
FC27	NF7	K1	V1	PA	15-mer	
+	−	−	−	−	−	11
−	−	−	+	−	−	1
−	−	−	−	+	−	16
−	−	−	−	−	+	5
+	−	−	+	−	−	1
+	−	−	−	+	−	2
+	−	−	−	−	+	1
+	−	−	+	−	+	10
+	−	−	+	+	−	2
+	−	−	−	+	+	3
+	−	−	+	+	+	3
+	+	+	+	+	+	1
−	+	−	+	+	+	1
−	−	−	+	−	+	8

These are the same individuals as in Table 2.2

effectively inhibited the growth of this isolate in vitro but the mechanism whereby antibodies to this soluble secreted antigen inhibit growth is not clear. African children were generally not re-infected with parasites of the same S-antigen serotype (Wilson et al 1975b) although without knowledge of the serotypes being transmitted at the time of follow-up it is not possible to come to a conclusion as to the significance of this finding. In the Madang study carried out by Forsyth et al (1989) longitudinal data were obtained on a sample of the study population. Although none of the 31 subjects studied longitudinally who had detectable FC27 S-antigenaemia at the initial survey was positive at later surveys the numbers were too low to be of significance. However, the data of Forsyth et al (1989) clearly show that in an endemic area the transmission of parasites of one particular S-antigen serotype is periodic. It remains to be established whether immune responses directed at S-antigens are responsible for reducing the transmission of one S-antigen serotype while the transmission of other serotypes increases.

Merozoite surface antigens

Considerable effort has been directed towards defining antigens on the surface of merozoites because of their potential as components of a malaria vaccine. The majority of the antigens that have been identified on the merozoite surface by surface radio-iodination derive from the proteolytic fragmentation of a large precursor polypeptide which has been given many names (reviewed by Holder 1988) but which we will refer to here as MSA 1. A number of laboratories have reported a small antigenic polypeptide on the merozoite surface that is not a fragment of MSA 1 (Stanley et al 1985, Ramasamy 1987, Epping et al 1988, Miettinen-Bauman et al 1988, Clark et al 1989). The reported characteristics indicated that these different laboratories are probably studying the same antigen (MSA 2) that we have recently cloned and sequenced (Smythe et al 1988).

MSA 1 and MSA 2, although very different sized polypeptides, have an interesting feature in common in that they are both post-translationally modified, probably by the attachment at the C-terminus of a glycosyl phosphatidylinositol moiety (GPI) which anchors the mature polypeptides into the surface membrane of the merozoite (Haldar et al 1985, Ramasamy 1987, Smythe et al 1988). This form of membrane anchoring is particularly common among surface membrane proteins of protozoa but the functional significance of the GPI anchors on the merozoite surface antigens is not clear (Ferguson & Williams 1988).

The variant surface glycoprotein (VSG) of the African trypanosome is also anchored in this way and cleavage of the GPI moiety by a phospholipase C of very restricted specificity results in release of the VSG from the trypanosome surface (reviewed in Englund et al 1988). Most of the fragments of MSA 1 are shed from the merozoite surface at the time of merozoite invasion (McBride & Heidrich 1987) but this presumably does not involve phospholipase acting on the GPI anchor of MSA 1 as the C-terminal fragment of MSA 1 remains attached to the invading merozoite (McBride et al 1987). There is no evidence that MSA 2 is proteolytically processed like MSA 1, nor can MSA 2 be detected in ring-stage parasites (Epping et al 1988, Miettinen-Bauman et al 1988, Smythe et al 1988, Clark et al 1989). Thus, MSA 2 may be released from the merozoite surface by the action of a phospholipase prior to, or at the time of, invasion.

Both MSA 1 and MSA 2 exist in antigenically diverse forms and the structural basis of this diversity is now understood as a result of extensive sequencing studies on a number of alleles for each of these polymorphic antigens. From a comparison of the available sequences for different MSA 1 alleles the polypeptide chain could be divided into 17 blocks of sequence that were conserved, semi-conserved or variable (Tanabe et al 1987, Peterson et al 1988a). Interestingly, the variable blocks occur in only two forms and there has been reassortment of these two types of variable sequence within the different alleles of MSA 1.

Thus, it appears that the existing alleles of MSA 1 have been generated largely as a result of intragenic recombination between two parental alleles. Cross-overs leading to intragenic recombination have apparently been restricted to the N-terminal constant regions (blocks 3 and 5) of MSA 1 as there has been no reassortment of the two types of variable regions on the C-terminal side of block 5 (Tanabe et al 1987, Peterson et al 1988a,b). This dimorphic model for the structure of MSA 1 does not explain all the diversity seen in MSA 1 as two isolates have been described which have a third form of variable block 2 (Certa et al 1987, Peterson et al 1988b). This region contains a set of degenerate tripeptide repeats and although the repeats in MSA 1 form a relatively small part of the polypeptide chain this region is the most variable part of the molecule. Studies with monoclonal antibodies have shown that MSA 1 contains both variable and constant antigenic epitopes (Hall et al 1984, McBride et al 1984, 1985, Pirson & Perkins 1985, Lyon et al 1987), but the epitopes for individual monoclonal antibodies have not yet been precisely mapped on to the known structure of the *P. falciparum* MSA 1. In contrast, the epitopes of monoclonal antibodies which provide passive protection to mice against infection with *P. yoelii* (Burns et al 1988) or *P. chabaudi* (Lew et al 1989) have been mapped on the MSA 1 of these species.

The antibodies which have been used to detect MSA 2 have usually been directed against epitopes that are variable (Stanley et al 1985, Ramasamy 1987, Epping et al 1988, Miettinen-Bauman et al 1988, Clark et al 1989). This reflects the fact that, as in the S-antigens, a very large proportion of the MSA 2 polypeptide chain varies among different isolates of *P. falciparum*. The sequences for 3 different alleles of MSA 2 have been determined (Smythe et al in press) and schematic diagrams of the gene structures are shown in Figure 2.3. Each of the sequences encodes a polypeptide with a molecular mass of approximately 28 kD with hydrophobic domains at both the N- and C-terminus which are presumed to

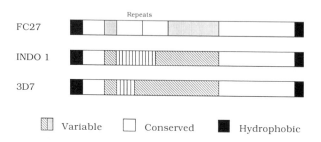

Figure 2.3 Schematic diagrams of the MSA 2 gene in different isolates of *P. falciparum*

be part of signal sequences for secretion and attachment of a GPI moiety, respectively. There are centrally located sequence repeats in each of the MSA 2 molecules but, as for the S-antigen repeats, there is variation in repeat sequence, length of the repeat unit and number of repeats.

In isolate FC27 the MSA 2 sequence encodes two identical copies of a 32-amino-acid sequence arranged in tandem. In contrast, the MSA 2 of the isolate Indochina 1 and the cloned line 3D7 contain 12 and 5 copies respectively of the sequence GGSA. Flanking the sequence repeats there are additional sequences which vary among the 3 known MSA 2 sequences. These flanking sequences are much more conserved between Indochina 1 and 3D7 than they are between FC27 and the other 2 isolates. The nucleotide sequences of the 3' flanking regions of Indochina 1 and 3D7 contain a second set of repeats which encode poly-threonine. Deletions in this region of the Indochina 1 sequence relative to the 3D7 sequence compensate for the longer sequence of GGSA repeats in Indochina 1 so that the overall size of the different forms of MSA 2 is preserved. At either end of the MSA 2 polypeptide chain there are very conserved sequences. The N-terminal 40 residues are identical in all 3 isolates and within the C-terminal 74 residues there is only one position where there is a difference (Smythe et al in press).

DNA probes for the sequences encoding the 32-amino-acid repeat of FC27 and the 4-amino-acid repeat of Indochina 1 and 3D7 have been used to probe DNA from other isolates after being amplified by the polymerase chain reaction. Although the DNA from the majority of isolates hybridized with either the 32- or 4-amino-acid repeat probes, some isolates failed to hybridize with either probe indicating that there are forms of MSA 2 containing other types of repeat sequences (Smythe et al 1989).

Monoclonal antibodies against MSA 2 are inhibitory to parasites growing in vitro (Ramasamy 1987, Epping et al 1988, Miettinen-Bauman et al 1988, Clark et al 1989). The epitope for one such antibody, recognizing the MSA 2 of FC27, has been identified by ELISA on a complete overlapping set of synthetic peptides for this antigen (Saul et al in press). The peptides that reacted with the monoclonal antibody contained the sequence STNS which occurs within the 32-amino-acid repeat and therefore occurs twice in the molecule. Human antibodies to MSA 2 have been assayed using either a glutathione S-transferase (GST) fusion protein containing most of the FC27 sequence or the synthetic peptide (GGSA)$_3$ coupled to bovine serum albumin (J Smythe & R F Anders unpublished results). Antibodies reacting with the GST/FC27 MSA 2 fusion protein were found in the majority of individuals, usually at high titre. There was an age-dependent increase in both the prevalence (Table 2.4) and titre of anti-FC27 MSA 2 antibodies. Antibodies reacting with the GGSA repeat were found in many individuals but were less prevalent and usually of lower titre than antibodies to the GST/FC27 MSA 2 fusion protein. Antibodies affinity-purified from human serum on (GGSA)$_3$ surprisingly reacted on an immunoblot with the MSA 2 of FC27 as well as the antigen in Indochina 1 and 3D7. Inspection of the 32-amino-acid repeat sequence in the FC27 MSA 2, which was considered unrelated to the GGSA repeat, revealed the sequence ASGS which may provide the cross-reacting epitope.

Table 2.4 Age-specific prevalence of antibodies to the MSA2 of isolate FC27

Age group	Number examined	MSA2 antibodies	
		Positive	Negative
1–3	14	6	8
4–9	26	18	8
10–14	17	15	2
15–20	22	22	0
21–30	21	20	1
31–40	13	13	0
>40	27	27	0

These are the same individuals as in Table 2.2

Antigens associated with the erythrocyte membrane

A number of different parasite protein antigens become associated with the membrane of the host erythrocyte at various stages of the asexual life cycle. The ring-infected erythrocyte surface antigen (RESA) (Brown et al 1985) and an M_r 105 000 rhoptry antigen (Sam-Yellowe et al 1988) are released from the apical organelles of the merozoite and transferred to the erythrocyte membrane at the time of merozoite invasion. Neither of these antigens is known to exhibit any diversity among different isolates of *P. falciparum* and other antigens located to the merozoite rhoptries are not notably diverse. This lack of diversity is surprising particularly because there is considerable evidence indicating that some of these antigens can induce protective immune responses (Holder & Freeman 1981, Perrin et al 1985, Collins et al 1986) and indicates that they must have critical functions.

Other antigens are transported out to the erythrocyte membrane from the maturing intra-erythrocytic parasite and are found associated with the membrane of erythrocytes containing mature trophozoites and schizonts (reviewed by Howard 1988a). Several of these antigens, including the mature parasite-infected erythrocyte surface antigen (MESA or Pf EMP 2) (Coppel et al 1986, Howard et al 1988), Pf 11.1 (Koenen et al 1984, Scherf et al 1988), and two histidine-rich proteins (KAHRP or HRP 1 and HRP 2) (Wellems & Howard 1986, Ardeshir et al 1987, Ellis et al 1987, Pologe et al 1987, Sharma & Kilejian 1987, Triglia et al 1987) have been cloned and extensively characterized. All these antigens contain sequence repeats and are polymorphic in size among different isolates of *P. falciparum*. Pf 11.1 contains 3 different sets of repeats, one of which is absent or very different in 2 of 7 isolates studied (Scherf et al 1988). Variation in the repeat structures undoubtedly underlies much of the size polymorphism in all these antigens but the extent to which variation in their repeat sequences leads to antigenic diversity is not established.

With the exception of HRP 2, which is secreted from the infected cell (Howard et al 1986b), these antigens all appear to associate with the cytoplasmic face of the erythrocyte membrane, presumably through interactions with components of the membrane skeleton. However, of particular interest as targets of protective responses are antigens exposed on the external surface of the infected erythrocyte. Antigens in this location have been detected with a variety of procedures including radio-iodination and immunoprecipitation (Aley et al 1984, 1986, Leech et al 1984, Magowan et al 1988), immunofluorescence microscopy (Hommel et al 1982, 1983, Mendis et al 1983, Marsh et al 1986), agglutination (Sherwood et al 1985, Marsh and Howard 1986, Howard et al 1988, Southwell et al in press) and antibody-mediated inhibition of cytoadherence (Udeinya et al 1983, Leech et al 1984, Howard et al 1988, Southwell et al in press). The antigen detected by radio-iodination and immunoprecipitation has been called Pf EMP 1 and is a large molecular mass polypeptide which is polymorphic in size and exhibits extensive antigenic diversity (Howard et al 1988). Considerable antigenic diversity is also a feature of the surface antigens detected by the other procedures and it has not been determined whether these different experimental approaches are all detecting the same antigen.

There is considerable evidence from experimental models of malaria that plasmodia can undergo antigenic variation whereby clonal populations of parasites can vary their antigenic phenotype (Barnwell et al 1983, McLean et al 1986, 1987, Handunnetti et al 1987), a process best described in African trypanosomes. The evidence points to the variant antigen of plasmodia being expressed on the surface of erythrocytes infected with mature parasites. Magowan et al (1988) have recently shown that when infected cells are fractionated by their ability to cytoadhere, size variants of Pf EMP 1 can be selected from clonal populations. The gene for Pf EMP 1 is yet to be cloned but when that is achieved it will be possible to determine whether the antigenic diversity in this molecule reflects the existence of multiple allelic genes or a mechanism of antigenic variation.

Antigens not expressed in some cultured isolates
Much of the progress in the characterization of antigens of the asexual blood-stages of *P. falciparum* has depended on the ability to grow these life-cycle stages in continuous culture in vitro. However, in studying parasites which have been adapted to growth in vitro it is important to be aware that there may have been changes in such characteristics as drug sensitivity, knob morphology, cytoadherence, phenotype, karyotype and antigen expression. As the asexual blood-stages of *P. falciparum* mature, they normally induce changes in the host cell membrane that lead to these cells adhering to the vascular endothelium and being sequestered out of the peripheral circulation (reviewed in Howard 1988b).

Electron-dense knobs in the erythrocyte membrane appear to be points of interaction between endothelial cells and the cytoadhering infected erythrocyte (Trager et al 1966, Luse and Miller 1971). During culture in vitro parasites often lose the ability to cytoadhere and this may be associated with loss of knobs (K$^-$) (Langreth et al 1979, Barnwell et al 1983, David et al 1983, Gritzmacher & Reese 1984). One of 3 histidine-rich proteins (KAHRP or HRP 1) described in *P. falciparum* has been located at the knob by immunoelectron microscopy (Ardeshir et al 1987, Culvenor et al 1987, Pologe et al 1987, Taylor et al 1987) and expression of this protein is lacking in K$^-$ parasites (Kilejian 1984). Failure to express one or other of the other two histidine-rich proteins (HRP 2 and HRP 3 or SHARP) has also been observed in some parasites growing in vitro (Stahl et al 1985, Kemp et al 1987, Wellems et al 1987, Pologe & Ravetch 1988). We affinity-purified human antibodies on HRP 3 expressed in *E. coli* and used these antibodies to probe immunoblots of several different *P. falciparum* isolates or clones. These antibodies reacted with both HRP 2 and HRP 3, which is not surprising given the sequence homology between these two antigens. Both these antigens were polymorphic in size among the different isolates but HRP 2 was not expressed in the FC27 clone D10, whereas HRP 3 was not expressed in the Honduras clone HB3 (Fig. 2.4).

Another antigen which *P. falciparum* growing in vitro can dispense with is RESA as this antigen is not expressed in the line of isolate FCR3 we obtained from Dr C. Newbold in Oxford (Cappai et al in press). As no field isolates have been observed lacking this antigen, loss of the ability to express RESA presumably occurred during culture in vitro. Thus a number of parasite proteins which interact with the erythrocyte membrane are not required for growth in vitro. The lack of a requirement to cytoadhere in vitro presumably would make redundant those molecules generating the knobs. We have proposed that RESA may have a function at the time of merozoite invasion but at least in FCR3 that cannot be so. It seems more likely that RESA in some way modifies the membrane of the parasitized erythrocyte to favour survival of this abnormal cell in the circulation of the infected host.

It has been observed that the genes for many of the antigens of *P. falciparum* are clustered near chromosome ends (reviewed by Kemp et al in press). The size of chromosomes in plasmodia is extremely polymorphic among isolates and these polymorphisms are generated by an apparently high frequency of recombination within subtelomeric repeats referred to as Rep 20 (Corcoran et al 1988, Patarapotikul & Langsley 1988). Deletions encompassing Rep 20 repeats completely explain the size differences seen in chromosomes 1 and 2 of *P. falciparum* (Fig. 2.5).

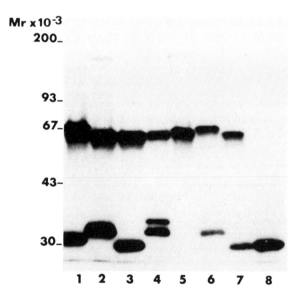

Figure 2.4 Immunoblots of antigens from different isolates of *P. falciparum* grown asynchronously in vitro, solubilized in SDS sample buffer and fractionated by 10% SDS-PAGE; lane 1, NF7; lane 2, K1; lane 3, FC27; lane 4, V1; lane 5, HB3; lane 6, 7G8; lane 7, E12; lane 8, D10. Antigens were identified by affinity-purified human anti-HRP 3 antibodies

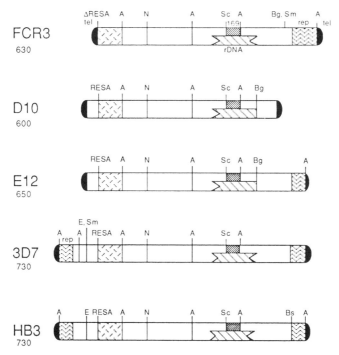

Figure 2.5 Physical map of *P. falciparum* chromosome 1 in 5 isolates. Starting with FCR3, the first time each marker occurs on a chromosome it is labelled with the name of the marker as defined in Corcoran et al (1988). When it reappears, lower in the figure, the region is identified by the shading pattern. The constructions of the maps for D10, E12,3D7 and HB3 have been previously described in Corcoran et al (1988) but the positions of the two leftmost ApaI sites shown in 3D7 have been revised. The position of the RESA gene is shown as a line, located at the point corresponding to the boundary of the deletion in FCR3 (Cappai et al in press). Sizes are shown at the left, in kbp. A = *Apa*I, Bg = *Bg*II, Bs = *Bss*HII, E = *Eag*I, N = *Nar*I, Sc = *Sac*II, Sm = *Sma*I

Similar deletions have been seen in parasites taken directly from patients so they are not only a feature of cultured isolates (Corcoran et al 1986, Biggs et al 1989). However, if the protein encoded by a particular gene is not required for growth in vitro these same processes may result in the deletion of genes or gene fragments. The lack of KAHRP expression in K⁻ parasites is due to the partial or total deletion of the KAHRP gene from the left end of chromosome 2 (Pologe & Ravetch 1986, Corcoran et al 1986, 1988, Tan-Ariya et al 1988) whereas the lack of RESA expression in FCR3 is due to the deletion of the first exon of the RESA gene from the left end of chromosome 1 (Cappai et al in press). It has been suggested that location of the antigen genes, many of them containing extensive repetitive structures, in these unstable subtelomeric regions may facilitate the rapid evolution that is a feature of some of these antigens (Kemp et al in press).

ACKNOWLEDGEMENTS

We thank Heather Saunders and Etty Bonnici for secretarial assistance. This work was supported by the Australian National Health and Medical Research Council, the John D. and Catherine T. MacArthur Foundation and the Australian Malaria Vaccine Joint Venture. Support was provided under the Generic Technology component of the Industry Research and Development Act 1986.

REFERENCES

Aley S B, Sherwood J A, Howard R J 1984 Knob-positive and knob-negative *Plasmodium falciparum* differ in expression of a strain-specific malarial antigen on the surface of infected erythrocytes. J Exp Med 160: 1585–1590

Aley S B, Sherwood J A, Marsh K, Eidelman O, Howard R J 1986 Identification of isolate-specific proteins on sorbitol-enriched *Plasmodium falciparum* infected erythrocytes from Gambian patients. Parasitology 92: 511–525

Anders R F, Brown G V, Edwards A E 1983 Characterization of an S-antigen synthesized by several isolates of *Plasmodium falciparum*. Proc Natl Acad Sci USA 80: 6652–6656

Ardeshir F, Flint J E, Matsumoto Y, Aikawa M, Reese R T, Stanley H 1987 cDNA sequence encoding a *Plasmodium falciparum* protein associated with knobs and localization of the protein to electron-dense regions in membranes of infected erythrocytes. EMBO J 6: 1421–1427

Barnwell J W, Howard R J, Coon H G, Miller L H 1983 Splenic requirement for antigenic variation and expression of the variant antigen on the erythrocyte membrane in cloned *Plasmodium knowlesi* malaria. Infect Immun 40: 985–994

Biggs B A, Kemp D J, Brown G V et al 1989 Subtelomeric chromosome deletions in field isolates of *Plasmodium falciparum* and their relationship to loss of cytoadherence in vitro. Proc Natl Acad Sci USA 86: 2428–2432

Brown G V, Culvenor J G, Crewther P E, Bianco A E, Coppel R L, Saint R B, Stahl H D, Kemp D J, Anders R F 1985 Localization of the Ring-infected Erythrocyte Surface Antigen (RESA) of *Plasmodium falciparum* in merozoites and ring-infected erythrocytes. J Exp Med 162: 774–779

Brown H, Kemp D J, Barzaga N, Brown G V, Anders R F, Coppel R L 1987 Sequence variation in S-antigen genes of *Plasmodium falciparum*. Mol Biol Med 4: 365–376

Burns J M, Daly T M, Vaidya A B, Long C A 1988 The 3′ portion of the gene for *Plasmodium yoeli* merozoite surface antigen encodes the epitope recognized by a protective monoclonal antibody. Proc Natl Acad Sci USA 85: 602–606

Cappai R, van Schravendijk M-R, Anders R F, Peterson M G, Thomas L M, Cowman A F, Kemp D J 1989 Expression of the RESA gene in *Plasmodium falciparum* isolate FCR3 is prevented by a subtelomeric deletion. Mol Cell Biol (in press)

Certa U, Rotmann D, Matile H, Reber-Liske R 1987 A naturally occurring gene encoding the major surface antigen precursor p190 of *Plasmodium falciparum* lacks tripeptide repeats. EMBO J 6: 4137–4142

Clark J T, Donachie S, Anand R, Wilson C F, Heidrich H-G, McBride J S 1989 46–53 Kilodalton glycoprotein from the surface of *Plasmodium falciparum* merozoites. Mol Biochem Parasit 32: 15

Collins W E, Anders R F, Pappaioanou M, Campbell G H, Brown G V, Kemp D J, Coppel R L, Skinner J C, Andrysiak P M, Favalaro J M, Corcoran L M, Broderson J R, Mitchell G F, Campbell C C 1986 Immunization of *Aotus* monkeys with recombinant proteins of an erythrocyte surface antigen of *Plasmodium falciparum*. Nature 323: 259–262

Coppel R L, Cowman A F, Lingelbach K R, Brown G V, Saint R B, Kemp D J, Anders R F 1983 Isolate-specific S-antigen of *Plasmodium falciparum* contains a repeated sequence of eleven amino acids. Nature 306: 751–756

Coppel R L, Culvenor J G, Bianco A E, Crewther P E, Stahl H D, Brown G V, Anders R F, Kemp D J 1986 Variable antigen associated with the surface of erythrocytes infected with mature stages of *Plasmodium falciparum*. Mol Biochem Parasitol 20: 265–277

Corcoran L M, Forsyth K P, Bianco A E, Brown G V, Kemp D J 1986 Chromosome size polymorphisms in *Plasmodium falciparum* can involve deletions and are frequent in natural parasite population. Cell 44: 87–95

Corcoran L M, Thompson J K, Walliker D, Kemp D J 1988 Homologous recombination within sub-telomeric repeat sequences generates chromosome size polymorphisms in *Plasmodium falciparum*. Cell 53: 807–813

Cowman A F, Saint R B, Coppel R L, Brown G V, Anders R F, Kemp D J 1985 Conserved sequences flank variable tandem repeats in two S-antigen genes of *Plasmodium falciparum*. Cell 40: 775–783

Culvenor J G, Langford C J, Crewther P E, Saint R B, Coppel R L, Kemp D J, Anders R F,

Brown G V 1987 *Plasmodium falciparum*: identification and localization of a knob protein antigen expressed by a cDNA clone. Exp Parasitol 63: 58–67

David P H, Hommel M, Miller L H, Udeinya I J, Oligino L D 1983 Parasite sequestration in *Plasmodium falciparum* malaria: spleen and antibody modulation of cytoadherence of infected erythrocytes. Proc Natl Acad Sci USA 80: 5075–5079

Ellis J, Irving D O, Wellems T E, Howard R J, Cross G A M 1987 Structure and expression of the knob-associated histidine-rich protein of *Plasmodium falciparum*. Mol Biochem Parasitol 26: 203–214

Englund P T, Hereld D, Krakow J L, Doering T L, Masterson W J, Hart G W 1988 Glycolipid membrane anchor of the trypanosome variant surface glycoprotein: its biosynthesis and cleavage. In: Englund P T, Sher A (eds) The Biology of Parasitism, Alan R Liss, New York, p 401

Epping R J, Goldstone S D, Ingram L T, Upcroft J A, Ramasamy R, Cooper J A, Bushell G R, Geysen H M 1988 An epitope recognized by inhibitory monoclonal antibodies that react with a 51 kilodalton merozoite surface antigen in *Plasmodium falciparum*. Mol Biochem Parasitol 28: 1–10

Ferguson M A J, Williams A F 1988 Cell surface anchoring of proteins via glycosyl-phosphatidylinositol structures. Annu Rev Biochem 57: 285–320

Forsyth K P, Anders R F, Kemp D J, Alpers M P 1988 New appraoches to the serotypic analysis of the epidemiology of *Plasmodium falciparum*. Phil Trans R Soc Lond B 321: 485–493

Forsyth K P, Anders R F, Cattani J A, Alpers M P 1989 Small area variation in prevalence of an S-antigen serotype of *Plasmodium falciparum* in villages of Madang, Papua New Guinea. Am J Trop Med Hyg 40: 344–350

Gritzmacher C A, Reese R T 1983 Reversal of knob formation on *Plasmodium falciparum*-infected erythrocytes. Science 226: 65–67

Haldar K, Ferguson M A J, Cross G A M 1985 Acylation of a *Plasmodium falciparum* merozoite surface antigen via sn-1,2-diacyl glycerol. J Biol Chem 260: 4969–4974

Hall R, Osland A, Hyde J E, Simmons D L, Hope I A, Scaife J G 1984 Processing, polymorphism, and biological significance of P190, a major surface antigen of the erythrocytic forms of *Plasmodium falciparum*. Mol Biochem Parasitol 11: 61–80

Handunnetti S M, Mendis K N, David P H 1987 Antigenic variation of cloned *Plasmodium fragile* in its natural host *Macaca sinica*. J Exp Med 165: 1269–1283

Holder A A 1988 The precursor to major merozoite surface antigens: structure and role in immunity. Prog Allergy 41: 72–97

Holder A A, Freeman R R 1981 Immunization against blood-stage rodent malaria using purified parasite antigens. Nature 294: 361–364

Hommel M, David P H, Oligino L D, David J R 1982 Expression of strain-specific surface antigens on *Plasmodium falciparum*-infected erythrocytes. Parasite Immunol 4: 409–419

Hommel M, David P H, Oligino L D 1983 Surface alterations of erythrocytes in *Plasmodium falciparum* malaria. J Exp Med 157: 1137–1148

Howard R J 1988a *Plasmodium falciparum* proteins at the host erythrocyte membrane: Their biological and immunological significance and novel parasite organelles which deliver them to the cell surface. In: Englund P T, Sher A (eds) The Biology of Parasitism, Alan R Liss, New York, p 111–145

Howard R J 1988b Malarial proteins of the membrane of *Plasmodium falciparum*-infected erythrocytes and their involvement in cytoadherence to endothelial cells. Prog Allergy 41: 98–147

Howard R J, Panton L J, Marsh K, Ling I T, Winchell E J, Wilson R J M 1986a Antigenic diversity and size diversity of *Plasmodium falciparum* antigens in isolates from Gambian patients. I. S-antigens. Parasite Immunol 8: 39–55

Howard R J, Uni S, Aikawa M, Aley S B, Leech J H, Lew A M, Wellems T E, Rener J, Taylor D W 1986b Secretion of a malarial histidine-rich protein (Pf HRP II) from *Plasmodium falciparum*-infected erythrocytes. J Cell Biol 103: 1269–1277

Howard R J, Barnwell J W, Rock E P, Neequaye J, Ofori-Adjei D, Maloy W L, Lyon J A, Saul A 1988 Two approximately 300 kilodalton *Plasmodium falciparum* proteins at the surface membrane of infected erythrocytes. Mol Biochem Parasitol 27: 207–224

Jeffrey G M 1966 Epidemiological significance of repeated infections with homologous and heterologous strains and species of *Plasmodium*. Bull WHO 35: 873–882

Kemp D J, Thompson J K, Walliker D, Corcoran L M 1987 Molecular karyotype of *Plasmodium falciparum*: conserved linkage groups and expendable histidine-rich protein genes. Proc Natl Acad Sci USA 84: 7672–7676

Kemp D J, Cowman A F, Walliker D 1989 Genetic diversity in *Plasmodium falciparum*. Adv Parasitol (in press)

Kilejian A 1984 The biosynthesis of the knob protein and a 65,000 dalton histidine-rich polypeptide of *Plasmodium falciparum*. Mol Biochem Parasitol 12: 185–194

Koenen M, Scherf A, Mercereau O, Langsley G, Sibilli L, Dubois P, Pereira da Silva L, Muller-Hill B 1984 Human antisera detect a *Plasmodium falciparum* genomic clone encoding a nonapeptide repeat. Nature 311: 382–385

Langreth S G, Reese R T, Moytl M R, Trager W 1979 *Plasmodium falciparum*: loss of knobs on the infected erythrocyte surface after long-term cultivation. Exp Parasitol 48: 213–219

Leech J H, Barnwell J W, Miller L H, Howard R J 1984 Identification of a strain-specific malarial antigen exposed on the surface of *Plasmodium falciparum*-infected erythrocytes. J Exp Med 159: 1567–1575

Lew A M, Langford C J, Anders R F, Kemp D J, Saul A, Fardoulys C, Sheppard M 1989 The protective monoclonal antibody recognizes a linear epitope in the precursor of the major merozoite antigens of *Plasmodium chabaudi adami*. Proc Natl Acad Sci USA 86: 3768–3772

Luse S A, Miller L H 1971 *Plasmodium falciparum* malaria. Ultrastructure of parasitized erythrocytes in cardiac vessels. Am J Trop Med Hyg 20: 655–660

Lyon J A, Haynes J D, Diggs C L, Chulay J D, Haidaris C G, Pratt-Rossiter J 1987 Monoclonal antibody characterization of the 195-kilodalton major surface glycoprotein of *Plasmodium falciparum* malaria schizonts and merozoites: identification of additional processed products and a serotype-restricted repetitive epitope. J Immunol 138: 895–901

McBride J S, Heidrich H-G 1987 Fragments of the polymorphic M_r 185,000 glycoprotein from the surface of isolated *Plasmodium falciparum* merozoites form an antigenic complex. Mol Biochem Parasitol 23: 71–84

McBride J S, Welsby P D, Walliker D et al 1984 Serotyping *Plasmodium falciparum* from acute human infections using monoclonal antibodies. Trans R Soc Trop Med Hyg 78: 32–34

McBride J S, Newbold C I, Anand R et al 1985 Polymorphism of a high molecular weight schizont antigen of the human malaria parasite *Plasmodium falciparum*. J Exp Med 161: 160–180

McLean S A, Pearson C D, Phillips R S 1986 Antigenic variation in *Plasmodium chabaudi*: analysis of parent and variant populations by cloning. Parasite Immunol 8: 415–424

McLean S A, Phillips R S, Pearson C D, Walliker D 1987 The effect of mosquito transmission of antigenic variants of *Plasmodium chabaudi*. Parasitology 94: 443–449

Magowan C, Wollish W, Anderson L, Leech J 1988 Cytoadherence by *Plasmodium falciparum*-infected erythrocytes is correlated with the expression of a family of variable proteins on infected erythrocytes. J Exp Med 168: 1307–1320

Marsh K, Howard R J 1986 Antigens induced on erythrocytes by *falciparum*: expression of diverse and conserved determinants. Science 231: 150–153

Marsh K, Sherwood J A, Howard R J 1986 Parasite-infected-cell-agglutination and indirect immunofluorescence assays for detection of human serum antibodies bound to antigens on *Plasmodium falciparum*-infected erythrocytes. J Immunol Methods 91: 107–115

Mattei D, Langsley G, Braun-Breton C, Guillotte M, Dubremetz J-F, Mercereau-Puijalon O 1988 The S-antigen of *Plasmodium falciparum* Palo Alto represents a new S-antigen serotype. Mol Biochem Parasitol 27: 171–180

Mendis K N, David P H, Hommel M, Carter R, Miller L H 1983 Immunity to malarial antigens on the surface of *Plasmodium falciparum*-infected erythrocytes. Am J Trop Med Hyg 32: 926–930

Miettinen-Baumann A, Strych W, McBride J, Heidrich H-G 1988 A 46000 Da *Plasmodium falciparum* merozoite surface antigen not related to the 185000–195000 Da schizont precursor molecule: isolation and characterization. Parasitol Res 74: 317–323

Nicholls S C, Hillman Y, Lockyer M J, Odink K G, Holder A A 1988 An S-antigen gene from *Plasmodium falciparum* contains a novel repetitive sequence. Mol Biochem Parasitol 28: 11–20

Patarapotikul J, Langsley G 1988 Chromosome size polymorphism in *Plasmodium falciparum* can involve deletions of the subtelomeric pPFrep20 sequence. Nucleic Acids Res 16: 4331–4340

Perrin L H, Merkli B, Gabra M S, Stocker J W, Chizzolini C, Richle R 1985 Immunization with a *Plasmodium falciparum* merozoite surface antigen induces a partial immunity in monkeys. J Clin Invest 75: 1718–1721

Peterson M G, Coppel R L, McIntyre P, Langford C J, Woodrow G, Brown G V, Anders R F, Kemp D J 1988a Variation in the precursor to the major merozoite surface antigens of *Plasmodium falciparum*. Mol Biochem Parasitol 27: 291–302

Peterson M G, Coppel R L, Moloney M B, Kemp D J 1988b Third form of the precursor to the major merozoite surface antigens of *Plasmodium falciparum*. Mol Cell Biol 8: 2664–2667

Pirson P J, Perkins M E 1985 Characterization with monoclonal antibodies of a surface antigen of *Plasmodium falciparum*. J Immunol 134: 1946–1951

Pologe L G, Ravetch J V 1986 A chromosomal rearrangement in a *P. falciparum* histidine-rich protein gene is associated with the knobless phenotype. Nature 322: 474–477

34

Pologe L G, Ravetch J V 1988 Large deletions result from breakage and healing of *P. falciparum* chromosomes. Cell 55: 869–874

Pologe L G, Pavlovec A, Shio H, Ravetch J V 1987 Primary structure and subcellular localization of the knob-associated histidine-rich protein of *Plasmodium falciparum*. Proc Natl Acad Sci USA 84: 7139–7143

Ramasamy R 1987 Characterisation of a novel merozoite membrane antigen of the human malaria parasite *Plasmodium falciparum*. Immunol Cell Biol 65: 419–424

Saint R B, Coppel R L, Cowman A F, Brown G V, Shi P T, Barzaga N, Kemp D J, Anders R F 1987 Changes in repeat number, sequence, and reading frame in S-antigen genes of *Plasmodium falciparum*. Mol Cell Biol 7: 2968–2973

Sam-Yellowe T Y, Shio H, Perkins M E 1988 Secretion of *Plasmodium falciparum* rhoptry protein into the plasma membrane of host erythrocytes. J Cell Biol 106: 1507–1513

Saul A, Cooper J, Ingram L, Anders R F, Brown G V 1985 Invasion of erythrocytes in vitro by *Plasmodium falciparum* can be inhibited by a monoclonal antibody directed against an S-antigen. Parasite Immunol 7: 587–593

Saul A, Geysen M, Lord R, Gale J, Epping R, Jones G, Smythe J, Ramasamy R 1989 Delineation of epitopes on a *Plasmodium falciparum* merozoite surface antigen using inhibitory monoclonal antibodies. In: Lasky L (ed) Technological Advances in Vaccine Development. Alan R. Liss, New York, (in press)

Scherf A, Hilbich C, Sieg K, Mattei D, Mercereau-Puijalon O, Müller-Hill B 1988 The 11–1 gene of *Plasmodium falciparum* codes for distinct, fast evolving repeats. EMBO J 7: 1129–1137

Schofield L, Tharavanij S, Saul A, do Rosario V, Kidson C 1985 A specific S-antigen of *Plasmodium falciparum* is expressed in a proportion of primary isolates in Brazil, Thailand and Papua New Guinea. Trans R Soc Trop Med Hyg 79: 493–494

Sharma Y D, Kilejian A 1987 Structure of the knob protein (KP) gene of *Plasmodium falciparum*. Mol Biochem Parasitol 26: 11–16

Sherwood J A, Marsh K, Howard R J, Barnwell J W 1985 Antibody mediated strain-specific agglutination of *Plasmodium falciparum*-parasitized erythrocytes visualized by ethidium bromide staining. Parasite Immunol 7: 659–663

Smythe J A, Coppel R L, Brown G V, Ramasamy R, Kemp D J, Anders R F 1988 Identification of two integral membrane proteins of *Plasmodium falciparum*. Proc Natl Acad Sci USA 85: 5195–5199

Smythe J, Peterson M G, Coppel R, Kemp D, Anders R 1989 Allelic variation of the M_r 45,000 merozoite surface antigen of *Plasmodium falciparum*. In: Brown F, Chanock R M, Lerner R A (eds) Vaccines 89. Cold Spring Harbor Laboratory (in press)

Southwell B, Brown G V, Forsyth K P, Smith T, Philip G, Anders R F 1989 Field applications of agglutination and cytoadherence assays with *Plasmodium falciparum* from Papua New Guinea. Trans R Soc Trop Med Hyg (in press)

Stahl H D, Kemp D J, Crewther P E, Scanlon D B, Woodrow G, Brown G V, Bianco A E, Anders R F, Coppel R L 1985 Sequence of a cDNA encoding a small polymorphic histidine- and alanine-rich protein from *Plasmodium falciparum*. Nucleic Acids Res 13: 7837–7846

Stanley H A, Howard R F, Reese R T 1985 Recognition of a Mr 56K glycoprotein on the surface of *Plasmodium falciparum* merozoites by mouse monoclonal antibodies. J Immunol 134: 3439–3444

Tanabe K, Mackay M, Goman M, Scaife J G 1987 Allelic dimorphism in a surface antigen gene of the malaria parasite *Plasmodium falciparum*. J Mol Biol 195: 273–287

Tan-Ariya P, Yang Y F, Kilejian A 1988 *Plasmodium falciparum*: Comparison of the genomic organization of the knob protein gene in knobby and knobless variants. Exp Parasitol 67: 129–136

Taylor D W, Parra M, Chapman G B, Stearns M E, Rener J, Aikawa M, Uni S, Aley S B, Panton L J, Howard R J 1987 Localization of *Plasmodium falciparum* histidine-rich protein 1 in the erythrocyte skeleton under knobs. Mol Biochem Parasitol 25: 165–174

Trager W, Rudzinska M A, Bradbury P C 1966 The fine structure of *Plasmodium falciparum* and its host erythrocytes in natural malarial infections in man. Bull WHO 35: 883–885

Triglia T, Stahl H D, Crewther P E, Scanlon D, Brown G V, Anders R F, Kemp D J 1987 The complete sequence of the gene for the knob-associated histidine-rich protein from *plasmodium falciparum*. EMBO J 6: 1413–1419

Udeinya I J, Miller L H, McGregor I A, Jensen J B 1983 *Plasmodium falciparum* strain-specific antibody blocks binding of infected erythrocytes to amelanotic melanoma cells. Nature 303: 429–431

Wellems T E, Howard R J 1986 Homologous genes encode two distinct histidine-rich proteins in a cloned isolate of *Plasmodium falciparum*. Proc Natl Acad Sci USA 83: 6065–6069

Wellems T E, Walliker D, Smith C L, do Rossario V E, Maloy W L, Howard R J, Carter R, McCutchan T F 1987 A histidine-rich protein gene marks a linkage group favored strongly in a genetic cross of *Plasmodium falciparum*. Cell 49: 633–642

Wilson R J M 1970 Antigens and antibodies associated with *Plasmodium falciparum* infections in West Africa. Trans R Soc Trop Med Hyg 64: 547–552

Wilson R J M 1980 Serotyping *Plasmodium falciparum* malaria with S-antigens. Nature 284: 451–452

Wilson R J M, McGregor I A, Hall P, Williams K, Bartholomew R 1969 Antigens associated with *Plasmodium falciparum* infections in man. Lancet ii: 201–205

Wilson R J M, McGregor I A, Williams K 1975a Occurrence of S-antigens in serum in *Plasmodium falciparum* infections in man. Trans R Soc Trop Med Hyg 69: 453–459

Wilson R J M, McGregor I A, Hall P J 1975b Persistence and recurrence of S-antigen in *Plasmodium falciparum* infections in man. Trans R Soc Trop Med Hyg 69: 460–467

Winchell E J, Ling I T, Wilson R J M 1984a A molecular basis for strain specificity in S-antigens of *Plasmodium falciparum*. J Immunol 133: 1702–1704

Winchell E J, Ling I T, Wilson R J M 1984b Metabolic labelling and characterisation of S-antigens, the heat-stable, strain-specific antigens of *Plasmodium falciparum*. Mol Biochem Parasitol 10: 287–296

Discussion of paper presented by R. F. Anders

Discussed by M. Hommel
Reported by G. A. T. Targett

The discussion began with a fairly fundamental challenge to much of the current research directed towards characterization of malarial antigens. Why expend so much time and effort on antigens that are so polymorphic? Why not concentrate on those that are protective and have a more conserved structure?

There are several answers. The extremely polymorphic nature of many antigens as revealed by a combination of sero-epidemiological and sequencing studies has been a surprise. The diversity of S-antigens was known but not that of, for example, merozoite surface antigens (MSA). Such diversity does, however, provide the best explanation for the fact that immunity in malaria is very slow to develop and is relatively unstable; a strong immunity is dependent on exposure to a large number of parasites which vary with respect to these highly polymorphic molecules.

There are studies in progress on conserved molecules like rhoptry proteins, and on the conserved regions of the polymorphic antigens like MSA 1 and MSA 2. The MSA 2 molecules fall into allelic families which are characterized by diverse repeat structures based on 4-, 8- or 32-amino-acid sequences but with a high degree of conservation outside the variable regions.

This degree of variability within repeat regions of molecules prompted questions on the effect this might have on the conformation of a protein. How does the molecule fold; are there important charge differences; what is the function and position of the conserved region? There are few data available at present and, because of likely difficulties in crystallizing antigens with hydrophilic repeats, information may come best from electron diffraction and n.m.r. studies, including two-dimensional n.m.r. on synthetic peptides. Anders found it difficult to envisage how a molecule with a 4-amino-acid sequence that repeats 13 times could have the same conformation as one with a 32-mer that repeats twice. However, it was pointed out that variant specific glycoproteins (VSGs) of Salivarian trypanosomes have no primary sequence homology whatsoever yet fold into the same packing shape. The VSG molecules are immunologically distinct from one another, which means that molecular shape and antigenicity may not be related. However, even small changes such as substitution of leucine for arginine in the 8-amino-acid repeat of the NF7 S-antigen produce a significant change in antigenicity and H-2 restriction.

Immune responses to the polymorphic antigens are determined primarily in terms of antibody and definition of T-cell epitopes of these asexual stage antigens is only just beginning. It should be noted, however, that most of the T-cell epitopes on the circumsporozoite protein (CSP) map within polymorphic regions that flank the repeat sequences.

Despite the variability of some of the asexual-stage antigens there are some cross-reactions between them, but experiments in progress, particularly with parasites like *P. fragile* in its natural (monkey) host, will show whether there are any protective effects. Cross-reactions at the level of species also occur but, again, the significance of this is unknown. One of the rhoptry antigens shows dramatic conservation of sequence between *P. falciparum* and *P. chabaudi*. In endemic areas where different *Plasmodium* species are common, cross-reactivity could be important.

The genes coding for polymorphic antigens that have been mapped are generally towards the telomere but are located on a number of different chromosomes. Of particular interest, a gene that is like RESA without its repeat region, is located on chromosome 11 while the RESA gene is on chromosome 1.

The discussion was widened by Hommel, to embrace other aspects of diversity. *P. falciparum* schizont-infected erythrocytes bind to a variety of cells because they express certain antigens on their surface (it is still uncertain which antigens are of key importance). Diversity in ability to cytoadhere has been shown and, in Bangkok, Singh, May Ho and White (unpublished data) found that amongst 30 patients, strains of the parasite which caused severe malaria all occurred within the group that was strongly cytoadherent.

Diversity can also be demonstrated with surface-binding antibodies. Immunofluorescence has been widely used, and Hommel outlined a highly reproducible immunogold technique that can be used on thin blood films (Hommel & Semoff 1988). With this technique, variance amongst populations of the Indochina strain of *P. falciparum* were demonstrated following infection of monkeys, and diversity was linked to protection.

A further aspect of diversity is being assessed by fingerprinting, using a biotin-labelled oligonucleotide probe based on a small portion of the consensus sequence of Rep20. Isolates have a characteristic pattern but, interestingly, serotypes of one isolate are identical, suggesting that the switch from one serotype to another does not involve major reorganization of the genome (Hughes & Crampton unpublished, Liverpool School of Tropical Medicine).

Anders described the loss of ability to express some antigens by parasites grown in vitro, and there was interest in the effect of this on growth in vivo. Experiments are in progress to compare growth in vivo of the uncloned FCR3 isolate of *P. falciparum* and a cloned line that does not express RESA. The expectation is that it will not grow, but if parasites do have the ability to dispense with some antigens, it would be an argument for no longer including them as vaccine candidates.

REFERENCE

Hommel M, Semoff S 1988 Expression and function of erythrocyte-associated surface antigens in malaria. Biol Cell 64: 183–203

3. From sporozoite to liver stages: the saga of the irradiated sporozoite vaccine

P. Druilhe and C. Marchand

The story starts forty years ago, when two important discoveries were made. The location in the liver of the exo-erythrocytic (EE) phase of the malaria life cycle was demonstrated for the first time (Shortt & Garnham 1948) and it was shown that UV irradiation of sporozoites made them no longer infectious, as animals inoculated with them were resistant to challenge with infectious parasites (Mulligan et al 1941). Twenty years later, R. Nussenzweig, in the laboratories of Meir Yoeli, extended this observation and began a systematic programme for the development of a sporozoite vaccine using first gamma-irradiation rather than UV as it was easier to deliver regulated doses and thereafter all tools of modern biology as soon as they became available (see review by Cochrane et al 1980).

In retrospect, it is amazing that a single observation, the effects of UV irradiation could give rise to such extensive studies, bringing with it high hopes, disillusionments and controversies. No attempt is made here to review the whole literature; rather we shall present a personal view of some of the critical steps of this fascinating story, and give some of our own recent results.

Ever since Garnham's discovery, the liver cycle has remained – particularly from an immunological standpoint – 'a big black box'. Little interest was shown in the antigens of that stage, and assessment of immunity induced by sporozoites was measured only by detection of erythrocytic stages. This impedes the interpretation of earlier experiments because there is no indication of what occurred in the stage between sporozoite and blood form, i.e. within the 'black box'. Therefore all the most critical and significant studies now need to be re-done with assessment of the fate of the parasites within hepatocytes.

Some of the initial experiments which led to the choice of the circumsporozoite protein (CS) as a major vaccine candidate need first of all to be recalled. Gamma-irradiated sporozoites (IRR-SPZ) proved protective to mice only when injected intravenously. It is important to stress that the protection achieved was total, allowing animals to resist challenge with millions of sporozoites. The same antigen (IRR-SPZ), injected by all other routes — intramuscularly, with or without a variety of adjuvants including Freund's complete adjuvant (FCA), intraperitoneally, subcutaneously, even orally — gave little protection, whatever the number of immunizing doses given. Conversely killed sporozoites injected intravenously, or by other routes, gave almost no protection (Table 3.1). The method of killing

Table 3.1 Immunization of mice against sporozoite challenge

Immunization regimen		Protection (%)		CS-precipitation
(i) X-irr. SPZ i.v.	⎫	90–100	⎫	+
(ii) Live SPZ + chloroquine	⎬		⎬	+
(iii) X-irr. SPZ i.m. + FCA	⎱			+
(iv) X-irr. SPZ s.c.				+
(v) X-irr. SPZ i.p.	⎬	0–25		+
(vi) Killed SPZ i.v.				+
(vii) Killed SPZ i.m./s.c.	⎰			+
(viii) SPZ antigens		0		+
(ix) No antigen		60–100		−
C. parvum/BCG/Poly I:C				

X-irr. = X-irradiated
SPZ = sporozoites
FCA = Freund's complete adjuvant

may influence the integrity of an antigen, but results were the same whether parasites were killed by heat, formaldehyde, glutaraldehyde, alcohol or iodoacetamide. In addition we are now aware that CS is a stable molecule, able to resist heating to 100°C. It is well established that antigen presentation to the immune system is crucial, but it seems difficult to explain the above discrepancy only in terms of antigen presentation, especially when one considers that, in the protected as in the non-protected animals, antibodies to the sporozoite surface were produced.

Another critical experiment was reported by Beaudoin and colleagues. It was shown that gamma-irradiated sporozoites are living organisms, able to invade hepatocytes and to transform into young trophozoites. They are unable to divide, probably because of DNA damage, do not develop and remain, at least in the mouse model, for unknown periods of time as uninucleate intrahepatic bodies (Ramsey et al 1982).

These data pose several questions. Irradiation may have modified the antigen physically, increasing its immunogenicity, but why is it ineffective when injected by routes other than intravenously? Furthermore, sporozoites exposed to higher doses of irradiation were no longer effective immunogens. Alternatively, the intrahepatic parasite resulting from injection of irradiated sporozoites and unable to continue its development, could constitute an antigen depot, increasing the immunogenicity. However, live non-attenuated sporozoites, injected into mice treated with chloroquine in order to prevent death due to the blood stages of infection, also induced a high degree of protection — as high as that due to irradiated sporozoites.

To analyse results which can be thought of as quantitatively but not qualitatively different it is also necessary to recall that sporozoite challenge can be to some extent combated by administration to mice of cytokine inducers such as polynucleotides (Poly I:C), C. parvum or BCG (Jahiel et al 1968) (Table 3.1). This may explain the partial protection achieved in some of the animals receiving, for example, sporozoites with FCA intramuscularly.

Since live sporozoites, either irradiated or non-irradiated, get into the liver, these experiments have been highly suggestive to us that it may be the newly formed liver trophozoite that is responsible for the immunity induced and more precisely the antigens appearing at that stage. In other words, it may be that the immunogenic molecule is not even carried by the sporozoite itself!

Let us now focus on a statement that has been encountered in more than one paper. 'Animals and man can be effectively protected against malaria by immunization with gamma-irradiated sporozoites'. We will also use this to illustrate the problem of models, which is certainly a very crucial one in the field of parasitology. As stated earlier, results in mouse models were excellent and protection achieved reached 100%. We even learned very recently that a single injection of only 1000 irradiated sporozoites, could induce protection in BALB/c mice for 5 months (Gordon et al 1989). In contrast, the results obtained in primate malarias, including humans, were far from being as convincing (see Table 3.2). Using *P. falciparum* sporozoites, 4 of 11 human volunteers injected were protected and only one of them resisted several challenges with various strains; 6–8 inoculations of irradiated sporozoites given intravenously were necessary to achieve this result which lasted for no more than 2 months. Four or fewer injections resulted in no protection. As in mice the intramuscular route was not effective (Bray 1976). Results obtained with *P. vivax* also highlight the problem of the number of doses: one group reported no protection in 3 volunteers receiving 4 doses of *P. vivax* IRR-SPZ, and another group protection in 2 volunteers receiving 7 inoculations. The results obtained with *P. cynomolgi* and *P. knowlesi* in monkeys were probably even worse. Up to 4×10^8 parasites have been injected in multiple doses for several months in monkeys to achieve either no protection or, in one experiment a low degree (20%) of protection (Table 3.2).

In contrast to mice which can be protected by 2 or 3 injections of non-irradiated sporozoites, data from the field suggest that the injection of live non-irradiated sporozoites in humans, does not induce any significant degree of protection whatever the number of injections. In areas of high endemicity, such as in the Congo, where individuals receive as much as 3 infective inoculations per day for life, that is nearly 100,000 immunizing doses of a few hundred sporozoites each,

Table 3.2 Comparison of protection achieved by immunization with attenuated or live sporozoites in various species

Hosts	*Plasmodium* spp.	Vaccine	Route and No. doses	Protection (% or n)	Duration (months)
Mice	*P. berghei/P. yoelii*	(i) X-irr. SPZ	i.v. × 2	100	6–20
		(ii) Live SPZ + chloroquine	i.v. × 3	90–100	
Monkeys	*P. cynomolgi/*	(i) X-irr. SPZ	i.v. × 5	0	
	P. knowlesi	(ii) X-irr. SPZ	i.v.–i.m. × 12	20	
Humans	*P. falciparum*	(i) X-irr. SPZ	i.v. × 3	0	
		,,	i.v. × 6–8	1–4/7	2
		,,	i.m. × 2	0	
		(ii) Live SPZ	i.v. × 10^{10}	±0	
	P. vivax	(i) X-irr. SPZ	i.v. × 7–10	2/2	
		,,	i.v. × 4	0/3	

X-irr. = X-irradiated
SPZ = sporozoites

the incidence of new blood infection is high; at any given time, blood-stage prevalence reaches about 60% in adults (Trape 1987).

At that time the increasing problems of malaria control led perhaps prematurely to all hopes being directed to a new vaccine.

Let us now examine how the effect of antibodies, and particularly the biological effect of monoclonal antibodies (MAbs), has influenced this research on a sporozoite vaccine. Based on a morphological alteration which appears as a tail-like precipitate, called the circumsporozoite precipitation reaction, but which can be seen only in a percentage of the sporozoites incubated with immune sera, it was thought that protection induced by irradiated sporozoites was antibody-mediated. Although the time course of protection and that of antibody production were not parallel, the biological effect of mAbs reinforced very strongly the idea that antibody could act either by destroying the sporozoite or by preventing its penetration into liver cells. However, it has now become clearer that on certain occasions the biological effects of a MAb cannot be reproduced by the polyclonal response to the corresponding antigen.

MAbs identified the CS as the sole antigen on the sporozoite surface and also established firmly the basis of an antibody-mediated effect which now appears debatable. This prevented a complete analysis of the antigenic content of the sporozoite which still has to be performed. In view of the undoubted blocking effect of mAbs, a report of successful protection induced in B cell-deficient mice by gamma-irradiated sporozoites (Chen et al 1977) and the much less significant effect in chimpanzee of MAbs to *P. falciparum* CS were not taken into consideration.

Since the amount of CS antigen in sporozoites was considered to be too limited to attempt any direct immunization with extracted proteins, vaccination trials had to await the identification of the corresponding gene and the production by recombination or synthesis of the mAb-defined epitopes. The problems which were later encountered in trying to raise an immune response to these molecules in man were in fact indicated by epidemiological studies of the immune response to the mAb-defined epitope. In several endemic areas of Africa, including the one quoted above, despite daily immunizations about 40–50% of the people did not mount an antibody response to the CS-repeats, or had extremely low titres (Brahimi et al unpublished results). The basis for this defective response was recently analysed at the molecular level by Good et al (1988).

Comparison of results obtained by sporozoite surface labelling in an immunofluorescent (IFA) 'wet' sporozoite assay, and CS-repeat recognition by ELISA, showed a clearcut discrepancy in about 30% of cases, indicating that antibodies to CS-repeats were only part of the whole antibody response to sporozoite surface epitopes. This was confirmed in competition assays using either synthetic or recombinant antigens or monoclonal antibodies to the repeats.

Finally, evidence for the occurrence in man of antibody to non-CS epitopes was obtained by producing human monoclonal antibodies by Epstein–Barr virus transformation of peripheral blood lymphocytes. HuMab have demonstrated the presence of several distinct epitopes on the sporozoite surface. Some parasites were defined by single human monoclonal antibody specificities (Galey et al submitted).

The low immune response recorded in individuals vaccinated with CS-repeats led to the study of its genetic restriction. However, this defective response prevented an evaluation of the degree of protection that can be expected if a proper anti-CS response is achieved, that is if means to overcome the genetic restriction are found. At that time our research on liver stages of *Plasmodium* led to the design of a culture method for *P. falciparum* in human hepatocytes. In such *in vitro* conditions the effect of antibody upon sporozoite penetration was found to be concentration-dependent up to a certain concentration, and thereafter remained high but never complete, even when using MAb concentrated 1000 to 10,000 times more than antibody concentrations reached in man (Mellouk et al 1986). Similarly, antibody from individuals exposed to daily infective bites and reaching IFA titres of 1/100,000 also showed an incomplete inhibitory effect in vitro. In vivo, despite these high antibody titres, at least some sporozoites managed to complete the exo-erythrocytic cycle since blood-stage infections occurred in the same individuals at the time of sampling for some of them, or during follow-up for the others.

The validity of this in vivo/in vitro comparison is also supported by recent results obtained with *P. yoelii* and *P. berghei*. Sera from mice receiving an anti-*P. yoelii* CS mAb, and fully protected, inhibited sporozoite invasion in vitro by 100%. Conversely, sera from mice immunized with several constructs based on a subunit CS vaccine, and not protected, were not fully inhibitory in vitro (Mellouk et al submitted). These experiments again show the difference between the rodent and the human models, full inhibition being achievable with mAbs in vivo and in vitro in one model and not in the other.

In view of the rather disappointing results obtained in man both with recombinant and with synthetic CS vaccines – we learned recently that more than 700 subjects were included in such immunization attempts – research has shifted progressively towards the study of cell-mediated immunity. The genetic restriction of T helper cell responses was demonstrated in mice and, in man, since T cells from adults in one endemic area did not respond in 40% of cases to any of the T epitopes of the CS-protein (Good et al 1988). Furthermore, antigenic diversity was found to occur between parasite strains within the T-cell epitopes identified. Cytotoxic lymphocyte (CTL) studies are now being undertaken, but CD8[+] T epitopes are again searched for only within the CS molecule. The effects of various cytokines on the pre-erythrocytic phase were investigated in vivo and in vitro in several models, and among them gamma-interferon was the one with the most profound effect. However, in rodents, and probably in man, the degree of inhibition achieved by IFN-γ would seem again to be incomplete. In endemic areas we found an overall prevalence of 85% of circulating IFN at levels of 60 IU/ml on average (Druilhe et al 1982), while about 60% of adults had a blood-stage infection suggesting a successful liver cycle.

These findings at least modified views about γ-IRR-SPZ induced immunity by introducing the liver stages. Liver forms became a likely target for CTL but it has not yet changed the view on the triggering antigen, the CS-protein with the known restrictions associated with its T-cell sites.

From the comparison of results obtained using living sporozoites given by the i.v. route, versus living sporozoites inoculated by other routes, and killed parasites

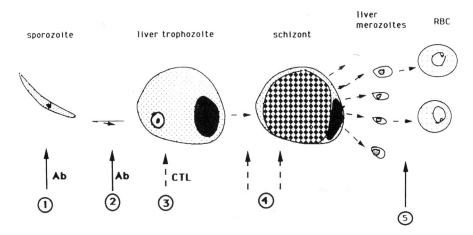

Figure 3.1 Schematic diagram of identified and non-identified but possible targets of defensive mechanisms to various stages of the pre-erythrocytic phase of malaria parasites

injected i.v., it always seemed likely to us that the transformation of sporozoites into liver forms was an obligatory requirement to achieve protection. In humans, this hypothesis was further reinforced by recent experiments. No protection was obtained in volunteers injected with sporozoites irradiated at 23 Krads instead of the 14 Krads used formerly (Herrington et al 1989). In vitro results obtained with sporozoites exposed at various irradiating doses demonstrate the lack of penetration of sporozoites exposed to the higher doses and therefore support our initial view that the production of young liver forms was critical in the induction of immunity.

For this and for other reasons we have focused our research on the characterization of liver stages or, more generally, on the pre-erythrocytic cycle (Fig. 3.1).

Despite initial progress which enabled production of *P. falciparum* liver forms both by in vitro and in vivo means, the output of those methods has remained too low to enable any immunochemical analysis (e.g. by electrophoresis), to have access to messenger RNA, or to induce an immune response in mice in order to prepare monoclonal antibodies. Human monoclonal antibodies specific for liver stages were produced but they turned out to be too unstable for screening purposes. The absence of probes for liver stage antigens (LSA), which was a major limitation, led us to use a more complex approach, which finally appears now to have been worthwhile.

We decided to try to select sera having mainly, and if possible only, antibodies directed against pre-erythrocytic antigens. Three sera from missionaries living in holoendemic areas, who had been taking uninterrupted chloroquine prophylaxis for 26 years, had very high titres of antibodies to sporozoite and liver stages while being almost negative for blood stages antigens. The screening of a genomic DNA library, cloned in an expression vector, by these sera allowed us to reject more than 85% of the antigen-expressing clones and to select about 120 clones thought to correspond to pre-erythrocytic stage antigens. We first picked up three of those most immunoreactive (Fig. 3.2). They encoded an epitope present only in

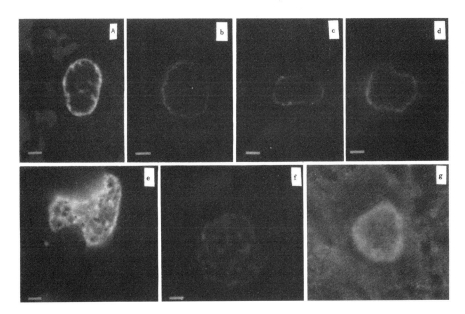

Figure 3.2 Reaction and localization of antibodies with liver-stage schizonts. *a*, Typical immunofluorescence using adult African serum diluted 1/2000 and reacted with 5-μm sections of Carnoy fixed liver fragments taken from *Cebus apella* monkeys infected with *P. falciparum*. Same antigen reacted with antibody eluted from protein expressed by: *b*, clone DG307; *c*, clone DG145; *d*, clone DG199, *e,f*, the same as *a* and *b*, using more mature schizonts to show the internal distribution of the antigen. *g*, Liver schizonts reacted with 1/250 dilution of a rabbit serum raised to clone DG307 fusion protein (one i.m. injection with FCA of the recombinant fusion protein isolated by preparative gel electrophoresis followed by four additional i.v. injections at 15-day intervals) (Marchand-Guerin et al, 1987, Nature 329: 164–167).

P. falciparum liver stages, made of 17-amino-acid repeats, organized in an α-helix, which was designated LSA (Marchand-Guerin et al 1987).

Further screening of the 120 clone-subset was performed by means of selected additional polyclonal sera, having high titres to sporozoite and liver stage native antigens, while being negative for CS and LSA. The pattern of reactivity with those sera allowed a first classification of clones into three categories.

One other means to select, preferentially, antigens well-conserved among isolates and with low, or no, restriction of immunogenicity, was to evaluate further the reactivity of each fusion protein with a complementary series of 8 immune sera, and retain the most consistently reactive.

Human affinity-purified antibodies were prepared from each clone and studied using as antigen, sporozoites, liver forms and blood forms of *P. falciparum* and from heterologous species, in order to determine the stage and species-specificity of the recombinant epitopes expressed. About 47 positive clones have been found so far.

One of them was called SALSA (sporozoite and liver stage antigen). The reactive epitopes are contained within an 87-amino-acid polypeptide which corresponds to a 70-kD protein in *P. falciparum* sporozoites.

The remaining clones were classified based on similarities in antigenic features and DNA structure. For the LSA 'family' and the SALSA clone a good correspondence between the two methods was found. Analysis of results from cross-immunological reactivity studies allowed us to distinguish three situations.

1. A first group of clones, negative with the selection sera, correspond only to the LSA family, and represents nearly 20% of the clones, an expected event since the 5-kbp gene is known to contain many 51-bp repeats.
2. A second group of clones, positive with each of the selection sera, corresponds to antigens mostly shared between sporozoites and liver stages, but probably distinct from SALSA.
3. In the third group, showing variable results with the 5 sera, we found mostly, if not only, sporozoite surface-specific antigens.

One of the important characteristics of some of the above proteins is their high and consistent immunogenicity when presented by the parasite to the human immune system. For example, in one area of very low endemicity in Africa, the prevalence of antibodies to CS-repeats was 27%, to LSA 80%, and to SALSA 93%. This may not appear surprising since the identification of these antigens is based on methods which are exactly opposite to those used previously for CS and for several blood stages antigens, that is mainly on the quality of the response they generate in man.

Thus, at least some information is coming from the formerly 'black box' liver phase. This phase is currently considered a likely target of CS-induced CTL which is MHC class I restricted. We believe that several more steps are now required in considering these antigens.

First, from the point of view of IRR-SPZ-induced immunity, there is evidence from several lines of investigation that additional, non-CS, antigens are present on sporozoites and one has been characterized. More important may be the newly formed antigens in young liver trophozoites which may be more relevant to the type of resistance induced by IRR-SPZ. From studies on mouse malaria, the mechanisms mediating protection were thought for a long time to be solely due to antibodies but now they are considered to be mostly by CTL. So far there is no indication of the possible mechanism prevailing in man and the history of model studies makes us cautious about extrapolation.

Second, the finding that irradiated sporozoites can induce protective immunity does not mean that other ways of inducing a protective immune response to pre-erythrocytic stages do not exist. The steps of transformation from liver trophozoite to liver schizont provide another interesting target, especially since an inflammatory reaction, with cellular infiltrates, is known to occur upon challenge of LS-primed animals. Also the steps of liver merozoite release into the blood stream and penetration of red blood cells are probably critical and, possibly, vulnerable ones.

Our continued interest in LS is also supported by results from epidemiological surveys performed using whole parasites as antigens which: (i) showed that LS-specific antigens were very immunogenic; (ii) suggested that the immune response to sporozoite surface antigens has a regulatory rather than a blocking effect on sporozoite penetration, modulating the proportion of sporozoites transforming into liver forms and dependent on the level of endemicity; (iii) As a consequence of this regulation of LS load by anti-CS immunity no epidemiological situation has allowed a maximal immunization with LS antigens. Therefore, the results of optimal immunization with such antigens cannot be derived, in contrast to sporozoites, from responses to naturally occurring challenges, and remain to be evaluated.

Until recently we were dealing with a single antigen triggering a single protective mechanism but now research has shifted towards liver stages and the range of antigens and of mechanisms is much wider. However, the lack of a relevant model, as is often the case in parasitology, is, in our opinion, likely to be the major limitation to vaccine development.

ACKNOWLEDGEMENTS

Some of the results quoted above are part of a team effort in which the following participated: B Galey, S Mellouk, E Bottius, K Brahimi, R L Beaudoin, A Londono, C Desgranges, O Puijalon, J F Trape. These studies were supported in part by WHO/UNDP/WB TDR programme, contract Nos. 840105 and 870121.

REFERENCES

Bray R S 1976 Vaccination against *Plasmodium falciparum*: a negative result. Trans R Soc Trop Med Hyg 70: 258
Chen D H, Tigelaar R E, Weinbaum F I 1977 Immunity to sporozoite-induced malaria infection in mice. 1. The effect of immunization of T and B cell-deficient mice. J Immunol 118: 1322–1427
Cochrane A H, Nussenzweig R S, Nardin E H 1980 Immunization against sporozoites. In: Kreier J (ed) Malaria, Academic Press, London, 3: 163–202
Druilhe P, Rhodes-Feuillette A, Canivet M, Gentilini M, Peris J 1982 Circulating interferon in patients with *Plasmodium falciparum, ovale* and *vivax*, malaria. Trans R Soc Trop Med Hyg 76: 422
Galey B, Druilhe P. Ploton, I et al. *Plasmodium falciparum:* evidence for diversity of sporozoite surface antigens derived from analysis of antibodies elicited in man. (submitted)
Good M F, Pombo D, Quakyi I A et al 1988 Human T-cell recognition of the circumsporozoite protein of *Plasmodium falciparum*: immunodominant T-cell domains map to the polymorphic regions of the molecule. Proc Natl Acad Sci USA 85: 1199–1203
Gordon D M, Egan J E, Arthur J D et al 1989 Subunit vaccines designed to induce protective antibodies against the circumsporozoite (CS) protein of *Plasmodium berghei*: Pre-erythrocytic stage malaria vaccine development: current status and future prospects, Bethesda 12–15 April, WRAIR/AID/WHO meeting. Am J Trop Med Hyg 1989 (in press)
Herrington D, Clyde D, Davis J et al 1989 Clinicals trials of sporozoite vaccine at the University of Maryland. Pre-erythrocytic stage malaria vaccine development: current status and future prospects. Bethesda 12–15 April, WRAIR/AID/WHO meeting. Am J Trop Med Hyg 1989 (in press)
Jahiel R I, Vilcek J, Nussenzweig R S, Vanderberg J 1968 Interferon inducers protect mice against *Plasmodium berghei* malaria. Science 161: 802–804
Marchand-Guerin C, Druilhe P, Galey B et al 1987 A liver stage antigen of *P. falciparum* characterized by gene cloning. Nature 329: 164–167
Mellouk S, Mazier D, Druilhe P, Berbiguier N, Danis M 1986 *In vitro* and *in vivo* results suggesting that anti-sporozoite antibodies do not totally block *Plasmodium falciparum* sporozoite infectivity New Engl J Med 315: 648
Mellouk S, Charoenvit Y, Berbiguier N, Beaudoin R L, Druilhe P 1989 High but sub-total inhibition of transformation of *P. falciparum* sporozoite to liver stage by monoclonal and human polyclonal antibodies to sporozoite surface antigens. (submitted)
Mulligan H W, Russell P F, Mohan B N 1941 Active immunization of fowls against *Plasmodium gallinaceum* by injections of killed homologous sporozoites. J Malar Inst India 4: 25–34

Ramsey J M, Beaudoin R L, Hollingdale M R 1982 Infection of tissue-culture cells with Co gamma-irradiated malaria sporozoites. In: Nuclear techniques in the study of parasitic infections, International Atomic Energy Agency, pp 19–25

Shortt H E, Garnham P C C 1948 Pre-erythrocytic stage in mammalian malaria parasites. Nature 161: 126

Trape J-F, Zoulani A 1987 Etudes sur le paludisme d'une zone de mosaïque forét-savane d'Afrique Centrale, la région de Brazzaville ll – Densités parasitaires. Bull Soc Path Ex 80: 84–99

Discussion of paper presented by P. Druilhe

Discussed by A. Holder
Reported by G. A. T. Targett

The discussion began by considering to what extent the nature of the immune responses in malaria has been revealed by how patients with agammaglobulinaemias or AIDS cope with infection. Agammaglobulinaemic patients are certainly highly susceptible but, so far, mechanisms of resistance to either pre-erythrocytic or blood stage infections have not been clarified from studies on groups of patients whose immune competence is impaired. With AIDS patients it was suggested that the group to examine is infants below 1 year when they are exposed to malaria infection and are beginning to respond immunologically.

Circulating gamma-interferon (IFN-γ) is demonstrable in malaria patients and the question of whether the levels are high enough to be (partly) responsible for symptoms was raised, as occurs with influenza-A. The levels detectable are, however, not so high and may last several months.

It is a common finding that attempts to prevent infection immunologically are never 100% effective. Druilhe had described experiments on blockade by monoclonal antibodies of liver cell invasion in which this was the case. Data recently presented by Anna Szarfman (NIH, Bethesda, USA) were described where sporozoites became non-reactive with an anti-CS protein monoclonal antibody, having shed the protein in a CSP reaction. This prompted questions on what happens to CS protein during and following invasion of liver cells, and how this is influenced by the presence or absence of high levels of anti-CS protein antibody. Druilhe found that sporozoites, either inside or outside cells, were detectable with the human monoclonal antibody tested. The incomplete protection occurred even when experiments were carried out with a cloned parasite, 7G8, which is evidence against the effect being due to polymorphism in antigenic structure. While sporozoites show some quantitative differences in their reactions with an anti-CSP monoclonal antibody, they are all labelled with it if the antibody concentration is sufficiently high.

A potentially important consequence of incomplete protection is the extent to which disease is dose dependent; what is the effect on parasitaemia or morbidity if 1, 10, 100 or hundreds of sporozoites successfully invade the liver? Clearly, if the parasite load in the blood can be reduced by 80–90%, the clinical situation will be improved. It has been claimed that reduction in the number of liver stage parasites would reduce the pathology, based on the hypothesis that a smaller load of

49

merozoites reaching the blood would allow the host to mount a more effective immune response. The evidence is generally against this view, and an infection induced by a single pre-erythrocytic parasite that had escaped effects of vaccination, would be as severe as the infection in those not vaccinated and caused by many more parasites. Also, first exposure to infection is not always the worst since many patients with cerebral malaria have a previous history of infection.

Claims that administration of the cytokines IL-1 or IFN-γ can be 100% effective against infection have been made. This appeared to be so from experiments by Schofield and colleagues (New York University Medical School) with IFN-γ where use of a DNA probe indicated 100% inhibition of parasite development in the liver. In due course, however, blood infections developed. The possibility that there are sites within the liver where parasites can escape the effects of cytokines should be considered.

The report, by Druilhe, of French missionaries from an endemic area who had taken chloroquine for 26 years prompted two questions, the first on the state of their retinas, and the second on their immunity to challenge infection. They were advised to stop using chloroquine prophylactically, and their immune status will be shown through exposure to natural challenge.

The exo-erythrocytic stages of *Plasmodium* express both sporozoite and asexual blood stage antigens and the discussant, Holder, described experiments in which the NANP repeat region of the *P. falciparum* CS gene was coupled to a C-terminus conserved region of the PMMSA (= MSA 1) merozoite antigen. This hybrid is immunogenic since it induced antibodies to both the CS sequence and the merozoite surface protein sequence (Holder et al 1988).

He described, too, a eukaryotic expression system used for the merozoite proteins and the hybrid, showing the importance of secretion of the construct protein on the surface of the eukaryotic cell. This can be achieved by removal of the anchor sequence. The conformation of the secreted protein was also important, underlining the need to consider very carefully not only which antigens to make but how they will be produced (Murphy et al in press).

REFERENCES

Holder A A, Lockyer M J, Hardy G W 1988 A hybrid gene to express protein epitopes from both sporozoite and merozoite surface antigens of *Plasmodium falciparum*. Parasitology 97: 373–382
Murphy V F, Rowan W C, Page M J, Holder A A 1989 Expression of hybrid malaria antigens in insect cells and their engineering for correct folding and secretion. Parasitology (in press)

4. Cerebral malaria

P.-H. Lambert and G. E. Grau

INTRODUCTION

The most severe complication of *Plasmodium falciparum* is the cerebral syndrome, from which more than 1 million children die annually in sub-Saharan Africa (Noguer et al 1976, Greenwood et al 1987). Recent estimations by the World Health Organization (WHO) indicate that more than 200 million people are infected by malaria every year. The pathogenesis of cerebral malaria remains incompletely understood (White 1986, Warrell 1987). In order to analyse the possible mechanisms involved in neurovascular lesions of malaria an experimental model was developed.

Using this model, we have conducted experiments aimed at the dissection of pathways of the immune system able to lead to pathology. More precisely, the interactions between T lymphocytes, macrophages and their mediators, the cytokines, have been studied. The respective role of each of these elements of the immune system has been analysed in relation to triggering of tissue lesions. These data are presented here together with recent observations in African children with severe falciparum malaria infection suggesting that cytokines may also have a role in human cerebral malaria.

HYPOTHESES FOR PATHOGENESIS OF CEREBRAL MALARIA

Cerebral malaria (CM) is the most common clinical presentation and cause of death in severe malaria, in some reports accounting for up to 10% of all cases of falciparum malaria admitted to hospital and for 80% of fatal cases (WHO Malaria Action Programme 1986). The mechanisms of this complication remain poorly understood, although several hypotheses have been proposed. The essential pathological feature of severe falciparum malaria is sequestration of erythrocytes containing mature forms of the parasite in deep vascular beds. Sequestration is greatest in the brain (MacPherson et al 1985), which may explain why coma is such a prominent feature. This condition is invariably fatal if untreated and is associated with a 20% mortality in treated patients. Three main pathogenic theories have been proposed for human cerebral malaria (reviewed in WHO Malaria Action Programme 1986):

(a) the *permeability theory*, originates from observations of increased blood–brain barrier permeability to ^{125}I-labelled albumin in *P. knowlesi*-infected rhesus monkeys, possibly mediated by kinins (Maegraith & Fletcher 1972). However, there are several experimental and clinical observations in man which argue against the permeability hypothesis. Opening pressures at lumbar puncture are usually normal, papilloedema is rare, computed tomography of the brain is normal in cerebral malaria, and in a large double-blind, placebo-controlled trial of dexamethasone there was no difference in mortality, but increased morbidity with dexamethasone.

(b) the *mechanical theory* states that the pathophysiology of severe falciparum malaria may be explained by microcirculation obstruction, with consequent local hypoxia and ischaemia. The reduced deformability of infected erythrocytes is proportional to the maturity of the intracellular parasite. Also, *P. falciparum*-infected erythrocytes have been shown to adhere specifically to endothelial cells. Studies of cerebral blood flow and metabolism in cerebral malaria patients have not indicated an absolute reduction in cerebral blood flow. However, lactate production is significantly higher in comatose patients.

(c) the *immunological theory*. The neuropathological findings in human cerebral malaria have been interpreted as resulting from a 'hyperergic' reaction of the central nervous system to the antigenic challenge of *P. falciparum* infection. The proposed mechanism for this is an immune complex vasculitis of the cerebral vessels. Epidemiological arguments also suggest that cerebral lesions in man could be favoured by immunopathological reactions. This complication occurs most frequently in children or in non-immune individuals. Its incidence is lower in malnourished children from endemic areas in whom a deficient cell-mediated immunity has been documented.

EPIDEMIOLOGICAL DATA

The pathological expression of malaria is dominated by features depending directly upon the proliferation of the parasites, and upon many secondary manifestations caused by various elements of the immune response of the host. In this respect, one should consider any aspect of humoral and cell-mediated immunity, including the release of mediators. Epidemiological aspects of these changes have been reviewed recently (Marsh & Greenwood 1986, Warrell 1987). The main aspects of malaria pathology in which immunopathological mechanisms have been suspected are renal disease, anaemia, thrombocytopenia, pulmonary oedema and cerebral malaria (Table 4.1).

We will discuss the extent to which the immune status of the host could be related to severe *P. falciparum* malaria and, in particular, to cerebral malaria. Other aspects of malaria immunopathology have been extensively reviewed by Marsh & Greenwood (1986).

The pathogenesis of CM is exceedingly complex. Numerous non-immunological factors are involved in the triggering of the neurovascular lesions (White 1986). As Warrell (1987) observed, elements of the immune response, such as mediators, are of potential relevance to the pathogenesis of severe falciparum malaria, but, so far,

Table 4.1 Examples of malaria pathology in which immunopathology has been suspected

Pathological condition	Immunological changes	
Renal disease	Glomerular Ig (IgG2), C and malarial antigen (*P. malariae*) deposits	(Ward & Conran 1969 Boonpucknavig et al 1972, Houba & Lambert 1974)
	IgM/IgG deposits	(Jerusalem et al 1983)
	HyperIg, low C', circulating immune complexes	(Bhamarapravati et al 1973, Boonpucknavig et al 1979)
	Electron-dense mesangial deposits	(Houba 1977)
Anaemia	RBC sensitization (IgG, C3d) (anti-schizont Ab) IgG1 subclass	(Facer et al 1979)
	Anti-RBC antibodies ? (direct agglutination test) Erythrophagocytosis (activated macrophages)	(Facer 1980)
Thrombocytopenia	IgM changes	(Beale et al 1972)
	High platelet-associated IgG, anti-platelet antibodies directed against malarial antigens	(Kelton et al 1983)
Pulmonary oedema	Damaged endothelium, WBC intravascular accumulation, role for mediators	(Duarte et al 1985 MacPherson et al 1985)
Cerebral malaria	Parallels with endotoxicosis and systemic inflammation role for mediators Ig, C' and malarial antigen deposits in brain capillary basement membrane Serum cytokines	(Maegraith 1948, (Maegraith & Fletcher 1972) (Oo et al 1987)
	High TNF levels are associated with high mortality	(Grau et al 1987c 1989b)

there has been no convincing evidence that they are responsible for CM in man. From an epidemiological point of view, only indirect arguments would suggest that the immune status of the infected individual is one of the factors leading to brain complications.

On the one hand, CM occurs most often in children and in non-immune adults. Thus, the development of this complication, or at least severe *P. falciparum* malaria, appears to be associated with a 'virgin' immune system, i.e. with a primary exposure to malaria. This is supported by the following observations:

1. The higher frequency of CM in children (most frequently 1–5 years old) versus adults in endemic areas. In such areas, humoral immunity develops slowly with increasing age, while prevalence of CM declines. Epidemiological analysis of humoral immune responses to malaria in Thailand indicates that patients who develop CM are less immune than those with acute uncomplicated malaria. Reduced humoral responses were found only in complicated CM patients (Tharavanij et al 1984). Thai patients developing CM were mainly adults, rather than children as in Africa; 65% of CM patients were not native of Chantaburi or

nearby endemic provinces but were immigrants from other parts of Thailand where malaria is not endemic.

2. CM frequency is also higher in visitors than in people living in endemic areas. Population movements (Ghana, Papua New Guinea, highlanders moving to the coast, Javan immigrants to West Irian, resettlement of Ethiopian highlanders (Warrell 1987)) are associated with more severe infections.

On the other hand, decreased cell-mediated immune responses can be associated with a decreased prevalence of CM. Indeed, malnourished children (protein and iron deficiency) are relatively protected against CM (Edington 1954, 1967, Hendrickse et al 1972, WHO-MAP 1986). Various aspects of cell-mediated immunity dysfunctions have been reported in relation to malnutrition (McMurray 1984). This can be intepreted as an indirect argument for a role of hyperreactivity of the immune system in CM.

The relationship of CM to immune status remains unclear, as the evidence for immunosuppression is the subject of continuing debate. However, one can note that the decrease in CM prevalence with age is paralleled by the development of immunity, but also by weaker T-cell reactivity (Weidanz 1982).

ANALYSIS OF AN EXPERIMENTAL MODEL OF CM

Description of the experimental model

It is obvious that animal models of malaria do not reproduce all the features of the human disease. However, the similarities which exist between defined antigens of human and rodent parasites as well as between immunopathogenic pathways in man and in mouse may justify the use of such models to orientate further investigations in man.

Our experimental model for CM is the neurovascular pathology induced by the infection with *Plasmodium berghei ANKA* asexual blood stages in genetically susceptible CBA/Ca mice. Six to 14 days after infection, we have observed a cumulative mortality of about 90% associated with a neurological syndrome. A particularly important feature of this model is that cerebral signs occurred when anaemia was moderate and the parasitaemia relatively low. The neurological manifestations include paralysis (mono-, hemi-, para- or tetraplegia), deviation of the head, ataxia and convulsions. In addition, several clinical and histopathological parameters are similar to those observed in patients with CM.

Essential role of CD4$^+$ T cells in neurovascular complications of experimental malaria

The immune status of the host appears to be critical for the development of cerebral complications in murine malaria, although in brain specimens from mice dying with clinically patent cerebral lesions, the sole classic morphological analysis would not have suggested any immune pathogenic mechanism. The absence of perivascular leucocyte infiltration parallels the observations in human cerebral malaria. It is in fact the same subset of T lymphocytes, namely the CD4$^+$ subset, which is involved both in protection and in the development of cerebral lesions.

Three lines of evidence indicate that helper T lymphocytes play a significant role in the development of murine cerebral malaria (Grau et al 1986).

First, we have demonstrated that the *in vivo* depletion in CD4$^+$ helper/inducer T cells, induced by treatment of *P. berghei*-infected mice with an IgG2b monoclonal antibody (MAb) directed against the CD4 molecule, completely prevented cerebral malaria, although there was no modification of the infection itself. No protective effect was seen after treatment of infected mice with a MAb of the same isotype directed against the CD8$^+$ T-cell subset. The effectiveness of this treatment by anti-CD4 mAb in infected mice has been demonstrated both phenotypically (depletion of the corresponding T-cell subset) and functionally (inhibition of the IgG antibody response to a T-dependent antigen, tetanus toxoid) (Grau et al 1986).

Second, experiments have been conducted in adult-thymectomized, irradiated and bone marrow-reconstituted (AT $\times$ BM) CBA mice which appear to be completely resistant to the development of neurological lesions upon infection with *P. berghei*. These results confirm and extend the results obtained using athymic nu/nu mice which suggest a role for T cells in the development of cerebral malaria. We have shown that T cells carrying the CD4 phenotype are particularly involved in this syndrome since reconstitution of AT $\times$ BM CBA mice with normal CD4$^+$ T cells renders these mice fully susceptible to the development of neurological complications. In contrast, AT $\times$ BM mice reconstituted with the CD8$^+$ T-cell subset did not die acutely with neurological signs but later developed severe anaemia and overwhelming parasitaemia (Grau et al 1986).

Third, there is an exacerbation of neurological signs and earlier mortality observed after transfer of CD4$^+$ CD8$^-$ T cells from mice with cerebral malaria into infected euthymic mice. This observation supports the hypothesis of an involvement of these cells in the pathogenesis of murine CM (Grau et al 1986).

These data indicate that murine cerebral malaria is most probably mediated by immune mechanisms. Indeed, the development of murine cerebral malaria is not directly related to the degree of anaemia and parasitaemia, but rather appears as the expression of immunopathological reactions of the infected host. The importance of the functional integrity of lymphoid cells expressing the CD4 phenotype (helper T cells) in the triggering of neurological complications is outlined in these studies. One should note that CD4$^+$ T cells of different specificities for malaria antigens may have different effects on the infection and particularly on the cerebral complications.

Various functional relationships between CD4$^+$ T cells and neurological lesions can be envisaged. The helper effect of CD4$^+$ T cells for the specific anti-plasmodium antibody response might be of particular importance, since we have observed that antibodies of certain specificities (against segmented schizont antigens) are consistently associated with the occurrence of cerebral malaria. This helper effect may also be exerted in a less specific manner: malaria-associated polyclonal B-cell activation appears indeed to be largely T-cell dependent. Second, CD4$^+$ T cells can also mediate delayed-type hypersensitivity (DTH). However, the existence of local DTH-like reactions in the cerebral compartment is not shown by histological studies since there was no accumulation of lymphocytes at the site of brain lesions. Third, the activation of T cells in the presence of properly presented malarial antigens results in the release of various lymphokines such as interleukin 2, interleukin 3, colony-stimulating factors and gamma-interferon. The production of gamma-interferon has been demonstrated in vitro by T cells in the presence of macrophages and parasitized erythrocytes. This is associated with the release of reactive oxygen species, participation of which has been documented in acute vascular changes and suggested in the pathogenesis of cerebral malaria. In addition, T-cell dependent macrophage activation leads to the release of a number of cytokines, including tumour-necrosis factor (TNF).

Identification of an endogenous mediator, tumour necrosis factor (TNF), as a key element in the pathogenesis of CM

TNF is a hormone produced principally by macrophages upon activation of these cells by various agents, the most potent of which is endotoxin (lipopolysaccharide, LPS) (Beutler & Cerami 1987). Besides its lytic effects on transformed cells and on parasites, TNF is able to interact with a vast array of host target cells, in a paracrine manner. It is able to potentiate its own synthesis by acting in an autocrine manner on the macrophage itself. In addition to its toxicity on a variety of tumour cells and its inhibitory effect on the enzyme lipoprotein lipase, this protein induces several changes in endothelial cells, including an increased adhesiveness for monocytes and polymorphonuclear leucocytes. Its injection in large amounts leads to a fatal state of shock, accompanied by severe haemorrhages and necrosis of viscera, especially intestine, kidney and lung (Tracey et al 1987).

The powerful effects of TNF on endothelial cells led us to explore the role of this molecule in CM. Indeed, endothelial cell alterations are a prominent feature of CM. Several gross and histological alterations of the brain have been described in murine cerebral malaria, and include haemorrhagic foci, most frequently in the meninges, cerebellum and olfactory bulbs. In the mice studied here, a striking feature of brain histological sections and 'brain smears' is focal accumulation of monocytes, often containing malaria pigment or phagocytosed erythrocytes within vascular lumina of capillaries and venules (Fig. 4.1) (Grau et al 1987c). Monocyte accumulation in this setting appears to be characteristic of murine cerebral malaria, since it is not present in brain vessels of infected mice which do not display neurological signs. At the level or in the vicinity of these monocyte accumulations, blood vessels showed ultrastructural signs of endothelial damage.

In order to investigate the relationship of murine cerebral malaria to the release of TNF by activated monocytes-macrophages, our first approach has been to study the serum levels of TNF at the time of the syndrome, as indicated by the appearance of the first neurological signs. While normal mice have undetectable levels, we have found that moderately elevated TNF concentrations are present in all malaria-infected mice. However, the serum TNF levels of the mice with CM were considerably higher than those of the other groups of mice without CM. It is of interest to note that the depletion in $CD4^+$ T cells, which prevents CM, also inhibits the rise in serum TNF levels (Grau et al 1987c).

To explore further the role of the increased TNF blood level in the pathogenesis of CM, we have attempted to modulate the syndrome by injecting a strongly neutralizing rabbit anti-mouse TNF antibody on day 4 or 7 after infection,

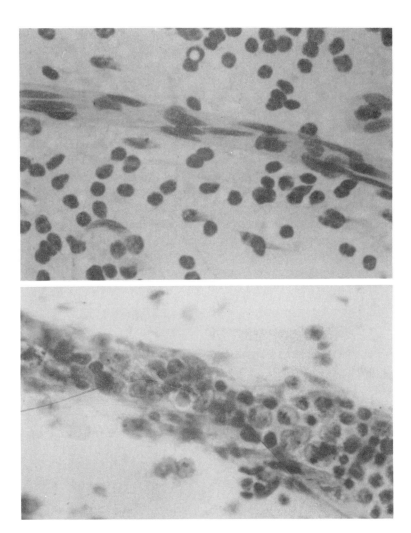

Figure 4.1 Anti-TNF antibody prevents neurovascular lesions in PbA-infected mice. Top: Absence of vascular plugging in a mouse protected against CM by a single injection of anti-TNF antibody, 4 days after infection with PbA. Bottom: Brain venule blocked by PbA-infected erythrocytes and monocytes in a mouse developing CM (brain impression smears on day 7 after infection)

i.e. before the appearance of neurological signs. Among the mice treated with anti-TNF IgG, only 8.3% developed CM, while 80–90% of the mice untreated or treated with non-specific IgG died of CM. The protective effect of the anti-TNF antibody against CM lasted until the animals died with severe anaemia. This treatment, indeed, does not influence the parasitaemia. In the sera of the treated animals, anti-TNF activity was still detectable up to 8 days after injection. Anti-TNF treatment significantly reduced the serum TNF levels in *P. berghei*-infected CBA/Ca mice and prevented all histological abnormalities including the focal arrest of monocytes and other circulating leucocytes within brain capillaries and venules (Grau et al 1987c). (Fig. 4.1.)

Another aspect of the role of TNF in CM is illustrated by immunohistochemical staining of brain smears and sections aimed at the detection of TNF at the site of lesions. The surface of capillary endothelial cells from mice developing CM, but not from malaria-infected mice without CM nor from normal mice, stain positively for TNF (Fig 4.2) (Grau et al unpublished observations). These observations could be interpreted as the presence of high levels of circulating TNF at the receptor site or, alternatively, as an increased production of TNF by activated endothelial cells.

Our observations may seem paradoxical with respect to the favourable role of T lymphocytes and macrophages in malarial infection. Indeed, TNF is shown here to mediate host tissue lesion although it is known to participate in the killing of malaria parasites. At least under these experimental conditions, a favourable role for TNF against the infection has not been demonstrated, since the parasitaemia curve is not changed by the injection of anti-TNF antibody. It is not difficult, however, to conceive that macrophages and their products may have both beneficial and deleterious effects depending on the degree of activation, timing and the location.

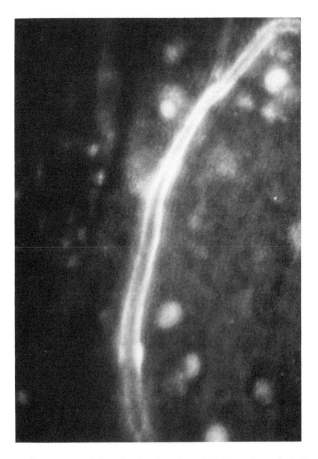

Figure 4.2 Immunofluorescent staining showing location of TNF on the endothelium in a mouse developing CM, 7 days after infection with *P. berghei* ANKA

ORIGIN AND PATHWAYS LEADING TO TNF OVERPRODUCTION IN CM

In an attempt to define the mechanisms which lead to in vivo TNF production, our attention has been focused on interleukin 3 (IL-3), granulocyte-macrophage colony stimulating factor (GM-CSF) and gamma-interferon (IFN-γ). We have found that IL-3 and GM-CSF play a role in the production of TNF during experimental neurovascular complications (Grau et al 1988b).

Interleukin 3 (IL-3) and GM-CSF are able to expand in vitro and in vivo the growth of granulocyte and macrophage precursors, and are known to enhance phagocytosis of opsonized bacteria in vivo. Continuous in vivo infusion of recombinant mouse IL-3 and GM-CSF has been shown by others to induce a marked leucocytosis. Repeated intraperitoneal injections of IL-3 have been shown to increase the number of macrophages in the peritoneal cavity. Since IL-3 and GM-CSF are both produced by activated T lymphocytes and since L3T4[+] T cells are involved in the triggering of CM, the possible role of these two molecules in CM lesions has been investigated, by using affinity-purified antibodies directed against recombinant IL-3 (rIL-3) and GM-CSF (rGM-CSF) in vivo.

Four groups of CBA-Ca mice, genetically susceptible to CM, have been infected with *P. berghei ANKA*. Three to 4 days later, these animals have been treated with either anti-rIL-3, anti-rGM-CSF, or both polyclonal antibodies, respectively. Similarly infected mice treated with normal rabbit IgG have been used as controls. The combined treatment with anti-rIL-3 and anti-rGM-CSF antibodies dramatically prevented the development of the neurological syndrome (Fig. 4.3). In contrast, each antibody injected separately had no significant effect compared with controls (Grau et al 1988b).

As a consequence of this beneficial effect on the development of CM in mice after *P. berghei* infection, the survival of mice receiving the dual treatment with

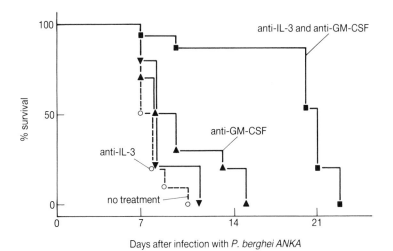

Figure 4.3 Prevention of murine cerebral malaria by combined treatment with anti-IL-3 and anti-GM-CSF antibodies

anti-IL-3 and GM-CSF was significantly prolonged. These mice died around the third week of infection, with severe anaemia and overwhelming parasitaemia but without CM. The interference with the development of CM by treatment with anti-IL-3 and anti-GM-CSF antibodies has been further demonstrated histologically. Microscopical examination of brain tissues on day 7 of infection showed that this combined treatment totally prevented the intravascular accumulation of mononuclear cells, which is characteristic of CM. More interestingly, the accumulation of macrophages in lymphoid organs, such as spleen red pulp and lymph nodes, which was consistently observed in mice developing CM, was significantly reduced upon treatment with both anti-IL-3 and anti-rGM-CSF antibodies. It is noteworthy that TNF was not detectable in the serum of mice treated with both antibodies and protected against CM (Grau et al 1988b).

These results suggest that IL-3 and GM-CSF are T-cell mediators involved in the production of TNF by macrophages in vivo. It is conceivable that the increase in the production of TNF by IL-3 and GM-CSF resulted from the capacity of these lymphokines to enlarge the pool of macrophages, i.e. the cells which were the main source of TNF. It is also likely that cells other than T lymphocytes were involved in the production of these mediators. Indeed, while IL-3 is essentially produced by T cells, it has been shown that GM-CSF can be produced by other cells than T lymphocytes. Among others, endothelial cells, which are a central element in the neurovascular lesions of experimental malaria, are able to produce GM-CSF under stimulation by TNF (Broudy et al 1986, Seelentag et al 1987). The blockade of this pathway by anti-GM-CSF antibody could also explain the protective effect on CM observed.

Another major lymphokine produced by activated T lymphocytes is IFN-γ. Recent experiments suggest that IFN-γ also plays a role in the development of CM and in the production of TNF in vivo. This contention is supported by preliminary observations which have shown that CM and its TNF overproduction could be prevented by treatment of *P. berghei*-infected mice with either polyclonal (recently produced in our laboratory) or monoclonal anti-IFN-γ antibodies (provided by Dr G. Milon, Pasteur Institute, Paris, and Dr A. Billiau, Rega Institute, Leuven, Belgium) (Grau et al in press).

In order to explain the production of TNF in vivo in CM, one may hypothesize the following (Fig. 4.4): on the one hand, IL-3 and GM-CSF would act by enlarging the pool of macrophages, and on the other hand, IFN-γ would be responsible for their activation resulting in the synthesis and release of excessive amounts of TNF.

Our current concept of the role of TNF in CM is that a sequence of the following pathological events is required for the development of neurovascular lesions: TNF is first produced systemically in excessive amounts, as the result of a cytokine cascade mediated by the immune response. As a second step, high levels of circulating TNF render the brain endothelial cells more sticky and favour the sequestration of parasitized erythrocytes and monocytes at this level. Thirdly, locally arrested monocytes also produce TNF which induces several auto-amplifying loops (among others, it induces endothelial cells to produce GM-CSF (Broudy et al 1986, Seelentag et al 1987)). Thus, high levels of TNF create a self-aggravating condition, which is rapidly fatal when occurring in the brain.

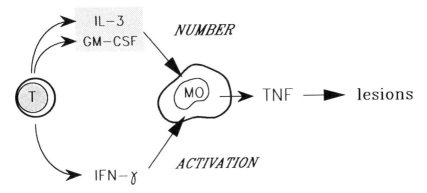

Figure 4.4 Interplay of cytokines leading to TNF overproduction in experimental cerebral malaria

In conclusion, the release of TNF, probably associated with various physio-pathological changes induced by malaria infection, appears to represent an important effector mechanism in the pathogenesis of murine CM. In human cases of cerebral malaria, accumulations of packed infected erythrocytes rather than macrophages are described in cerebral vessels. However, both phenomena may result from a similar mechanism, such as an increased endothelial adhesiveness, which might reflect TNF-mediated vascular alterations. Therefore, TNF may also be of pathogenic significance in human cerebral malaria and that possibility was evaluated.

RECENT OBSERVATIONS IN HUMAN CEREBRAL MALARIA: POSSIBLE PATHOGENIC ROLE OF TNF

Elevated concentrations of TNF have been noted in the serum of malaria patients (Scuderi et al 1986, Grau et al 1987c, VanderMeer et al 1988), and treatment with anti-TNF antibodies protects mice from the cerebral complications of *P. berghei ANKA* infection (Grau et al 1987c). However, the relationship between serum TNF concentration and human cerebral malaria has not been analysed.

We have studied malaria-infected Malawian children, in collaboration with Malcolm E. Molyneux (Liverpool School of Tropical Medicine, Liverpool, UK), Terrie Taylor (College of Osteopathic Medicine, Michigan State University), and Jack J. Wirima (Kamuzu Central Hospital, Lilongwe, Malawi). This study has been carried out with the permission of the Malawi Health Sciences Research Committee between January and June 1988 in the Department of Paediatrics at the Queen Elizabeth Central Hospital in Blantyre, Malawi. Parents or guardians had given informed consent for the participation of children in this study.

Sixty-five children, presenting with asexual *P. falciparum* parasitaemia and requiring treatment with parenteral quinine, either because of altered conscious-ness or persistent vomiting, were eligible for inclusion in the study. Children were excluded if an additional cause of fever, altered consciousness or vomiting could be found on physical examination, if the cerebrospinal fluid (CSF) contained >5 leucocytes/mm^3, or if blood culture yielded a pathogen.

The *P. falciparum* infections varied in severity and were associated with varying degrees of neurological manifestations. The concentrations of TNF were measured in the serum and in the CSF during the acute stage of the illness, and one month later in survivors. The results were then analysed in relation to the clinical course and outcome of the illness, and to known indicators of severity of falciparum malaria in children, with particular attention to hypoglycaemia (Grau et al 1989b).

Patients had been evaluated at least every 2 h until they recovered or died. Levels of consciousness were assessed using a modification of the Glasgow Coma Scale (Teasdale) developed for use with pre-verbal as well as verbal children (Taylor et al 1988). Survivors were discharged when they had recovered fully, and had been requested to return for a follow-up visit 1 month later. A venous blood sample had been collected at that time for measurements of parasitaemia and TNF. TNF concentrations were determined using a sensitive immunoradiometric assay (IRMA) from IRE-Medgenix, Fleurus, Belgium. All assays were performed without knowledge of the patients' clinical status.

In this study, the presence of markedly elevated serum levels of TNF during the acute phase of cerebral malaria was reported in a group of Malawian children. Serum concentrations of TNF were elevated in many children with severe *P. falciparum* infection (148 ± 25 pg/ml, mean $\pm$ s.e.m.) but were within normal range 1 month after discharge from hospital in the same patients (15.7 ± 3 pg/ml; $n = 38$: paired samples: $p < 0.0005$, 95% CI = 70 126). A significant correlation existed between the serum TNF level on admission and the severity of the illness: the mean concentrations of TNF were higher, on admission, in patients who died (709 ± 312 pg/ml, $n = 10$) than in the 55 survivors (184.7 ± 31.5 pg/ml; $p = 0.012$, 95% CI = 30 328), and in those with four or more falciparum malaria risk factors (929 ± 33 pg/ml) than in those patients possessing fewer than four risk factors (158.7 ± 21.7 pg/ml; $p = 0.0003$, 95% CI = 145 1 240) (Grau et al 1989b). Furthermore, the development of sequelae was associated with high TNF levels. Of the nine risk factors identified (Taylor et al 1988), three correlated with serum TNF concentrations: hypoglycaemia, hyperparasitaemia and age less than 3 years. The highest TNF concentrations (2300 and 2800 pg/ml) were seen in hypoglycaemic patients who died shortly after the blood samples had been obtained. The relation between serum TNF level on admission and outcome has been analysed. While patients with admitting levels under 100 pg/ml had a mortality of less than 5%, the mortality increased with serum TNF level and was 100% in the 2 patients with serum levels above 1500 pg/ml (Fig. 4.5).

TNF concentrations in the CSF during the acute neurological phase were found to be slightly but not significantly elevated (22.1 ± 5.4 pg/ml, $n = 17$). However, the highest CSF TNF level was seen in the only lethal case among those studied for CSF. The evolution of serum TNF levels, monitored in some patients during the first 24 h after admission, indicated that most of the patients had fairly stable TNF levels immediately on admission, but 3, 12 and 24 h later the TNF level was moderately elevated. There was nonetheless a gradual decrease in patients with high admitting level of TNF who recovered fully. In one case, there was a low admitting TNF level and then a gradual increase in serum TNF level over the first 24 h. This patient died.

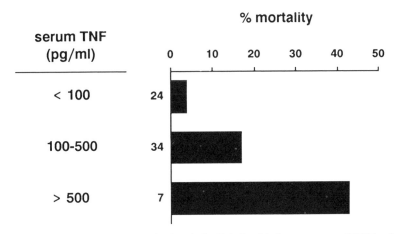

Figure 4.5 Malawian children with cerebral malaria. Relationship between serum TNF level on admission and outcome (Reproduced with permission of N Engl J Med)

There have been very few reports of TNF levels in human diseases. Elevated concentrations of TNF have been reported particularly in patients with meningococcal infections (Waage et al 1986, Girardin et al 1988). Indeed, Gram-negative bacterial endotoxin is the most potent known stimulator of TNF release. Elevations in the serum concentrations of this cytokine have been reported in patients with leishmaniasis and malaria, but the relation to the neurological syndrome has not been analysed (Scuderi et al 1986, Grau et al 1987c, Vander-Meer et al 1988). In the present study, we describe TNF concentrations in human cerebral malaria, we demonstrate an association with the severity of the disease, and document a return of TNF concentrations to normal in convalescence.

A relationship between TNF and malaria pathology can be envisaged with respect to the symptomatology and the lesion of the disease. In vivo, TNF has been shown to produce a wide variety of biological effects (Warren et al 1987, reviewed in Beutler & Cerami 1987), some of which are parallel to symptoms observed in children with severe *P. falciparum* infections: hyperpyrexia, hypoglycaemia and hypercortisolism. On the other hand, paediatric malaria patients rarely demonstrate a clinical picture entirely consistent with endotoxaemic shock: hypotension, acute renal failure, and disseminated intravascular coagulation are not prominent features of the paediatric syndrome in Africa (Taylor et al 1988) nor in south-east Asia (Warrell 1987). Of interest is the wide overlap in serum TNF concentrations among patients who died and those who survived. A similar wide range of variations in TNF effects has been noted in a study of the acute metabolic effects of TNF administration in humans (Warren et al 1987). It may be that these patients differ in their sensitivities to TNF, or develop a tolerance to it. The half-life of TNF is particularly short (Beutler et al 1986), and some of the apparent variations in serum concentrations between individuals may result from transient fluctuations in the course of the illness.

The origin of TNF should be questioned. Protozoan parasites can activate macrophages to produce cachectin/TNF-related activity in vivo (Hotez et al 1984), and TNF production during malaria infection has been documented (Taverne et al

1986, Grau et al 1989a). Causes other than malaria infection itself are potentially able to induce TNF release and should be envisaged in the patients studied here. Since Gram-negative bacteraemia is a known complication of severe falciparum malaria, blood cultures were performed but all were found negative in the patients of this study. Infections by other parasites could also be involved in the elevated TNF levels but this is unlikely, as TNF levels returned to normal in the convalescent phase. Another possible source of TNF is the immune system itself. Malaria infection leads to prominent activation of lymphocytes and macrophages (Wyler & Oppenheim 1974, Wyler 1976). This might result in an inappropriate TNF secretion.

In human cases of cerebral malaria, accumulations of packed infected erythrocytes have been described in cerebral vessels (MacPherson et al 1985), but there is no prominent macrophage accumulation as observed in an experimental model of malaria-induced neurovascular lesions (Grau et al 1987). However, both phenomena may result from a similar mechanism, such as an increased endothelial adhesiveness, which might reflect TNF-mediated vascular alterations. In human cerebral malaria, the major role of knob-associated structures in the adhesion of infected erythrocytes to endothelial cells has been documented (Aikawa et al 1980). Cytoadherence appears to involve histidine-rich proteins (Rock et al 1987), other membrane proteins, and thrombospondin (Sherwood et al 1987). In normal haemodynamic conditions, this could nevertheless be insufficient to arrest infected erythrocytes in brain vessels. When released in large amounts, TNF could modulate the adhesiveness of endothelial cells for parasitized erythrocytes (as has been shown for leucocytes) (Fig. 4.6).

In experimental malaria, the immune status of the host appears to be critical for the development of cerebral complications. However, in brain specimens from

CEREBRAL MALARIA

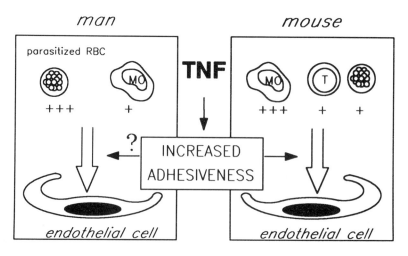

Figure 4.6 Schematic representation of the possible role of TNF in the triggering of experimental and human cerebral malaria

mice dying with clinically patent cerebral lesion, the sole classic morphological analysis would not have suggested any immune pathogenic mechanisms. The absence of perivascular leucocyte infiltration in this model parallels the observations in human cerebral malaria (MacPherson et al 1985).

Although a clear association is described here between TNF and the severity of human cerebral malaria, the role of this cytokine in the pathogenesis of the syndrome remains to be evaluated. In an experimental model of cerebral malaria, reproducing some features of the human disease, a pathogenic role for TNF in the triggering of neurological lesions has been demonstrated (Grau et al 1987c). TNF has some properties of particular relevance for the neurovascular lesions of cerebral malaria, such as its effects on endothelial cells (reviewed in Grau et al 1989a). If TNF plays a role in the pathogenesis of cerebral malaria in children, further studies will be required to elucidate the nature of its selective effects. The prevention of endotoxaemic shock (Tracey et al 1987) and experimental cerebral malaria (Grau et al 1987c) by pretreatment with anti-TNF antibodies as well as the amelioration of TNF-related symptomatology and biochemical changes by cyclooxygenase inhibitors (Talmadge et al 1987, Michie et al 1988) suggest that new therapeutic options may be promising in settings where TNF has a major pathophysiological effect.

The data presented here suggest that serum TNF levels can have a predictive value for outcome in cerebral malaria. Further studies are warranted to define more clearly the significance of this cytokine in acute cerebral malaria.

RELEVANCE OF THE MURINE EXPERIMENTAL MODEL TO HUMAN CEREBRAL MALARIA

The study of experimental models of malaria infection allows a further appraisal of the role of the immune system in the pathogenesis of major complications. Antimalarial antibody responses are T-cell dependent (Jayawardena et al 1977), and the involvement of several humoral immunity alterations in malarial immunopathology has been suggested (Table 4.1). However, as stated by Jerusalem et al (1983), the early occurrence of cerebral syndromes in clinical and experimental malaria (6 days) points against the role of circulating immune complexes in the pathogenesis of the cerebral lesion. Humoral factors may have an aggravating influence rather than be the cause. Also, one can certainly rule out an involvement of DTH-like reactions in the development of neurovascular lesion of CM, since no inflammatory cell infiltration has ever been observed (MacPherson et al 1985, Oo et al 1987).

This has been taken as an argument against immune mechanisms in CM. However, consistent absence of perivascular infiltration is also typical of the lesion of experimental CM (MacKey et al 1980, Rest 1983, Grau et al 1986, 1987). Indeed, in the *P. berghei* model of CM, histopathological analysis *per se* would not have suggested immune mechanisms, even though the importance of the immune status had been demonstrated (Rest 1982, Finley et al 1982, Grau et al 1986, 1987). The production of TNF and the interplay of other cytokines such as IFN-γ, IL-3, and GM-CSF in the triggering of experimental CM has been shown (Grau et al 1989a). In this model, the prevention of CM by low-dose cyclosporin A (Grau et al 1987b) is an additional argument for the role of T-cell dependent immunopathology. Beneficial effects of cyclosporin A have also been observed in human malaria (J F Borel personal communication).

The relevance of this murine model should be questioned. In Tables 4.2 to 4.4, we review several parameters of cerebral malaria. Both immunological and non-immunological parameters, as well as characteristics of the lesion itself are listed and are compared with what is observed in the model of *P. berghei* infection in the mouse.

Malaria infection is known to induce a considerable macrophage activation, partly through cytokines such as IFN-γ, released by activated T cells. A recent study of neopterin (a product of activated macrophages) levels in Tanzanian and Thai patients with malaria confirms that macrophage reactivity parallels the course of acquired specific antimalarial immunity (Reibnegger et al 1987). Indeed, Tanzanian children during their first years of life show extremely high neopterin levels compared with older children and adults. Also, patients from Bangkok, where malaria is not fully endemic, have higher neopterin levels than Tanzanians of comparable age, inhabiting an area where malaria is highly endemic. Thus, macrophage reactivity is highest in those patients who are most likely to develop CM.

Besides their capacity to produce cytokines, macrophages can also be directly

Table 4.2 Non-immunological parameters in cerebral malaria. Comparison between an experimental model, *P. berghei ANKA* (PbA) infection in mouse and human disease

Non-immunological parameters	Exp (PbA)	Human	Ref (Human)
Hyperparasitaemia	−	−	Warrell 1987
Severe anaemia	−	−	Warrell 1987
Diffuse symmetrical upper motor neurone lesions	+	+	Warrell 1987
Hypoglycaemia	+	+	White 1986
Disseminated intravascular coagulation	−	−	Warrell 1987

Table 4.3 Immunological parameters in cerebral malaria. Comparison between experimental model and human disease

Immunological parameters	Exp (PbA)	Human	Ref (Human)
Hyper Ig	+	+	Adam et al 1981
Circulating immune complexes	+	+	Adam et al 1981
T-cell dependency	+	+[*]	Edington 1954
Ig, C3, malarial antigen brain deposits	+	+/−	Oo et al 1987 (+) MacPherson et al 1985 (−)
Perivascular inflammatory cells	−	−	MacPherson et al 1985
High serum IFN-γ	+	+	Ojo-Amaize et al 1981 Tharavanij et al 1984 Rhodes-Feuillette et al 1985
High serum TNF	+	+	Scuderi et al 1986 VanderMeer et al 1988 Grau et al 1987c

(*) = indirect evidence

Table 4.4 Histopathology of neurovascular lesions in cerebral malaria. Comparison between experimental model and human disease

Histopathology	Exp (PbA)	Human	Ref(Human)
Brain sequestration knobs[+] pRBC	−	+	Aikawa et al 1980
pRBC	+	+ + +	MacPherson et al 1985
Leucocytes	+ + +	+	Warrell 1987
Perivascular leucocyte infiltration	−	−	MacPherson et al 1985
Perivascular haemorrhages	+	+	MacPherson et al 1985
Endothelial cell pseudopodia (free radical-mediated damage)	+	+	MacPherson et al 1985
Permeability changes	+	−	Warrell et al 1986
Brain oedema	+	+/−	Warrell et al 1986

involved in lesions of severe falciparum malaria. Indeed, in adult respiratory distress syndrome (ARDS)-like syndrome associated with malaria, monocytes/macrophages were found occluding the lumen of lung capillaries (Duarte et al 1985). This lesion is very similar to the brain lesion in murine CM.

The parallels between endotoxicosis or meningococcaemia and severe malaria have led Maegraith to speculate that the elements leading to systemic inflammation could explain several manifestations of severe malaria (Maegraith 1948). Various mediators of inflammation, such as kinins were believed to be involved in CM (Maegraith & Fletcher 1972). Other mediators possibly involved are undoubtedly lymphocyte- and monocyte-derived cytokines. In 1978, Clark rightly hypothesized that monokines, and particularly TNF, could be secreted during malaria and contribute to the illness it causes (Clark 1978, 1981 et al, 1982a, 1982b, 1987a, 1987b, reviewed in 1987c). TNF has been demonstrated as a key mediator in experimental CM (Grau et al 1987c).

Several questions remain unanswered, the major one being: why all children with knob-positive parasitized erythrocytes do not die of CM? It is conceivable that the triggering of the neurovascular lesion requires not only the adherence of knob-bearing parasitized erythrocytes to brain endothelia, but also some factors related to lymphocyte and monocyte activation, such as cytokines or other mediators. Several aspects of malarial pathology can be viewed as the results of interplay between TNF and other mediators, such as IFN-γ, reactive oxygen species, prostaglandins, PAF, leukotrienes. These mediators are able to modulate vascular adhesiveness phenomena and to enhance endothelial cell damage (reviewed in Grau et al 1989a, Fajardo 1989). The possibility that cytokines could modulate the adhesiveness of parasitized erythrocytes to endothelial cells, by modulating the expression of adhesion molecules, is under current investigation in our laboratory (Fig. 4.6).

The association of pathological manifestations with the immune response to plasmodial antigens has been frequently reported. Obviously, such manifestations may often result from a combined effect of the parasitic infection with a particular expression of the immune response to the parasite. The conditions in which such manifestations occur and a better knowledge of their pathogenesis should also help us in evaluating the relative risk of increasing their incidence after active immunization against some malarial antigens.

SUMMARY

A natural body protein is probably a major cause of the deadliest complication of malaria, a finding that could point towards new methods of treatment. Studies in an experimental model indicate that tumour necrosis factor (TNF), a protein also known as cachectin, is an essential element in highly fatal cerebral malaria. This contention is supported by the following observations.

First, during the course of an infection by *P. berghei ANKA* strain, mice of a CM-susceptible strain expressed markedly elevated levels of TNF in their serum at the time when neurological signs were evident.

Second, in contrast, mice from non-susceptible strains, susceptible strains depleted of $CD4^+$ T lymphocytes, or susceptible mice inoculated with malaria organisms incapable of producing CM all failed to express high serum TNF activity.

Third, passive immunization against mouse TNF significantly prolonged the survival of *P. berghei*-infected CBA/Ca mice, and prevented the development of neurological signs to an extent that is highly significant. Treatment with the anti-TNF antibody also prevents the histopathological lesions which are characteristic of CM, i.e. plugging of cerebral vessels by macrophages, lymphoid cells and parasitized erythrocytes.

We have recently shown that this increased TNF release and macrophage accumulation are schematically made of two components, each mediated by different cytokines presumably released by stimulated $CD4^+$ T lymphocytes: (a) a quantitative component: increased accumulation of macrophages results from the concomitant release of IL-3 and GM-CSF, and (b) a qualitative component: macrophage numbers have not only to be raised, but macrophages need to be activated by IFN-γ. Thus, CM appears to be the result of a cytokine cascade mediated by the immune response.

TNF might also be involved in the pathogenesis of human cerebral malaria. Indeed, we have recently shown that in African children with severe falciparum malaria, elevated serum concentrations of this molecule are associated with severe neurological involvement and fatal outcome.

ACKNOWLEDGEMENTS

Excellent technical assistance of D. Gretener and C. Gysler is gratefully acknowledged. This work was supported by grants No. 3.803.0.86 and 3.650.0.87 from the Swiss National Foundation, by the Sandoz Research Foundation and by the United Nations Development Program/World Bank/World Health Organization Special Programme for Research and Training in Tropical Diseases.

REFERENCES

Adam C, Geniteau M, Gougerot-Pocidalo M, Verroust P, Lebras J, Gilbert C, Morel-Maroger L 1981 Cryoglobulins, circulating immune complexes and complement activation in cerebral malaria. Infect Immun 31: 530–535

Aikawa M, Suzuki M, Gutierrez Y 1980 Pathology of malaria. In: Kreier J P (ed) Malaria. Pathology, vector studies, and culture. Academic Press, New York 2: 47–102

Beale P J, Cormack J D, Oldrey T B N 1972 Thrombocytopenia in malaria with immunoglobulin (IgM) changes. Br Med J 1: 345–349

Beutler B, Cerami A 1987 Cachectin: more than a tumor necrosis factor. New Engl J Med 316: 379–385

Beutler B, Milsark I W, Cerami A C 1986 Passive immunization against cachectin/tumor necrosis factor protects mice from lethal effects of endotoxin. Science 229: 869–871

Bhamarapravati N, Boonpucknavig V, Boonpucknavig S, Yaemboonruang C 1973 Glomerular changes in acute *Plasmodium falciparum*-infection. Arch Pathol 96: 289–293

Boonpucknavig V, Boonpucknavig S, Bhamarapravati N 1972 Immunopathological studies in *Plasmodium berghei*-infected mice. Arch Pathol 94: 322–330

Boonpucknavig V, Boonpucknavig S, Bhamarapravati N 1979 *Plasmodium berghei*-infected mice. Focal glomerulonephritis in hyperimmune state. Arch Pathol Lab Med 103: 567–572

Broudy V C, Kaushansky K, Segal G M, Harlan J M, Adamson J W 1986 Tumor necrosis factor type alpha stimulates human endothelial cells to produce granulocyte/macrophage stimulating factor. Proc Natl Acad Sci USA 83: 7467

Clark I A 1978 Does endotoxin cause both the disease and parasite death in acute malaria and babesiosis? Lancet i: 75–77

Clark I A 1982a Correlation between susceptibility to malaria and babesia parasites and to endotoxicity. Trans R Soc Trop Med Hyg 76: 4–7

Clark I A 1982b Suggested importance of monokines in pathophysiology of endotoxin shock and malaria. Klin Wochenschr 60: 756–758

Clark I A, Virelizier J L, Carswell E A, Wood P R 1981 Possible importance of macrophage-derived mediators in acute malaria. Infect Immunol 32: 1058–1066

Clark I A 1987a Monokines and lymphokines in malarial pathology. Ann Trop Med Parasitol 81: 577–585

Clark I A 1987b Cell-mediated immunity in protection and pathology of malaria. Parasitol Today 3: 300–305

Clark I A, Cowden W B, Butcher G A, Hunt N H 1987a Possible roles of tumor necrosis factor in the pathology of malaria. Am J Pathol 129: 192–199

Clark I A, Hunt N H, Butcher G A, Cowden W B 1987b Inhibition of murine malaria (*P. chabaudi*) in vivo by recombinant interferon gamma or tumor necrosis factor, and its enhancement by butylated hydroxyanisole. J Immunol 139: 3493–3496

Duarte M I S, Corbett C E P, Boulos M, Amato Neto V 1985 Ultrastructure of the lung in falciparum malaria. Am J Trop Med Hyg 34: 31–35

Edington G M 1954 Cerebral malaria in the Gold Coast African: four autopsy reports. Ann Trop Med Parasitol 48: 300–306

Edington G M 1967 Pathology of malaria in West Africa. Br Med J 1: 715–718

Facer C A 1980 Direct Coombs' antiglobulin reactions in Gambian children. II. Specificity of erythrocyte-bound IgG. Clin Exp Immunol 39: 279–288

Facer C A, Bray R S, Brown J 1979 Direct Coombs reactions in Gambian children with *Plasmodium falciparum* malaria. I. Incidence and class specificity. Clin Exp Immunol 35: 119–127

Fajardo L F 1989 The complex physiology of endothelial cells and its implication in radiobiology. Amer Jnl Clin Pathol 92: 241–250

Finley R W, Mackey L J, Lambert P H 1982 Virulent *P. berghei* malaria: prolonged survival and decreased cerebral pathology in cell-deficient nude mice. J. Immunol 129: 2213–2218

Girardin E, Grau G E, Dayer J M, Roux-Lombard P, J5 study group, Lambert P H 1988 Tumor necrosis factor and interleukin 1 in the serum of children with infectious purpura. New Engl J Med 319: 397–400

Grau G E, Piguet P F, Engers H D, Louis J A, Vassalli P, Lambert P H 1986 L3T4[+] T lymphocytes play a major role in the pathogenesis of murine cerebral malaria. J Immunol 137: 2348–2354

Grau G E, Del Giudice G, Lambert P H 1987a Host immune response and pathological expression in malaria: possible implications for malaria vaccines. Parasitology 94: S123–S137

Grau G E, Gretener D, Lambert P H 1987b Prevention of murine cerebral malaria by low-dose cyclosporin A. Immunology 61: 521–525

Grau G E, Fajardo L F, Piguet P F, Allet B, Lambert P H, Vassalli P 1987c Tumor necrosis factor/cachectin as an essential mediator in murine cerebral malaria. Science 237: 1210–1212

Grau G E, Piguet P F, Gretener D, Vesin C, Lambert P H 1988a Immunopathology of thrombocytopenia in experimental malaria. Immunology. 65: 501–506

Grau G E, Kindler V, Piguet P F, Lambert P H, Vassalli P 1988b Prevention of experimental cerebral malaria by anti-cytokine antibodies. Interleukin 3 and granulocyte-macrophage colony-stimulating factor are intermediates in increased tumor necrosis factor production and macrophage accumulation. J Exp Med 168: 1499–1504

Grau G E, Piguet P F, Vassalli P, Lambert P H 1989a Involvement of tumor necrosis factor and other cytokines in immune-mediated vascular pathology. Int Arch Allergy Appl Immunol 88: 34–39

Grau G E, Taylor T E, Molyneux M E, Wirima J J, Vassalli P, Hommel M, Lambert P H 1989b Tumor necrosis factor and disease severity in children with falciparum malaria. N Engl J Med 320: 1586–1591

Grau G E, Heremans H, Piguet P F, Pointaire P, Lambert P H, Billiau A, Vassalli P 1989c Monoclonal anti-gamma interferon antibodies prevent experimental cerebral malaria and its TNF overproduction. Proc Natl Acad Sci USA (in press)

Greenwood B M, Bradley A K, Greenwood A M, Byass P, Jammen K, Marsh K, Tulloch S, Oldfield F S, Hayes R 1987 Mortality and morbidity from malaria among children in a rural area of The Gambia, West Africa. Trans R Soc Trop Med Hyg 91: 478–486

Hendrickse R G, Adenyi, Edington G M, Glasgow E F, White R H R, Houba V 1972 Quartan malarial nephrotic syndrome. Lancet i: 1143–1148

Hotez P J, LeTrang N, Fairlamb A H, Cerami A 1984 Lipoprotein lipase suppression in 3T3-L1 cells by a haemoprotozoan-induced mediator from peritoneal exudate cells. Parasite Immunol 6: 303–309

Houba V 1977 Immunopathological mechanisms in protozoal infections. Am J Trop Med Hyg 26: 233–239

Houba V, Lambert P H 1974 Immunological studies on tropical nephropathies. Adv Biosci 12: 617

Jayawardena A N, Targett G A T, Carter R L, Leuchars E, Davies A J S 1977 The immunological response of CBA mice to P. yoelii. I. General characteristics, the effects of T cell deprivation and reconstitution with thymus grafts. Immunology 32: 849

Jerusalem E, Polder T, Wijers-Rouw P, Heinen U, Eling W, Osunkoya B O, Trinh P 1983 Comparative clinical and experimental study on the pathogenesis of cerebral malaria. Contr Microbiol Immunol 7: 130–138

Kelton J G, Keystone J, Moore J, Denomme G, Tozman E, Glynn M, Neame PB, Gauldie J, Jensen J 1983 Immune mediated thrombocytopenia of malaria. J Clin Invest 71: 32–836

MacKey L J, Hochman A, June C H, Contreras C E, Lambert P H 1980 Immunopathological aspects of Plasmodium berghei infection in five strains of mice. II. Immunopathology of cerebral and other tissue lesions during the infection. Clin Exp Immunol 42: 412–420

McMurray D N 1984 Cell-mediated immunity in protein calorie malnutrition. Prog Food Nutr Sci 8: 193–228

MacPherson G G, Warrell M J, White N J, Looaresuwan S, Warrell D A 1985 Human cerebral malaria. A quantitative ultrastructural analysis of parasitized erythrocytes sequestration. Am J Pathol 119: 385–401

Maegraith B 1948 Pathological processes in malaria and blackwater fever. Blackwell, Oxford

Maegraith B G, Fletcher A 1972 The pathogenesis of mammalian malaria. Adv Parasitol 10: 49–75

Marsh K, Greenwood B M 1986 Immunopathology of malaria. Clin Trop Med Commun Dis 1: 91–125

Michie H R, Manogue K R, Spriggs D R et al 1988 Detection of circulating tumor necrosis factor after endotoxin administration. New Engl J Med 319: 1481–1486

Noguer A, Wernsdorfer W H, Kouznetsov R 1976 The malaria situation in 1975. WHO Chronicle 30: 486–493

Ojo-Amaize E A, Salimonu L S, Williams A I O, Akinwolere O A O, Shabo R, Alm G V, Wigzell H 1981 Positive correlation between degree of parasitaemia, interferon titers and natural killer cell activity in P. falciparum-infected children. J Immunol 127: 2296–2300

Oo M M, Aikawa M, Than T, Aye T M, Myint P T, Igarashi I, Schoene W C 1987 Human cerebral malaria: A pathological study. J Neuropathol Exp Neurol 46: 223–231

Reibnegger G, Fuchs D, Hausen A, Schmutzhard E, Werner E R, Wachter H 1987 The dependence of cell-mediated immune activation in malaria on age and endemicity. Trans R Soc Trop Med Hyg 81: 729–733

Rest J R 1982 Cerebral malaria in inbred mice. I. A new model and its pathology. Trans R Soc Trop Med Hyg 76: 410–415

Rest J R 1983 Pathogenesis of cerebral malaria in golden hamsters and inbred mice. Contrib Microbiol Immunol 7: 139–146

Rhodes-Feuillette A, Bellosguardo M, Druilhe P, Ballet J J, Chousterman S, Canivet M, Peries J 1985 The interferon compartment of the immune response in malaria. II. Presence of serum interferon gamma following the acute attack. J Interferon Res 5: 169–178

Rock E P, Marsh K, Saul A J, Wellems T E, Taylor D W, Maloy W L, Howard R J. 1987 Comparative analysis of the *Plasmodium falciparum* histidine-rich proteins HRP-I, HRP-II, and HRP-III in malaria parasites of diverse origin. Parasitology 95: 209–227

Scuderi P, Steriling K E, Lam K S, Finley P R, Ryan K J, Ray C G, Petersen E, Shymen D J, Salmon S E 1986 Raised serum levels of tumor necrosis factor in parasitic infections. Lancet ii: 1364–1365

Seelentag W, Mermod J J, Montesano R, Vassalli P 1987 Additive effects of interleukin 1 and tumor necrosis factor alpha on the accumulation of the three granulocyte and macrophage colony stimulating factor mRNAs in human endothelial cells. EMBO J 6: 2261

Sherwood J A, Roberts D D, Marsh K, Harvey E B, Spitalnik S L, Miller L H, Howard R J 1987 Thrombospondin binding by parasitized erythrocyte isolates in falciparum malaria. Am J Trop Med Hyg 36: 228–233

Talmadge J E, Bowersox O, Tribble H, Lee S H, Shepard H M, Liggit D 1987 Toxicity of tumor necrosis factor is synergistic with gamma interferon and can be reduced with cyclooxygenase inhibitors. Am J Pathol 128: 410–425

Taverne J, Treagust J D, Playfair J H L 1986 Macrophage cytotoxicity in lethal and non-lethal malaria and the effect of vaccination. Clin Exp Immunol 66: 44–51

Taylor T E, Molyneux M E, Wirima J J, Fletcher K A, Morris K 1988 Blood glucose levels in Malawian children before and during the administration of intravenous quinine for severe falciparum malaria. N Engl J Med 319: 1040–1047

Tharavanij S, Warrell M J, Tantivanich S, Tapchaisri P, Chongsa-Nguan M, Prasertsiriroj V, Patarapotikul J 1984 Factors contributing to the development of cerebral malaria. 1. Humoral immune responses. Am J Trop Med Hyg 33: 1–11

Tracey K J, Fong Y, Hesse D G, Manogue K R, Lee A T, Kuo G C, Lowry F, Cerami A 1987 Anticachectin/TNF monoclonal antibodies prevent septic shock during lethal bacteremia. Nature 330: 662–664

VanderMeer J W M, Endres S, Lonnemann G, Cannon J G, Ikejima T, Okusawa S, Gelfand J A, Dinarello C A 1988 Concentrations of immunoreactive human tumor necrosis factor alpha produced by human mononuclear cells in vitro. J Leuk Biol 43: 216–223

Waage A, Halstenstein A, Espevik T 1986 Association between tumor necrosis factor in serum and fatal outcome in patients with meningococcal disease. Lancet i: 355–357

Ward P A, Conran P B 1969 Immunopathology of renal complications in Simian malaria and human quartan malaria. Milit Med 134: 1228–1236

Warrell D A, Looaresuwan S, Phillips R E, White N J, Warrell M J, Chapel H M, Areekul, Tharavanij S 1986 Function of the blood–cerebrospinal fluid barrier in human cerebral malaria: rejection of the permeability hypothesis. Am J Trop Med Hyg 35: 882–889

Warrell D A 1987 Pathophysiology of severe falciparum malaria in man. Parasitology 94: S53–S76

Warren R S, Starnes H F, Gabrilove J L, Oetigen H F, Brennan M F 1987 The acute metabolic effects of tumor necrosis factor administration in humans. Arch Surg 122: 1396–1400

Weidanz W P 1982 Malaria and alterations in immune reactivity. Br Med Bull 38: 167–172

White N J 1986 Malaria pathophysiology. Clin Trop Med Commun Dis. Vol 1: Malaria. W D Saunders, London 1: 55–90

World Health Organization – Malaria Action Programme 1986 Severe and complicated malaria. Trans R Soc Trop Med Hyg 80: S1–S50

Wyler D J 1976 Peripheral lymphocyte subpopulations in human falciparum malaria. Clin Exp Immunol 23: 471–476

Wyler D J, Oppenheim J J 1974 Lymphocyte transformation in human *Plasmodium falciparum* malaria. J Immunol 113: 449–454

Discussion of paper presented by G. E. Grau

Discussed by W. Peters
Reported by G. A. T. Targett

The experimental cerebral malaria (CM) model described shows a very marked genetic restriction, developing in only a few strains of mice. It is not H-2 related, and there is little evidence of the nature of the genetic control except an indication that susceptibility to CM might be linked to capacity for TNF (cachectin) production. Thus mice such as NZB × WF1, which are low TNF producers, are totally resistant to the triggering of CM, while high producers of TNF, such as CBA/Ca mice, are very susceptible. However, TNF production even within one strain is very variable and some mice behaving as high TNF producers are not susceptible to CM. The capacity for TNF production appears to be only one aspect of CM induction.

The site of production of TNF was discussed, especially since monocytes are involved in the experimental lesion but not in human cerebral malaria. Endothelial cells can produce TNF but whether this occurs in vivo is still uncertain. TNF bound to endothelial cells has been shown both with the CM model and in association with lesions of human CM but whether this is circulating TNF that has bound to the cells or is derived from the endothelium has to be resolved. The possibility that a membrane-bound form of TNF, which has recently been described, is produced and might give rise to a secreted form, was discussed.

Northern blot analysis showed increased TNF mRNA production in the spleen and the lung but not in the brain during the syndrome. Polymerase chain reaction did give evidence of increased production in the brain but did not indicate where. It is not known whether, on the one hand, splenectomy would protect CM-sensitive strains from developing the syndrome, or on the other hand whether activation of macrophages of CM-resistant mice by injection of C. parvum or BCG, would render them susceptible to cerebral blockage.

There is pharmacological evidence for marked differences between endothelial cells taken from different capillary beds. However, the vascular plugging seen in the mouse brain was also demonstrable in the lungs and the skin. Endothelial cell lines from various organs of both susceptible and resistant strains of mice are being tested, and possible markers of activation within brain vessels are being investigated.

The importance of TNF in induction of the cerebral lesion was demonstrated by Grau and his colleagues by TNF administration. It was infused either by minipump or by i.v. injection into CM-resistant animals with malaria. The first effect was a reduction in parasitaemia, indicating that TNF has a protective as well as a pathogenic effect. After several days of infusion, cerebral lesions like those in susceptible mice developed. TNF given in this way to CM-sensitive mice not infected with malaria induced rather similar lesions, the main difference, apart from absence of parasitized erythrocytes, being the presence of polymorphs.

Sublethal doses of endotoxin have been shown to protect an animal from a subsequent lethal dose and might be expected here to make mice resistant to CM or TNF. It was tested but failed. Nor did high doses of LPS induce the experimental cerebral malaria.

Human populations include both high and low responders to TNF and it was suggested that stimulating peripheral blood monocytes with LPS might indicate associated susceptibility to cerebral malaria. This is in fact being done by Kwiatkowski et al in the Gambia, and there seemed justification too for supplementing therapy of severe malaria infections with anti-TNF antibody. Trials have been started already, not in malaria but in patients with septic shock.

Granuloma formation in experimental tuberculosis was shown to be abrogated by treatment with anti-TNF antibodies. Grau saw two important differences. First the BCG granuloma formation is a chronic process whereas cerebral malaria is acute. Second, although the granuloma is an immunopathological lesion, it is involved in defence against infection (by the mycobacteria). TNF is not detectable in sera of BCG-infected mice and a general conclusion is that at appropriate (low) levels TNF acts as a cytokine involved in protective responses but when produced in excess, as in CM, it becomes deleterious to the host.

Sequestration of parasitized erythocytes in cerebral capillaries involves adhesion to the endothelium, with strong evidence that this is mediated by parasite-derived ligands. It is known that many adhesion molecules are up-regulated by TNF and there is very recent (unpublished) information that one parasite molecule involved in cytoadherence is TNF-inducible.

The experimental CM syndrome is $CD4^+$ T-cell dependent and there was discussion on how this equates with cerebral malaria in AIDS patients. The data are conflicting because in some parts of Africa (e.g. Zambia) there are claims of an increase in cerebral malaria in AIDS patients, while elsewhere, such as in Zaire, the reverse is true. It is difficult, too, to interpret results when there are problems of differential diagnosis between cerebral malaria and HIV-associated brain pathology.

Patients in coma with cerebral malaria usually recover fully after treatment, with no sequelae. The infected mice also became comatose but it was not possible to treat them successfully. However, the small numbers that survived recovered fully.

Peters questioned the validity of the *P. berghei*/mouse syndrome as a model for human cerebral malaria and emphasized the great complexity of the pathophysiological cascade in falciparum malaria. He wondered too whether any of the observations described were relevant to the sequestration of parasitized erythrocytes in the placenta, especially as this may not be associated with cerebral or indeed very severe malaria. Finally, he stressed the importance of new methods of therapy or control being integrated with established programmes.

Plenary Lecture II

Chairman: S. R. Norrby

5. The role of the plasma membrane in the response of parasites to stress

M. Mogyoros   E. Calef and C. Gitler

INTRODUCTION

Parasites live under continuous assault by the hostile surroundings where their different life stages have to develop. Stress responses of varying types must be present in the parasites which allow them to surmount deleterious conditions and continue with their development. In the host tissues, we refer to 'activation' as the normal stress response of different monocytes to the presence of foreign organisms. In addition, all cells studied respond to insult by the induction of heat shock or stress proteins. Likewise, parasites must undergo continual 'activation' or stress responses when faced with the varied host defences. The ability of the parasite to develop means to attenuate the stress by either adapting or overcoming the pressure can in a broad sense be referred to as its virulence. Pathogenicity would then define the genetic framework in which the phenotypic stress-related responses occur. If stress conditions are of such magnitude that they endanger its life, the parasite may then differentiate into forms, for example cysts, that will allow it to seek a new, more benign environment. Growth of parasites in vitro creates conditions in which stress is diminished. This could lead to phenotypic changes which alter the behaviour of the parasite when tested within the host.

This paper focuses on the role of membranes in various mechanisms used by parasites to respond to stress. We will concentrate in our examples on the behaviour of *Entamoeba histolytica*. There is no evidence to date that infection by this parasite can be limited by the human host. Therefore, the classic approaches of immunology cannot be followed. If adaptation to host attack in this parasite is so effective, the only hope we have to eradicate it may be to interfere with some of the mechanisms involved in the stress responses of the amoebae.

AXENIC GROWTH, VIRULENCE AND COMPLEMENT RESISTANCE
OF *Entamoeba histolytica*

It is generally accepted that in vitro growth of *E. histolytica* and many other parasites in axenic media results in the loss of virulence. The goal in the design of an in vitro growth medium is to maximize growth by decreasing nutritional and other stress factors. It is likely, therefore, that in vitro grown parasites will not express stress-response-related phenotypic characteristics which are present in the same parasite growing in a hostile environment. If the characteristics involved in virulence are not constitutive, the more successful the in vitro growth medium, the lower the retention by the parasite of the capacity to respond to the host defences and to cause disease. Growth in vitro may introduce unique stress situations that may differ from those occurring in the host. Clearly, amoebae growing in axenic media must adapt to the ingestion of nutrients by pinocytosis, in contrast to amoebae in their natural habitat, where phagocytosis is the basis for nutrient acquisition. Our experience with virulence and complement resistance of *E. histolytica* helps to illustrate the above analysis. HM-1:IMSS trophozoites, the most commonly used pathogenic amoebae, were isolated from a patient's liver abscess and were cloned and grown in TYI-S-33 axenic growth medium (Diamond et al 1978). Patients with liver abscesses have high titres of humoral C'-activating antibodies directed against many surface components of the amoebae. Therefore, HM-1 trophozoites had to be complement resistant to survive within the host. When HM-1:IMSS trophozoites which had been axenically grown for extended periods (referred to as Ax-HM-1), were tested for complement resistance (Table 5.1), they were found to be highly susceptible to the alternative complement pathway (ACP). Intraperitoneal injection of high numbers (1.2×10^6) of Ax-HM-1 trophozoites into 2-month-old hamsters, resulted in abscess formation in only $10 \pm 4\%$ of the animals (Gitler et al 1985, Mogyoros et al 1986). Lower numbers failed to induce abscess formation. Therefore, axenic growth resulted in loss of C'-resistance and a markedly reduced virulence. In contrast, when trophozoites were isolated from hamster liver abscesses induced by high numbers of Ax-HM-1, and grown axenically for short periods, the amoebae which had passed through the liver (P-Ax-HM-1) were highly resistant to the alternative (Table 5.1) or direct complement pathways (DCP) (Mogyoros et al submitted). In addition, injection of 0.1×10^6 or 1.2×10^6 P-Ax-HM-1 trophozoites into hamsters resulted in liver abscess formation in $64 + 11\%$ and $92 + 2\%$ of the hamsters, respectively (Gitler

Table 5.1 Complement resistance of *Entamoeba histolytica*. Effect of axenic growth conditions and modification of surface thiols

Amoebae	Treatment	Trophozoite lysis (%)	Eosin (+) trophozoites[d] (%)
Ax-HM-1[a]	None	89 ± 5	10 ± 5
Ax-HM-1[b]	None	79 ± 3	12 ± 2
P-Ax-HM-1[a]	None	26 ± 11	45 ± 13
P-Ax-HM-1[b]	None	27 ± 20	9 ± 7
C-Ax-HM-1[a]	None	0	40 ± 2
C-Ax-HM-1[b]	None	5 ± 2	2 ± 2
Ax-HM-1[b]	Leupeptin (1 mmol/l)	0	42
Ax-HM-1[b]	Cysteine (1 mmol/l)[c]	3 ± 2	25 ± 7
Ax-HM-1[b]	Dithiothreitol (0.25 mmol/l)[c]	0	15 ± 2

Conditions for complement assay: 40% fresh human serum in a volume of 0.4 ml was incubated for 15 min with [a]62 000 trophozoites or [b]500 000 trophozoites
[c]Cells were pre-incubated for 5 min and then washed before testing for complement resistance
[d]Cells stained by 0.1% eosin

et al 1985). However, with increased time of axenic growth, P-Ax-HM-1 lost their high virulence and complement resistance and tended to behave like Ax-HM-1.

COMPLEMENT STRESS IN VITRO RESULTS IN COMPLEMENT RESISTANCE AND HIGH VIRULENCE

Removal of stress in the axenic medium (in this case, complement attack), appeared to be responsible for loss of both C'-resistance and virulence. We therefore tested the effect of a continual complement challenge in the axenic medium (growth of HM-1 trophozoites in the presence of 20% of normal bovine serum as a source of active complement). After an initial period of high trophozoite mortality, trophozoite growth continued at a level equivalent to that attained with the medium containing heat-inactivated bovine serum (Mogyoros et al submitted). Lysis due to complement decreased from 80–90% in Ax-HM-1 to 37, 12 and 3% within 2, 4 and 6 days, respectively, of growth with active complement. The amoebae growing in the presence of active complement (referred to as C-Ax-HM-1) not only were highly resistant to complement (Table 5.1), but had a high virulence in the hamster liver abscess model, equivalent to that of recently isolated P-Ax-HM-1 (Mogyoros et al 1986).

There is additional evidence to suggest that adaptation to complement may not be a specific response of the amoebae but, rather, a general 'activation' occurring in the trophozoites. Thus, complement resistance can also be elicited by growing trophozoites in the presence of heat-inactivated immune sera (Calderon & Tovar-Gallegos 1980). Furthermore, Reed et al (1986) have shown that amoebae isolated from patients retain their original complement resistance if grown in a monoxenic medium (one containing live organisms) containing bacterial flora (Robinson's medium). These same amoebae lose complement resistance if they are adapted to grow in axenic medium (in the absence of bacteria). While Calderon & Tovar-Gallegos (1980) did not test the virulence of the trophozoites made C'-resistant by growth in the presence of anti-amoebae antibodies, Bracha & Mirelman (1984) have demonstrated enhanced virulence of trophozoites grown in the presence of bacteria. The nature of the common mechanism(s) that may be elicited in the varying stress situations, which endow amoebae with complement resistance, are discussed below.

DISULPHIDE EXCHANGE AND COMPLEMENT RESISTANCE

The above findings that conditions in the axenic growth medium can drastically change complement resistance and virulence of *E. histolytica*, suggest that other factors in the medium might also play a role in the behaviour of the parasite. The literature contains contradictory conclusions about the supposed redox potential requirements for *quasi*-anaerobic growth of this parasite (Mehlotra & Shukla 1988). Thus, Gillin & Diamond (1980, 1981) found that the high levels of cysteine (CYSH) and ascorbic acid in the medium, apparently required to keep a low redox potential, could be substituted by equivalent levels of cystine (CYSSCY) without affecting *E. histolytica* growth, attachment and resistance to oxygen toxicity. Furthermore, because of the high Fe^{3+}-content of the medium, even when cysteine was added to the medium, it was rapidly oxidized to cystine during medium preparation. In all cases, therefore, the trophozoites grew in a medium in which the only reducing capacity came from ascorbic acid. Cystine can readily undergo disulphide exchange reactions with plasma membrane protein monothiols and vicinal thiols (Fig. 5.1).

The reaction with monothiols (1) to form mixed disulphides can block catalytic functions but can also facilitate interaction with host proteins having free thiols (see below). In the case of vicinal thiols (2), the initial formation of a mixed disulphide results in the subsequent intramolecular thiol-disulphide exchange to liberate a second molecule of cysteine and form the protein-disulphide (Fig. 5.1). This modification of the surface sulphydryls can be considered a form of oxidation stress that could affect many functions related to solute and electron transfer, as well as interaction with host proteins.

Treatment of Ax-HM-1 trophozoites with fresh cysteine or dithiothreitol (DTT), should result in the removal of the cysteines present as mixed sulphides and in the reduction of reactive disulphides. This could modify the behaviour of the parasite, for example, with respect to complement-mediated lysis. When this was tested, the surprising finding was that pre-incubation for 5 min of Ax-HM-1 with cysteine or DTT resulted in trophozoites which were completely resistant to lysis by the alternative complement pathway (Table 5.1) (Mogyoros & Gitler (a) in preparation). These results indicated that the artificial nature of the axenic medium modified the amoebae surface rendering the Ax-HM-1 amoebae incapable of resisting complement attack. However, C-Ax-HM-1 trophozoites grown in the same high cystine-containing medium, but with added active complement, were found to be highly resistant to complement lysis. If the mechanism of resistance in C-Ax-HM-1 is the same as that of Ax-HM-1 plus cysteine or DTT, then C-Ax-HM-1 must have an intrinsic mechanism that reduces the number of mixed disulphides present on the surface of the trophozoites.

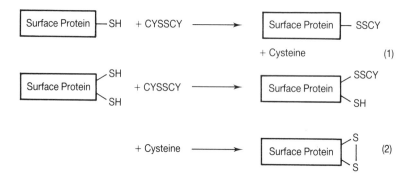

Figure 5.1 Reaction of cystine with surface protein-thiols. Reaction with monothiols (1) results in mixed disulphides. Reaction with vicinal thiols (2) results in disulphide formation

IDENTIFICATION OF THE SURFACE THIOL-CONTAINING PROTEINS

A direct demonstration that the axenic medium affected the plasma membrane thiols of *E. histolytica*, was achieved by labelling with a newly developed thiol-specific reagent (Mogyoros & Gitler (b) in preparation). N-α-Iodoacetyl-[^{125}I]-3-iodotyrosine (IAIT) can be made with specific radioactivity of up to 1000 Ci/mmol. It labels specifically the surface thiols when added to intact amoebae at pH 7.0 in isotonic phosphate-buffered saline (PBS). The exclusive labelling of surface thiols was demonstrated by the absence of labelling (Fig. 5.2, lane C) in

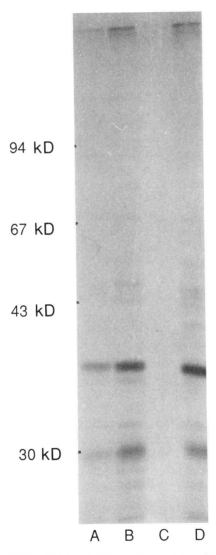

Figure 5.2 Labelling by IAIT of thiol-containing surface proteins of *Entamoeba histolytica*. Ax-HM-1 (lane A); Ax-HM-1 treated with dithiothreitol (lane B); AX-HM-1 treated with DTNB (lane C); and C-Ax-HM-1 (lane D) (From Mogyoros & Gitler submitted)

D

trophozoites pretreated with the impenetrant, thiol-specific reagent 5,5'-dithiobis(2-nitrobenzoic acid) (DTNB). Trophozoites grown in the axenic media in the absence of active complement (Ax-HM-1), showed low label incorporation into surface protein thiols (Fig. 5.2, lane A), which was markedly increased following pretreatment of the amoebae with DTT (Fig. 5.2, lane B). However, even after this treatment, label incorporation was less than that noted in C-Ax-HM-1 (Fig. 5.2, lane D) – the trophozoites grown in the presence of active complement.

In passing, it is of interest to note that IAIT labelling of intact parasites should allow the identification of a series of functionally important surface proteins. Thus, the glucose transporter and the Na^+/K^+ ATPase, among others, are very sensitive to non-penetrant mercurials and other non-penetrant thiol-reagents. Gillin et al (1984) have shown that *Giardia* and *E. histolytica* are rapidly killed by treatment with non-penetrant thiol-specific reagents. Isolation of the proteins involved, following IAIT-labelling, appears to be a straightforward project.

MECHANISM OF COMPLEMENT RESISTANCE IN *Entamoeba histolytica*

It is generally accepted that the final stage in the complement lysis of cells involves the formation of C5b–C9n membrane attack complexes (MAC). The same terminal stages occur whether activation results from the direct or alternative pathways. The formation of the MAC is a cooperative, concerted process that can be interrupted in many stages prior to the formation of a poly C9 transmembrane pore. Reed et al (1986) and Mogyoros et al (1986, submitted) showed that complement-resistant amoebae consume complement (including C9) to a greater extent than C'-sensitive trophozoites. Thus, resistance is not due to the interruption of the complement cascade but, rather, C'-resistance appears to involve inhibition of poly C9 formation. Mogyoros et al (submitted) have shown that no lysis or enhanced permeability to eosin ensued when amoebae were exposed to human serum depleted of C9. The results presented in Table 5.1 indicate that in all cases studied, C'-resistance was associated with inhibition of lysis even though enhanced permeability to eosin was observed.

Measurement of C9 incorporation into the different amoebae (Mogyoros et al submitted) indicated that resistant trophozoites incorporated significantly lower amounts of the terminal complement component. Furthermore, the enhanced permeability to eosin was a transient phenomenon. It peaked 15 min after exposure to the serum. By 30 min the trophozoites had regained their original impermeability to eosin. These results suggest that C'-resistant amoebae interfered with the formation of lytic poly C9 and rapidly removed any C9 incorporated into their plasma membrane. Even though the actual mechanism is unknown, it is of interest to speculate on the nature of the processes which might be involved because they represent membrane reactions that can be of relevance to other parasite stress responses.

Nucleated cells are known to be much more resistant to complement lytic action than erythrocytes. It is generally agreed that resistance results from an enhanced capacity to remove the MACs from the cell surface. Elimination of the MACs depends on an increase in cytosolic calcium brought about both by influx of external Ca^{2+} and by the mobilization of internal stores (Morgan & Campbell 1985). The latter reaction is believed to be mediated by inositol triphosphate released from phosphorylated phosphatidylinositol by phospholipase C (Berridge & Irvine 1984). The elimination of the MACs occurs mainly by the formation of small vesicles that are released to the extracellular medium from the cell surface. These vesicles are devoid of cytoskeletal proteins but are enriched in MAC complexes and contain representative plasma membrane proteins. The mechanism leading to vesicle formation is not completely understood. However, it appears to involve calcium-mediated release of the attachment of the plasma membrane from the underlying cytoskeleton (Fig. 5.3). Release can be the result of activation of protein kinase C with phosphorylation of key regulatory proteins, equivalent to band 4.1 in the erythrocyte, that may modulate the attachment of spectrin-like

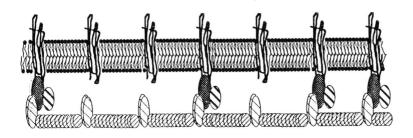

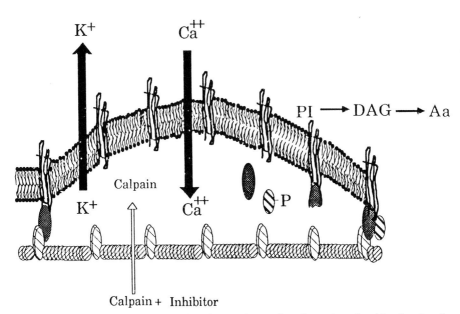

Figure 5.3 Schematic representation of the factors that mediate formation of vesicles that detach from the cell surface

proteins to transmembrane integral proteins. In addition, activation of calpain, the calcium-activated thiol protease, can result in proteolysis of the anchoring proteins. Furthermore, oxidation of thiols in the cytoskeletal proteins is known to enhance vesiculation in ageing erythrocytes and in sickle cells. Allan & Thomas (1981) conducted a detailed kinetic analysis of vesicle formation in the human erythrocyte induced by the Ca-ionophore A23187. Extensive vesicle formation, as much as 20% of the membrane lipid being released, occurred on exposure to this agent. They found that neither transaminidase-mediated cross-linking nor proteolysis of polypeptides 2.1 (ankyrin) or 4.1 appeared to be required for vesiculation to take place. Microvesicles were released only when the intracellular rise in Ca^{2+} stimulated KCl efflux leading to cell shrinkage, and when polyphosphoinositides were broken down (activation of protein kinase C). In nucleated cells, vesiculation to the extracellular medium predominated over endocytosis. The Ca^{2+}-activated K^+ efflux (Gardos effect), leading to cell shrinkage could result in the formation of blebs at the cell surface that favoured release. Quinine, an inhibitor of potassium efflux should then potentiate complement lysis. Ankyrin, the erythrocyte protein believed to mediate inter-action of band 3 with spectrin, has been found to be fatty acid acylated (Staufenbiel & Lazarides 1986). Modulation of the fatty acid attachment may be another means of regulating cytoskeletal attachment.

Morgan et al (1987) have made the intriguing suggestion that cell lysis may result from the endocytosis of C5b–C9n-containing vesicles that fuse with lyso-somes. This could result in the release into the cytoplasm of lysosomal enzymes mediating the consequent autolysis.

Therefore, C'-resistant cells have to inhibit the formation of the poly C9 pore, which is large enough to allow passage of proteins, if lysis is to be inhibited. One possibility could be that resistant cells have a proteolytic enzyme that can cleave C9. This is an appealing mechanism in the case of *E. histolytica*, because this parasite contains a very active thiol-protease which can be activated by cysteine or DTT. However, no differences in the fraction of the enzyme that is active nor in the total activity could be found between C'-resistant or labile trophozoites.

Furthermore, exposure of Ax-HM-1 to leupeptin (which completely inhibits in vitro the thiol protease) resulted in complement resistance (Table 5.1). This is the opposite of what would have been predicted if proteolysis of C9 was a key step in resistance to complement. External cysteine or DTT did not activate intracellular protease activity. However, one cannot ignore the possibility that proteases may be activated in the vicinity of MACs.

Another intriguing possibility of how *E. histolytica* escapes complement attack relates to the role of free thiols on the amoeba surface. The current views of how complement C9 transfers from solution to insert and polymerize in a target membrane to form large transmembrane channels have been summarized by Stanley et al (1986). A diagrammatic representation of this two-step insertion model is shown in Figure 5.4. The binding to the cell surface of the C5b–C8 complex leads, in some cells, to a slow increase in the permeability to calcium. However, in the amoebae, C9 depleted serum did not induce enhanced eosin permeability. There is evidence from photolabelling experiments that C8 is

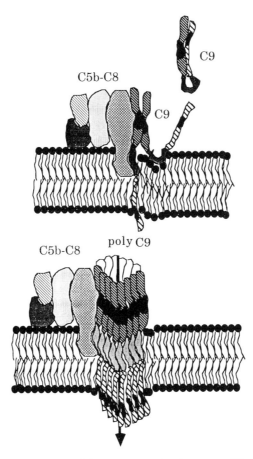

Figure 5.4 Schematic representation of the two-step mechanism responsible for the formation of the C9 complement transmembrane channel (Based on Stanley et al 1986)

inserted into the lipid core. The initial insertion of C9 leads within seconds to a rapid influx of calcium, this occurs faster than the times required for the large poly C9 pore to be formed (see Stanley et al 1986 for a detailed discussion). It was shown in Figure 5.2 that Ax-HM-1 (grown under normal axenic conditions) has a much lower number of free thiols than the same cells pretreated with DTT or in C-Ax-HM-1 trophozoites grown in media containing active complement. Yamamoto et al (1982, 1983) have shown that C9 polymerization may require initial nucleation, involving the opening of C9 disulphides, to form the disulphide-linked C9 dimers. Figure 5.5 shows how such dimers could form. Recently, Katz and Kossiakoff (1986) completed a study of previously described protein X-ray crystal structures which revealed that some disulphide cross-links in naturally occurring proteins exist in high-energy configurations. Dihedral strain energies as high as 4.7 kcal were noted. Plasma contains free GSH in.amounts of 35 µmol/l in mice and rats and 1–3 µmol/l in humans. Yamamoto et al (1982) found that GSH could catalyse poly C9 formation (Fig. 5.5b). Amoebal free surface thiols could compete with GSH and bind to the exposed reactive disulphides. This could inhibit

a)

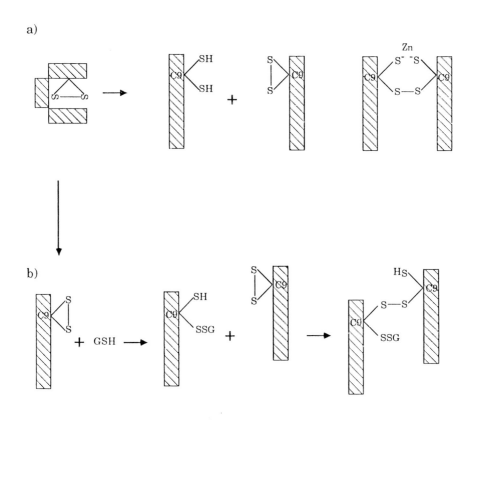

b)

c)

Membrane | Reducing Activity

Figure 5.5 Possible role of thiols in the formation of C9 dimers

polymerization by steric hindrance. Another possibility is that C'-resistant amoebae have a high surface disulphide reductase activity that could impair nucleation by reducing the reactive C9 disulphide (Fig. 5.5c). The presence of an active disulphide reductase in the amoebae could explain why C-Ax-HM-1 has a high surface free thiol concentration even though these trophozoites are also grown in media containing high levels of cystine.

SURFACE REDUCTASE OF *Entamoeba histolytica*

Only one reductase reaction has been described in *E. histolytica* which could meet the requirements of a surface disulphide reductase. This is the nitroblue tetrazolium (NBT) reductase reaction first described by Aust-Kettis et al (1982). They found that intact trophozoites had a high basal activity that can be enhanced when amoebae ingest bacteria or surface immune complexes. This is of interest because as mentioned before, Calderon & Tovar-Gallegos (1980) have shown that C′-sensitive axenized amoebae become C′-resistant on exposure to immune sera in the absence of complement. Furthermore, Reed et al (1983, 1986) have shown that amoebae grown in the presence of bacteria retain their original C′-resistance. We examined the activity of the NBT-reductase and found that the C′-resistant C-Ax-HM-1 has almost twice the reductase activity of Ax-HM-1 (Fig. 5.6). The NBT-reductase activity is higher in the absence of oxygen and under these conditions, it is not inhibited by superoxide dismutase (SOD). The activity observed in the presence of oxygen is reduced by some 60% in the presence of SOD. Thus, like xanthine oxidase, direct and more efficient reduction occurs in the absence of O_2. However, reduction can also occur by the O_2^- anion when oxygen is the competing electron acceptor. Amoebae can reduce external cytochrome C. Thus the reductase activity, as in monocytes and macrophages, is present in the plasma membrane and can react with external substrates. However, in trophozoites the activity is not cryptic since it can be detected in the absence of stimuli. Thus, basal activity is equivalent to that of stimulated polymorphonuclear leucocytes (Fig. 5.6).

Neutrophils and other phagocytes produce superoxide by the one electron

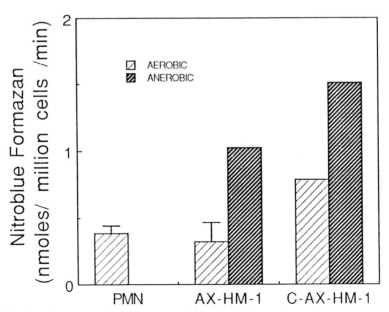

Figure 5.6 Nitroblue tetrazolium reduction by different amoebae and stimulated polymorphonuclear leucocytes. The methodology used was that of Aust-Kettis et al (1982)

reduction of oxygen at the expense of NADPH, which is mainly generated by the hexose monophosphate shunt. Amoebae lack glucose-6-phosphate dehydrogenase; they also lack haemoproteins. The amoebal activity is clearly different from mammalian burst oxidases in which cytochrome b_{558} has been suggested as an acceptor in a short electron transport chain resembling the cytochrome P_{450}–P_{450} reductase system. *E. histolytica* contains an electron transport chain in which electrons derived from the conversion of pyruvate to acetyl CoA by pyruvate synthase are transferred to a non-haem iron-containing amoebal ferredoxin (Reeves et al 1977). The gene for this ferredoxin has recently been cloned (Huber et al 1988). The deduced amino acid sequence of *E. histolytica* ferredoxin shows that the 59 amino acid polypeptide contains its eight cysteine residues in an arrangement that is characteristic of the conserved cysteine sequence of clostridial ferredoxins. It is likely that amoebal ferredoxin contains 2[4Fe–4S] electron transport centres, coordinated by each set of 4 cysteines of the polypeptide chain. This allows it to have a high negative redox potential to accept electrons from pyruvate as donor. Weinbach (1981) found that ethanol and, particularly, 2-propanol enhance oxygen consumption by the amoebae. The NADPH-dependent alcohol dehydrogenase of *E. histolytica* was also found to have 2-propanol as its most active substrate. In addition, an NADPH:flavin oxidoreductase was purified to homogeneity by Lo & Reeves (1980). The enzyme does not contain firmly bound flavin. Aerobically, the purified enzyme passed the reduced equivalents from reduced flavin to oxygen to form H_2O_2. However, intact amoebae do not form peroxide when they respire. These results suggest that electron flow can occur in the amoebae from either pyruvate or NADPH flavin mononucleotide (FMN) to ferredoxin and then to oxygen to form O_2^-. All of these components have been shown to be present in the cytosol. The question then remains of how reduction of extracellular cytochrome C can occur. Weinbach (1981) has suggested that the amoebae contain two different iron-sulphur centres. One of these would have to be present in the membrane to accomplish the release of extracellular superoxide. Knowledge regarding these electron transport systems is of interest because two of the drugs that effectively kill amoebae, namely quinacrine and metronidazole, act by inhibiting flavins and by functioning as single electron acceptors, respectively. A tentative scheme depicting the amoebae electron transport systems is shown in Figure 5.7.

The superoxide anion can function as a reducing agent. Murray et al (1981) showed that HM-1 trophozoites are susceptible to H_2O_2 but not to superoxide. The sensitivity to peroxide decreased as the numbers of trophozoites in the assay were increased. This implies that amoebae contain systems that inactivate peroxide. The high levels of lipopeptidoglycan present in amoebae may function as radical scavengers. Sonicates of amoebae displayed low levels of SOD (0.45 ± 0.31 U/mg). They were reported to contain low, but measurable amounts of glutathione peroxidase. However, the relevance of this activity is difficult to assess because the amoebae have no glutathione (Fahey et al 1984). Cysteine appears to be the main intracellular thiol in the trophozoites. About 75% was found to exist in the reduced form. Thus amoebae must contain a cystine reductase, since as mentioned, the axenic growth medium contains high levels of cystine and other unidentified thiols are also found mainly in the oxidized state.

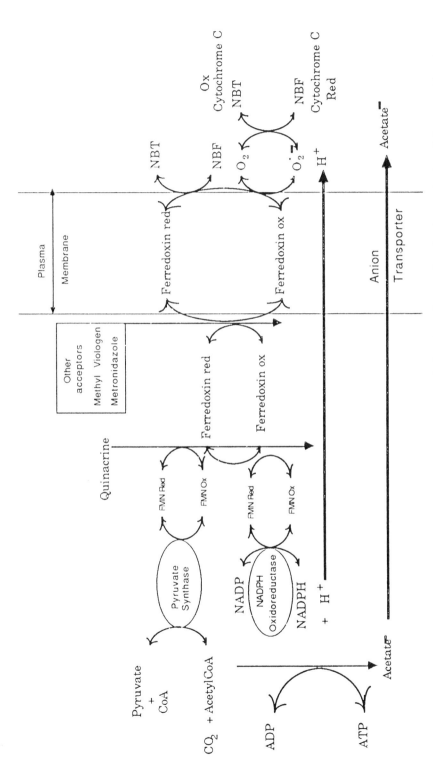

Figure 5.7 Schematic representation of the electron transport systems of *Entamoeba histolytica* that may be related to production of the superoxide anion

89

CONTACT KILLING BY *Entamoeba histolytica*

It is likely that one of the reasons that *E. histolytica* can resist attack by the host resides in its remarkable capacity to kill cells that it contacts. Interestingly, amoebae were the first eukaryotic organisms in which an ion-channel forming protein was implicated in the mechanism of contact killing. The identification of amoebapore (Lynch et al 1980, 1982, Young et al 1982, Gitler et al 1984) preceded the description of perforins (Stanley and Luzio 1988) in natural killer cells and some granule-containing lymphocytes. Amoebapore was found to be present in the trophozoites in a highly aggregated form. It was apparently not enclosed by a membrane within the amoebae and yet it was liberated to the extracellular medium when amoebae were stimulated by addition of concanavalin A or the calcium ionophore A23187. The material released from cells was also present in a highly aggregated state which could be sedimented at high speed. After sodium dodecyl sulphate (SDS) treatment, the monomer had a molecular weight of 14 000. Two isoforms of molecular weight 28 000 were detected by dissociation with salts, low pH or repeated cycles of freeze-thaw. These had isoelectric points of 5.3 and 6.7 respectively (Rosenberg et al in press). Addition of amoebapore to cells results in a rapid depolarization. Thus the pore-forming material incorporates spontaneously into the plasma membrane of target cells. The channels formed by amoebapore did not release proteins but allowed ions like calcium to diffuse rapidly down their concentration gradients.

Several aspects were difficult to understand. How was particulate amoebapore released from cells since it was not contained within a secretory vesicle? One possible explanation is that upon interaction of amoebapore with the endofacial surface of the plasma membrane, the induced calcium flow into the amoebae results in vesiculation and release into the medium in a manner equivalent to that discussed for the complement pore. We have discussed (Gitler et al 1984) that an ion-channel, even one with the high unit conductance of amoebapore (1600 pS), was unlikely to kill target cells. Macrophages and lymphoblasts, although they were initially depolarized, recovered their surface potential after a period of about 60 min. Thus, amoebapore may participate in an initial stage of contact killing, but other factors must play a role leading to cell death.

One aspect which is of interest in the above discussion, is the fact that amoebae produce high amounts of external superoxide. The low levels of superoxide dismutase in the trophozoites imply that peroxide would not accumulate in these cells. On the other hand, host cells would be expected to form high levels of peroxide because they contain both cytoplasmic and mitochondrial superoxide dismutases. When low levels of peroxide (100 µmol/l for 15 min), which are below those that would be produced by amoebae, were added to cells, there was (i) a rapid fragmentation of DNA which developed within 20 s and reached a maximal effect in minutes. When lymphocytes were exposed to neutrophils activated with phorbolmyristate acetate, DNA damage was prevented by catalase but not by superoxide dismutase; (ii) a marked loss in cellular ATP due both to direct inhibition of glyceraldehyde-3-phosphate dehydrogenase and depletion of NAD due to activation of poly(ADP-ribose) polymerase active in DNA repair; (iii) formation of blebs that led to microvesiculation of the plasma membrane. This was probably the result of oxidation of thiols in cytoskeletal proteins; (iv) cell death ensued with an ED_{50} of 500 μmol/l peroxide when cells were exposed for a period of 15 min (Cochrane et al 1988).

The cellular changes observed following exposure to peroxide are remarkably similar to those detected in cells following contact with virulent *E. histolytica* (or killer lymphocytes). This may imply that the combined effect of amoebapore and superoxide production may underlie the exceptional capacity of amoebae to kill target cells. This hypothesis can be readily tested because 3-aminobenzamide, an inhibitor of the poly(ADP-ribose) polymerase, inhibited the fall in NAD and ATP levels of cells exposed to peroxide and also markedly decreased cell death (Cochrane et al 1988).

ANION TRANSPORT, AN ALTERNATIVE DETOXIFICATION MECHANISM

The response of parasites to drugs can be considered another form of stress-response which enables these organisms to survive under adverse conditions. Hydrophobic drugs having aromatic rings and the tendency to be positively charged at neutral pH, have been shown to be eliminated from cells, including parasites, by a multidrug transport protein, known as P-glycoprotein or P170, which is encoded by the MDR1 gene in the human (Gottesman & Pastan 1988). Colchicine, doxorubicin (adriamycin), actinomycin D or vinblastin are some of the drugs eliminated from the cell by the P-glycoprotein. However, little attention has been given to the elimination of drugs having a net negative charge. This is surprising because one of the main detoxification systems in the cell, the glutathione S-transferase, results in the formation of mercapturic acids which are negatively charged. Little is known about the membrane transport systems that handle these molecules.

We became interested in this subject when trying to develop procedures to covalently label parasites with fluorescent dyes in order to study their distribution within the host. Our strategy was to administer to amoebae derivatives of diacetylfluorescein which contained reactive moieties that could attach covalently to intracellular components. Because of their insolubility in water, these derivatives partitioned very rapidly into the membrane lipid core. This prevented covalent attachment to the outer surface components of the cell. Within most cells, there are acetyl- or butyryl-specific hydrolases which remove the acetyl moieties forming fluorescein-reactive-moiety derivatives that are trapped within the cell. The derivatives used were diacetylfluorescein-5-isothiocyanate (DAFITC), diacetyl-5 and 6-carboxyfluorescein succinimidyl ester (DACFSE) (Bronner-Fraser 1985).

The derivatives dissolved in acetone were added to the trophozoites so that the final acetone was $> 1\%$ and the fluorescein derivative was about 1 μmol/l. Within 10 min, cells became loaded with concentration in the range of 0.4 mmol/l. No labelling could be detected in the outer surface by means of fluorescein-specific antibodies. The surprising finding was that, irrespective of the reagent used, the majority of the fluorescent label was lost from the cells with a half-life of about 1 h. By 24 h, the fluorescent derivatives that remained within the cells were in the order of 4–6% for the isothiocyanate and 12–16% for the hydroxysuccinimide ester. Comparison of the doubling times of fluorescently labelled with unlabelled cells indicated that cells were not affected by the labelling procedure. This allowed tracing of the original trophozoites and their progeny, for at least 3 divisions (Calef & Gitler in preparation).

Since the reactive derivatives could, in addition to being hydrolysed, attach covalently to small molecules such as amino acids and glutathione, it was surprising that the removal from the cells of the different fluorescent products occurred with essentially the same exit rates. To test further whether a transport system might be present which removes anions we loaded cells with different diacetylfluorescein derivatives that had no reactive moieties, but differed in the nature and the number of anionic groups. We loaded trophozoites with 2 µmol/l diacetylfluorescein (DAF), diacetyl-5 and 6-carboxyfluorescein (DACF) and diacetylfluorescein-5-thiocarbamyltaurine (DAFT). Fluorescein, carboxyfluorescein and fluorescein-5-thiocarbamyltaurine were removed from cells with a t_{1M2} of 28.2, 50 and 61 min, respectively. Loading with lower concentrations of the diacetyl derivatives resulted in faster exit rates. Thus, with 0.2 µmol/l DAF, the rate of fluorescein exit had a t_{1M2} of 11.3 min. Equivalent exit rates were observed for the exit of BCECF, a fluorescent pH indicator. Attempts to load amoebae with fluorescein failed even at mmol/l external concentrations. The efflux was inhibited by lowering the temperature. Below 20°C, the rates of exit were negligible. In addition, exit rates were inhibited by energy deprivation (Prosperi et al 1986). Thus the process appears to involve a unidirectional, energy-dependent active transport. Parallel studies with L1210 lymphoblasts, showed that exit of the fluorophores involved exchange with external anions, the order of preference being nitrate > chloride > bromide > sulphate > gluconate. In addition, in the lymphoblasts, exit was inhibited by probenecid and ethacrynic acid. No such exchange or inhibition by probenecid or ethacrynic acid was observed in the amoebae. The fluorescent anions are not modified within the cell in order to be excreted. In addition, we found no inhibition by surface depolarization, inhibitors such as 4,4'-diisothiocyanostilbene-2, 2'-disuphonic acid (DIDS) and 4-acetamido-4'-iso-thiocyanatostilbene-2, 2'-disulphonic acid (SITS) that inhibit the anion exchange in erythrocytes or by monensin (Calef & Gitler in preparation).

These results are, in general terms, similar to those reported by Steinberg et al (1987) for macrophages. They suggest that non-specific unidirectional anion transporters are present in many cells. It will be of interest to determine whether cellular elimination of mercapturic acids and other anionic drugs occurs by the same transport systems.

CONCLUSIONS

E. histolytica infections do not appear to be limited by the host. The only strategy that seems available at present to attempt to prevent this disease, involves the perturbation of the mechanisms used by the amoebae to overcome the host defences. We have discussed different facets of how the parasite responds to stress.

The further definition of these processes might identify key reactions that may be used as targets for the development of vaccines or more effective drug therapies.

ACKNOWLEDGEMENT

This work was supported by a Grant from the John D. and Catherine T. MacArthur Foundation.

REFERENCES

Allan D, Thomas P 1981 Ca^{2+} induced biochemical changes in human erythrocytes and their relation to microvesiculation. Biochem J 198: 433–440

Aust-Kettis A, Jarstrand C, Urban T 1982 The nitroblue tetrazolium (NBT) reduction of *Entamoeba histolytica* during endocytosis of *E. coli* and homologous antibodies. Arch Invest Med (Mexico) 13: (suppl 3): 261–264

Berridge M J, Irvine R F 1984 Inositol triphosphate, a novel second messenger in cellular signal transduction. Nature (Lond) 312: 315–321

Bracha R, Mirelman D 1984 Virulence of *Entamoeba histolytica* trophozoites. Effects of bacteria, microaerobic conditions, and metronidazole. J Exp Med 160: 353–368

Bronner-Fraser M 1985 Alterations in neural crest migration by monoclonal antibody that affects cell adhesion. J Cell Biol 101: 610–618

Calderon J, Tovar-Gallegos G R 1980 Resistance to immune lysis induced by antibodies in *Entamoeba histolytica*. In: Van den Bosch H (ed) The host invader interplay. Elsevier, Amsterdam pp 227–230

Calef E, Gitler C 1989 The anion transporter of *Entamoeba histolytica* and L1210 lymphoblasts (in preparation)

Cochrane C G, Schraufstatter I U, Hyslop P, Jackson J 1988 Cellular and biochemical events in oxidant injury. In: Halliwel B (ed) Oxygen radicals and tissue injury (Proceedings of an Upjohn Symposium) Federation of American Societies for Experimental Biology, Bethesda

Diamond L S, Harlow D R, Cunnick C C 1978 A new medium for the axenic cultivation of *Entamoeba histolytica* and other *Entamoeba*. Trans R Soc Trop Med Hyg 72: 431–432

Fahey R C, Newton G L, Arrick B, Overdank-Bogart T, Aley S B 1984 *Entamoeba histolytica*: a eucaryote without glutathione metabolism. Science 224: 70–72

Gillin F D, Diamond L S 1980 Attachment of *Entamoeba histolytica* to glass in a defined maintenance medium: specific requirement for cysteine and ascorbic acid. J Protozool 27: 474–478

Gillin F D, Diamond L S 1981 *Entamoeba histolytica* and *Giardia lamblia*: Growth responses to reducing agents. Exp Parasitol 51: 382–391

Gillin F D, Reiner D S, Levy R B, Henkart P A 1984 Thiol groups on the surface of anaerobic parasitic protozoa. Mol Biochem Parasitol 12: 1–12

Gitler C, Calef E, Rosenberg I 1984 Cytopathogenicity of *Entamoeba histolytica*. Phil Trans R Soc (Lond) B307: 73–85

Gitler C, Mogyoros M, Calef E, Rosenberg I 1985 Lethal recognition between *Entamoeba histolytica* and the host tissues. Trans R Soc Trop Med Hyg 79: 581–587

Gottesman M M, Pastan I 1988 The multidrug transporter, a double-edged sword. J Biol Chem 263: 12163–12166

Huber M, Garfinkel L, Gitler C, Mirelman D, Revel M, Rozenblatt S 1988 Nucleotide sequence analysis of an *Entamoeba histolytica* ferredoxin gene. Mol Biochem Parasitol 31: 27–34

Katz B A, Kossiakoff A A 1986 The crystalographically determined structures of atypical strained disulphides engineered into subtilisin. J Biol Chem 261: 15480–15485

Lo H S, Reeves R E 1979 *Entamoeba histolytica*: Flavins in axenic organisms. Exp Parasitol 47: 180–184

Lo H S, Reeves R E 1980 Purification and properties of NADPH: flavin oxidoreductase from *Entamoeba histolytica*. Mol Biochem Parasitol 2:23–30

Lynch E C, Harris A, Rosenberg I, Gitler C 1980 A natural protozoan-derived ionophore: a possible mechanism of cytotoxicity by *Entamoeba histolytica*. Biol Bull 159: 496–497

Lynch E C, Rosenberg I, Gitler C 1982 An ion channel forming protein produced by *Entamoeba histolytica*. EMBO J 1: 801–804

93

Mehlotra R K, Shukla O P 1988 Reducing agents and *Entamoeba histolytica*. Parasitol Today 4(3): 82–83

Mogyoros M, Calef E, Gitler C 1986 Virulence of *Entamoeba histolytica* correlates with the capacity to develop complement resistance. Isr J Med Sci 22: 915–917

Mogyoros M, Gitler C (a) The role of trophozoite surface protein-thiols in the resistance of *Entamoeba histolytica* to complement lysis (in preparation)

Mogyoros M, Gitler C (b) Differential labelling of protein mono- and vicinal-thiols (in preparation)

Mogyoros M, Fishelson Z, Gitler C 1989 Axenically grown complement sensitive and resistant pathogenic *Entamoeba histolytica* differ in their regulation of the membrane-attack complex. (submitted)

Morgan B P, Campbell A K 1985 The recovery of human polymorphonuclear leucocytes from sublytic complement attack is mediated by changes in intracellular free calcium. Biochem J 231: 205–208

Morgan B P, Dankert J R, Esser A F 1987 Recovery of human neutrophils from complement attack: Removal of the membrane attack complex by endocytosis and exocytosis. J Immunol 138: 246–253

Murray H W, Aley S B, Scott W A 1981 Susceptibility of *Entamoeba histolytica* to oxygen intermediates. Mol Biochem Parasitol 3: 381–391

Prosperi E, Croce A C, Bottiroli G, Supino R 1986 Flow cytometric analysis of membrane permeability properties influencing intracellular accumulation and efflux of fluorescein. Cytometry 7: 70–75

Reed S L, Sargeaunt P G, Braude A I 1983 Resistance to lysis by human serum of pathogenic *Entamoeba histolytica*. Trans R Soc Trop Med Hyg 77: 248–253

Reed S L, Curd J G, Gigli I, Gillin F D, Braude A I 1986 Activation of complement by pathogenic and nonpathogenic *Entamoeba histolytica*. J Immunol 136: 2265–2270

Reeves R E, Warren L G, Suskind B, Lo H S 1977 An energy-conserving pyruvate-to-acetate pathway in *Entamoeba histolytica* pyruvate synthase and a new acetate thiokinase. J Biol Chem 252: 726–731

Rosenberg I, Bach D, Loew L M, Gitler C 1989 Amoebapore: isolation, characterization and partial purification of a transferable membrane channel produced by *Entamoeba histolytica*. Mol Biochem Parasitol (in press)

Stanley K K, Luzio J P 1988 A family of killer proteins. Nature 334: 475–476

Stanley K K, Page M, Campbell A K, Luzio J P 1986 A mechanism for the insertion of complement component C9 into target membranes. Mol Immunol 23: 451–458

Staufenbiel M, Lazarides E 1986 Ankyrin is fatty acid acylated in erythrocytes. Proc Natl Acad Sci USA 83: 318–322

Steinberg T H, Newman A S, Swanson J A et al 1987 Macrophages possess probenecid-inhibitable organic anion transporters that remove fluorescent dyes from the cytoplasmic matrix. J Cell Biol 105: 2695–2702

Weinbach E C 1981 Biochemistry of enteric parasitic protozoa. Trends Biochem Sci 6: 254–257

Yamamoto K, Migita S 1983 Mechanisms for the spontaneous formation of covalently linked polymers of the terminal membranolytic complement protein (C9). J Biol Chem 258: 7887–7889

Yamamoto K, Kawashima T, Migita S 1982 Glutathione-catalyzed disulphide-linking of C9 in the membrane attack complex of complement. J Biol Chem 257: 8573–8576

Young J D-E, Young T M, In L P, Unkeless J C, Colin Z A 1982 Characterization of a pore-forming protein from *Entamoeba histolytica*. J Exp Med 156: 1677–1690

Discussion of paper presented by C. Gitler

Introduced by M. Pereira
Reported by S. R. Norrby

Gitler's paper raised several important questions, one being whether the acquisition of complement resistance is the result of a selection of a subpopulation which differs genetically in being complement resistant or if complement resistance results from phenotypic variation. Gitler argued in favour of the latter theory. Thus, if *E. histolytica* cells are exposed to antibodies against their surface antigens or to complement alone, they become complement resistant. Also, encysted amoebas seem to be complement sensitive which they should not be if complement resistance is the result of a genotypic variation.

In the discussion it was also pointed out that amoebiasis in HIV-infected homosexual men in Western Europe and North America tends to be a rather benign disease with few if any cases of liver abscesses or amoebomas. That could either be the result of interaction between the HIV infection and the amoeba parasites or of a genotypic variation between amoeba strains infecting patients in various parts of the world. Several findings support the latter theory. First, HIV-positive homosexuals in Mexico tend to have very active amoebic infections with no noticeable differences in comparison with other groups of patients with amoebiasis. Second, there are now preliminary studies indicating differences in the DNA base sequences when *E. histolytica* strains from the Third World and from Western countries are compared. Gitler's group is looking at commensal isolates of *E. histolytica* to see if there are mutants which lack the ability to become complement resistant and which should therefore be less pathogenic and unable to cause invasive infections.

Pereira, pointed out that complement–complement receptor interaction is important also with other parasites such as *Leishmania major* and *Trypanosoma cruzi*. He also emphasized the fact that this type of interaction is only one of several types of receptor–ligand interaction known to be of importance in parasitic infections. One example of such interactions is the *T. cruzi* neuraminidase which is a lipoprotein receptor as summarized in Figure 5.8. The discovery of a developmentally regulated neuraminidase activity in *T. cruzi* was made in the early 1980s. Pereira and co-workers later found a specific inhibitor of the neuraminidase activity in plasma of non-infected individuals. When purified and amino-acid sequenced, the inhibitor was found to be high-density lipoprotein (HDL). It could subsequently be demonstrated that both HDL and low-density lipoprotein (LDL) are potent inhibitors of the neuraminidase activity of *T. cruzi*.

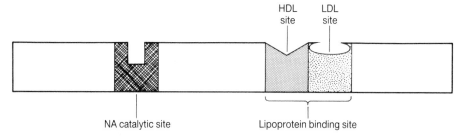

HDL   LDL
site   site

NA catalytic site   Lipoprotein binding site

Figure 5.8 Structure–function relationship of the *T. cruzi* neuraminidase, emphasizing three functional domains of the enzyme: the catalytic site and sites for HDL and LDL

As shown in Figure 5.8, the enzyme molecule is unique in that it has one domain containing the catalytic site and two other domains for binding of HDL and LDL, respectively.

The biological function of the interaction between HDL and LDL on the one hand and the *T. cruzi* neuraminidase on the other hand is summarized in Figure 5.9. Inhibition of enzyme activity in the trypomastigote will enhance infectivity while in the non-infectious epimastigote inhibition seems to enhance growth as indicated by the fact that epimastigotes cannot multiply in vitro unless the medium contains HDL or LDL.

Pereira then summarized the state of knowledge about lipoprotein receptors in parasites (Table 5.2). Such receptors have been described in *Trichomonas vaginalis*, *Trypanosoma brucei*, *Schistosoma mansoni* and *T. cruzi*. Both pathogenic and non-pathogenic protozoa, e.g. *Tetrahymena*, have cholesterol on their membrane. However, while the former are incapable of synthesizing cholesterol, the non-pathogenic organisms make their own cholesterol or cholesterol analogues. Parasites may acquire cholesterol for membrane biogenesis through receptor mechanisms analogous to the mechanisms present in vertebrate cells. If that is the case, there should be analogues to the neuraminidase receptor also in other parasites. Pereira and his group have obtained interesting results both with *Leishmania* and malaria. In an effort to study similarities between *T. cruzi* and malaria, the ability of sera from 200 patients with vivax or falciparum malaria to immunoprecipitate or immunoblot *T. cruzi* proteins was investigated. The only

Table 5.2 Lipoprotein receptors in parasites

Organism	Receptor	Cholesterol biosynthesis	Sterol nutritional requirement
Trypanosoma cruzi	Neuraminidase MW = 120–205 kD	No	Yes
Trypanosoma brucei	Receptor-mediated endocytosis of LDL MW = ?	No	Yes
Trichomonas vaginalis	MW = <250 kD	No	Yes
Schistosoma mansoni	MW = 45 kD	No	Yes
Tetrahymena pyriformis	ND	Yes[a]	No

[a]*T. pyriformis* is not a pathogen, lives in water, and synthesizes tetrahymanol, a cholesterol analogue

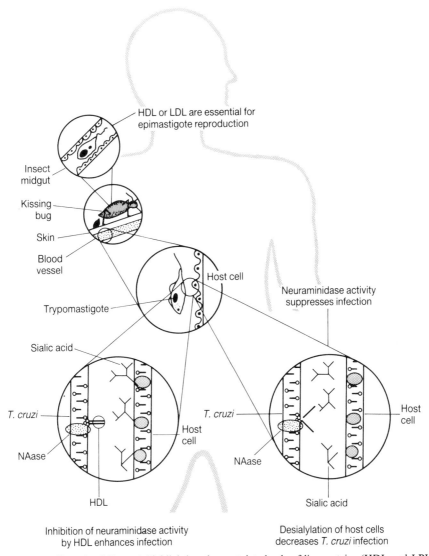

Figure 5.9 Life cycle of *T. cruzi*, highlighting the postulated role of lipoproteins (HDL and LPL) in epimastigotes multiplication in the insect vector and trypomastigote infection in the mammalian host

positive finding was that about 25% of the sera contained antibodies to the *T. cruzi* neuraminidase. *T. cruzi* neuraminidase, purified by affinity chromatography was insolubilized on a solid support to purify the reactive antibodies. The affinity-purified antibodies were then used to locate the structural analogue of the *T. cruzi* neuraminidase on *Plasmodium falciparum* parasites. Fluorescence microscopy showed that the antibodies reacted both with merozoites and schizonts. Further studies demonstrated that the antibodies interacted with the so-called electrodense granules in the merozoites, with schizonts and also with the surface of infected erythrocytes. The presence of antibodies to the *T. cruzi* neuraminidase raises the possibility that malaria parasites contain a neuraminidase, a lipoprotein receptor or both. Preliminary results have indicated that *P. falciparum* has neuraminidase activity as shown with a fluorescent substrate and by peanut haemagglutination.

Section II: Trypanosomes

Chairman: L. Hudson

6. African trypanosomes: an elusive target

J. D. Barry

INTRODUCTION

Elusiveness and adaptability are fundamental to African trypanosomes. Many features encountered in their life cycle render them vulnerable to potential control measures: they are extracellular, inhabit accessible niches in their hosts, encounter rapid and extreme environmental changes and must cope with all of this with a relatively simple genome. It is, therefore, a measure of their supreme elusiveness and adaptability that there is little hope for an immunological approach to control. Paradoxically, the large volume of research into trypanosomes has merely emphasized the ineffectiveness of current control measures, and it is difficult to escape the impression that chemotherapy is the main hope for the future. Indeed, the extent to which the trypanosome differs biochemically from its hosts is such that prospects for chemical control look reasonably good. Hence, we should continue to search for alternative approaches to control.

The African trypanosomes' hosts include humans, and game and domestic animals, causing sleeping sickness-type diseases (Hoare 1972). There are several pathogenic species: *Trypanosoma congolense* and *T. vivax* are major animal pathogens whereas, within the *T. brucei* group, *T. b. rhodesiense* causes acute sleeping sickness, generally in East Africa and *T. b. gambiense* is responsible for chronic sleeping sickness, generally in West Africa, while *T. b. brucei* does not infect humans. The *T. brucei* group has been the one used the most extensively for research and is the subject of the major part of this review.

Trypanosomes are protozoa with a well-organized and economical development cycle in tsetse flies and mammals (Vickerman 1985) characterized by a series of stages with specific roles (Fig. 6.1). In the mammal, the long slender form undergoes mitosis, invades and transforms to the non-dividing stumpy form, the role of which is to be transmitted to tsetse flies. In the fly gut, the stumpy form develops to the procyclic stage, which divides repeatedly, establishing infection. Within weeks, the infection spreads to the salivary glands, in which the epimastigote form arises. It is attached to the gland and generates a monolayer from which develops, through cell division, the free-swimming metacyclic form; the only fly stage with mammal infectivity. This does not divide, but is pre-adapted to survival and development in the mammal.

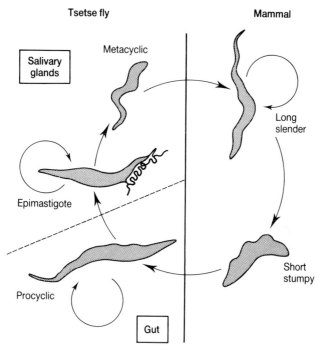

Tsetse fly

Mammal

Metacyclic

Salivary glands

Long slender

Epimastigote

Short stumpy

Procyclic

Gut

Figure 6.1   The life cycle of *Trypanosoma brucei*. The main role of each stage is indicated. Thus, the long slender, procyclic and epimastigote stages multiply by division and develop to the next stages, while the transient short stumpy and metacyclic stages are pre-adapted for transmission between hosts and subsequent development

Recent advances in two areas of research are discussed here. In the first, antigenic variation, we are now beginning to understand molecular mechanisms. The second area is the developmental cycle, where the trypanosome displays remarkable adaptability in overcoming rather dramatic environmental changes. This area raises several important questions, including how the trypanosome can respond promptly to these rapid changes and the relative degrees to which its growth and development are intrinsically controlled within a genetically determined developmental programme or are subject to external signals.

ANTIGENIC VARIATION

Antigenic variation in the mammal

The trypanosome population induces humoral immunity and radical reduction in parasite numbers ensues (Vickerman & Barry 1982) (Fig 6.2). Survival is ensured by antigenic variation, the continual switching of the variant surface glycoprotein (VSG), the only antigen accessible to antibodies on the organism's surface (Cross 1975). This is organized as the surface coat, which contains $> 10^7$ VSG molecules (Turner 1985). Only one VSG is expressed by each trypanosome at a time, except during switching and in a few cases in in vitro culture when double expression has been detected (Esser & Schoenbechler 1985, Baltz et al 1986). Double expressors

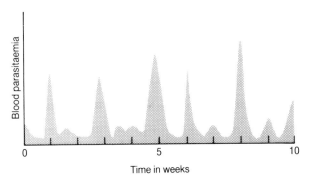

Figure 6.2 Variation in the number of trypanosomes in the blood of a patient infected with *Trypanosoma brucei* based on the classic observations of Ross and Thomson (1909). There were regular fluctuations in the number of parasites in the blood of a patient infected with African trypanosomiasis. The fluctuations were independent of intermittent drug therapy which was, in any case, ineffective.

It is now known that each peak population represents an immunologically distinct population of parasites. As the immune response eliminates each peak population new, antigenically distinct parasites arise. Antigenic variation therefore represents one of the most elegant (and successful) mechanisms of immune avoidance. In the absence of chemotherapy, the patient would die of infection even in the face of massive immune response

are selected against in vivo (Baltz et al 1986), perhaps because mixed coats are structurally abnormal. It is unlikely that the VSG has any specific biochemical role, as reflected in the diversity in its variable domain, and its importance resides in its dense packing on the cell surface (to block access of antibodies to other surface molecules), its effect on surface charge (thwarting non-specific immune mechanisms) and perhaps also in its immunogenicity (helping maintenance of parasitaemia at sublethal level). The VSG molecule is discussed in detail elsewhere in this volume (Ch. 7).

A minority of trypanosomes, which have switched to a new variable antigen type (VAT), continue multiplying until they, in turn, invoke an immune response (Vickerman & Barry 1982). It is generally thought that, in a clonal infection, several hundred different VATs can arise. Despite this large number, there is a degree of order in their expression, probably resulting mainly from an order of gene switching (Capbern et al 1977, Barry 1986) and it is believed that, for optimum parasite transmission, this is in delicate balance with the kinetics of the immune response. Thus, too many parasites may prematurely kill the host, whereas an insufficient number may lead to elimination or to decreased opportunity for ingestion by the fly. Presence of only one VSG on each trypanosome prolongs use of the antigen repertoire. Expression is hierarchical, as there is a range in probabilities of expression within the repertoire (Liu et al 1985, Capbern et al 1977, Barry 1986), and this seems a very effective way of prolonging infection and of avoiding an overwhelming initial parasitaemia. Divergence in switching (Miller & Turner 1981) and lack of total predictability in sequence lead to the presence of more than one VAT in the population at a time, preventing termination of infection due to pre-existing antibodies.

As a result of recent re-examination, our concept of one fundamental aspect of

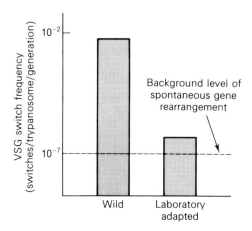

Figure 6.3 Rates of switching of VSG genes in 'wild' and laboratory-adapted *Trypanosoma brucei.*
It has been suggested that the rate of switching in wild lines is about 1 in 100
switches/trypanosome/generation, a much greater frequency than previously suspected from the
study of laboratory-adapted lines (between 10 000 and 10 000,000). It is possible that there is a
background level of spontaneous gene rearrangement which contributes to antigenic switching
(below dashed line) but, more importantly, a driven, specific system (above dashed line). The
background level may have achieved disproportionate significance in laboratory-adapted lines and,
in reality, be of no significance.

antigenic variation must be changed. The rate of switching has been estimated at
between 10^{-4} and 10^{-7} switches per trypanosome per generation (Van Meirvenne
et al 1975, Myler et al 1985, Lamont et al 1986). In each case this involved
trypanosome lines adapted to laboratory rodents through extensive syringe
passaging, but such lines have a greatly reduced switching rate. Study of a more
natural line has now revealed a much higher rate, of 10^{-2} to 10^{-3} switches per
trypanosome per generation (Turner & Barry in press) (Fig. 6.3). This has a very
important implication: switching appears to be a driven system, with a specific
molecular mechanism, rather than resulting from a background level of gene
rearrangements as is generally believed.

The trypanosome genome and the genes for variant surface glycoproteins
Although much has been discovered about the structure, organization and
expression of VSG genes (reviewed by Donelson 1988, Pays & Steinert 1988), key
areas which remain poorly understood include which molecules are involved in
switches, the promoter for the VSG transcription unit, whether there are
regulatory genes, how exclusivity of expression is achieved and how the VSG gene
repertoire evolves. In the absence of DNA transformation and of a usable genetic
system, experimentation in these areas is difficult.

There is a separate gene (or small gene family) for each VSG, and the repertoire
numbers slightly more than 1000 in the diploid genome (Van der Ploeg et al
1984a). The majority are in long tandem arrays within chromosomes and, as such,
are never expressed (Van der Ploeg et al 1984a). These silent basic copy (BC) genes
possess common flanking regions on either side. The upstream flank contains a
series of repeats approximately 70 base pairs (bp) long, followed by a spacer
region (Liu et al 1983, Aline et al 1985). At the 3' end of the gene, there is similarity

of sequence extending from within the coding region to about 100 bp downstream, in the non-translated region of the transcript (Michels et al 1983). For expression, these genes have to be copied into specific expression sites (ES), which are located at telomeres (Kooter et al 1987, Pays et al 1989). By gene conversion, an extra expression linked copy (ELC) of the BC is inserted into the ES, destroying the VSG gene which is already resident (see Fig. 6.4). The common 5′ and 3′ flanks mark the limits of the converted sequence; the ES telomeres which act as recipients in conversion generally possess long arrays of the 5′ 70-bp repeats and the 3′ flank is present in the resident ELC (Michels et al 1983, Shah et al 1987).

Another set of BC genes are located permanently at telomeres (Donelson 1988) and there is a large pool of telomeres due to the presence of about 100 minichromosomes per diploid genome (Van der Ploeg et al 1984a,b). These chromosomes contain no detectable genes apart from telomeric VSG genes and are apparently composed mainly of highly repetitive sequence (Van der Ploeg et al 1984a). The tendency of telomeres to participate in recombinational events possibly lends greater fluidity to the VSG gene repertoire: exchange and sequence conversion between telomeres have been recorded (De Lange et al 1983, Pays et al 1985). Both can lead to an antigenic switch, if a new VSG gene is inserted into a transcriptionally active telomere. The most common route of switching, however, is that telomeric genes are activated in situ when their telomere becomes turned on as an ES, the previously active telomere being switched off independently (Bernards et al 1984). For example, one particular telomere has been shown to be activated in 50% of all switches (Liu et al 1985), although expression patterns may not be that predictable (Myler et al 1988). Because we now know that switching is more common than was believed, some of the rarely recorded switch mechanisms (translocation between telomeres, ELC formation mediated by sequence other than 70-bp repeats) recede in importance, and can be considered as resulting from a background level of spontaneous gene rearrangement (Fig. 6.3).

Ploidy and the VSG gene repertoire

By patterns of separation in pulsed field gel electrophoresis (PFGE), trypanosome chromosomes can be divided into four size classes (Van der Ploeg et al 1984a). Although VSG genes are detectable in all classes, all other genes examined map only within the two classes containing the largest chromosomes. Only VSG genes, their flanks, the major satellite sequence and standard telomere repeats have been found in chromosomes of the two smaller chromosome classes. The implication is that the larger chromosomes are essential, while the smaller ones probably are not. This is evident in genetic crosses, where the former display Mendelian behaviour at meiosis, whereas the latter do not and are probably aneuploid (Sternberg et al 1988), and from the diversity in number and length of smaller chromosomes observed between trypanosome stocks (Van der Ploeg et al 1984b). It is predictable that VSG genes in the smaller classes would be unstable in the genome, being susceptible to loss through random segregation.

At least some VSG genes are haploid within the diploid genome (Bernards et al 1984, Donelson 1988). This would not cause problems with their inheritance during mitosis, as each haploid gene that segregated normally would still be replicated, at least for those genes contained within the larger chromosomes.

There are, perhaps, some benefits to the parasite arising from haploidy in a diploid genome. There may in fact be twice the expected number of VSG genes in each trypanosome. There may be only one copy of each ES, perhaps relieving the parasite of the need for an allelic exclusion mechanism during expression, although recent indications are that one ES may exist simultaneously as active and inactive alleles (Pays et al 1989). Diversification of the VSG repertoire arising from trypanosome mating may be greatly enhanced over that for diploid genes.

It is not difficult to envisage how such a haploid state may have arisen, if the gene repertoire is considered as a class of repetitive DNA (containing repetitive copies of the common 5′ and 3′ flanks of the genes) which happens to accommodate coding sequences, rather than as a set of normal genes occupying distinct loci. The repetitive regions would thus occupy the same large regions on homologous individual chromosomes but, within these regions, classic allelism of coding sequences would be meaningless. Intra- and interchromosomal recombination, mediated by the common flanks, could easily occur, leading to a steady reorganization within the repertoire.

The mechanism of VSG gene conversion
Virtually all VSG gene conversions involve the 70-bp repeat region at the 5′ limit (Aline et al 1985, Shah et al 1987). The 3′ limit is usually within the common flank of the VSG gene (Michels et al 1983), although when the conversion is between two telomeric genes, it involves instead the repeat motif of the telomere itself (De Lange et al 1983). Specificity of conversion is therefore provided by the 70-bp region. Two recent developments now provide clues to possible mechanisms. First, the high rate of switching predicts a specific mechanism. Second, a flank containing less than two 70-bp repeats has been mapped consistently as the 5′ conversion limit in the frequent generation of ELCs from one telomeric VSG gene (Shiels et al submitted). This telomere is acting only as a donor in gene conversion (although trypanosomes in which it has acted as a recipient would be difficult to detect), which raises the possibility of an inverse relationship between the number of 70-bp repeats and the capacity to act as a donor. A mechanism similar to that in the classic DNA double-strand break repair model (Fincham & Oliver 1989) would be consistent with these findings. This would operate via a 70-bp specific double-strand endonuclease, with a capacity to bind and cut in direct proportion to the number of repeats. The cut telomere would then act as the recipient of information, as observed for events with this telomere. This model involves an element of randomness in the selection of individual 70-bp regions, so to avoid an excess of double-strand breaks in the genome, the enzyme would have to be present at only a low level in any switching cell and to act probably once only. There would also be a bias towards telomeres being selected by the enzyme. Several of these predictions are testable.

VSG gene expression sites
Besides containing just the VSG gene, its conserved flanks and a promoter, ES include a series of other genes, termed expression site associated genes (ESAGs) (Cully et al 1985, 1986) (Fig. 6.4). So far, three bloodstream ES have been analysed in detail. They are long, comprising respectively about 60, 45 and 40

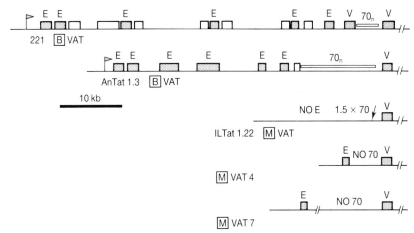

Figure 6.4 VSG gene expression sites. Two bloodstream ES (top 2 lines) and three metacyclic ES. V, VSG genes; the upstream VSG gene in the 221 site is a pseudogene; 70 bp, 70-bp repeat region; E, expression site associated gene. Filled boxes are genes identified by more than one criterion (DNA hybridization, DNA sequence, stable RNA product, protein product identified); open boxes are potential ESAGs identified by single criteria. Flags represent transcriptional start areas. Map lengths from VSG genes to the end of the chromosome are variable, and the distance from the M-VAT 7 gene to the ESAG gene is not known. Data are from, for 221, Kooter et al (1987); for AnTat 1.3, Pays et al (1989); for ILTat 1.22, Shiels et al (submitted); for M-VATs 4 and 7, Son et al (1989)

kilobase pairs (kbp) (Johnson et al 1987, Kooter et al 1987, Borst 1989, Pays et al in press). There seems to be a total of 7 different ESAGs in individual ES, most of them apparently encoding membrane-type proteins. One shares significant homology, in the predicted amino-acid sequence, with the catalytic site of yeast adenylate cyclase (Pays et al in press). This enzymatic activity has been identified on the plasma membrane, in the organism's flagellar pocket (Walter & Opperdoes 1982). ESAGs are shared by different ES, the best studied case being two ES in the same trypanosome, which have the same set of ESAGs in perhaps the same order (Borst personal communication). It has been suggested, from the copy number of different ESAGs, that there may be about 20 potential ES in each trypanosome, although this does not take account of duplication within an individual ES or of non-telomeric ESAG copies (Kooter et al 1987). As to the role of ESAG products, it may be that they are functionally associated with VSG synthesis or coat assembly, or they may have independent functions, merely using ES to achieve stage-specific transcription, although not all copies appear to fall into this category (Pays et al in press). Those ESAGs which are predictably present in different ES may have been selected because of a phenotypic link with the VSG.

There is indirect evidence that ES are transcribed, rather unusually, by RNA polymerase I (pol I), which is normally used for ribosomal RNA genes. First, there is the classic pol I character of insensitivity to the inhibitor alpha-amanitin (Kooter & Borst 1984). Second, within ES some gaps in transcription occur, with re-initiation apparently occurring at sequences resembling trypanosome ribosomal promoters (Shea et al 1987, Alexandre et al 1988, Pays et al in press, Borst personal communication). However, it is important to note that the authentic regions of transcription start in these telomeres do not resemble pol I promoters, when either active or inactive (Borst personal communication). If pol I is used, the possibility arises that ES are transcribed within the nucleolus; the usual or main location of pol I. Should this be so, it could be that selective ES expression results from competition amongst the different telomeres for inclusion in the nucleolus. Other ideas about why telomeres are used as ES are discussed by Pays & Steinert (1988).

Antigen expression by the metacyclic stage

Expression of VSG genes ceases in the tsetse fly, being resumed only as the infective metacyclic stage develops. In many respects, the patterns of expression in the metacyclic population are different from those in the bloodstream. This population uses only a small and specific subset of the VSG repertoire, known as the metacyclic VAT (M-VAT) repertoire, which consists of some 12 VATs in *T. congolense* (Crowe et al 1983) and no more than 27 in *T. b. rhodesiense* (Turner et al 1988). Remarkably, the M-VAT repertoire is very predictable in content, regardless of the VAT(s) expressed by the trypanosomes originally ingested by the fly (Hajduk & Vickerman 1981). Such predictability does not easily fit with the general concept that VSG expression is essentially a system of great diversification. The M-VSG repertoire does change slowly, however, probably ruling out its exploitation for vaccination (Barry et al 1983).

M-VSGs are expressed in the fly by a system distinct from that used in the mammal. In the first few days of infection following transmission by flies there is a continued expression of, and switching between, M-VSGs even though the trypanosomes transform rapidly to mammalian stages (Barry et al 1985), and in this period M-VSG expression takes precedence over bloodstream VSG expression (Hajduk et al 1981, Turner et al 1986). Labelled antibodies have been used to examine initiation of VSG synthesis directly in the fly, while the coating metacyclic cells are still attached to the gland epithelium. This has shown that the same individual VSG is activated repeatedly, using a stochastic mechanism which operates as the surface coat is first synthesized (Tetley et al 1987).

In keeping with prediction, all seven M-VSG genes examined do seem to have a special location, namely at the telomeres of the largest chromosomes (Cornelissen et al 1985, Lenardo et al 1986, Delauw et al 1987), and, calculating from the few data available (Van der Ploeg et al 1984a), there may be enough chromosomes in this set to accommodate all the M-VSG gene repertoire, as well as some non M-VSG genes, at telomeres. Given the telomeric location, the question arises whether these genes are activated in the fly in situ, or by duplication into another telomere, which may be a metacyclic-specific expression site. The former seems more likely, as it would be a one-step process, whereas the latter would require not only specific selection of the M-VSG genes, but also the existence of a specific ES. As very few metacyclic cells are available, studies have been performed only on the whole population of bloodstream trypanosomes in the early days following fly transmission, when metacyclic-type VSG expression persists. However, this approach has problems, due to the polyclonal activation of genes in the fly and switching between M-VSGs in the bloodstream. Indeed, it has been concluded from two separate studies that activation in the tsetse fly is mediated in situ (Lenardo et al 1986) or by duplication (Delauw et al 1987). These problems have now been overcome by use of a virulent parasite line which yields antigenically relatively stable metacyclic-derived trypanosome clones. This has revealed not only that the two M-VSG genes studied are probably activated in situ in the fly but also strongly supported the view that there are fundamentally different expression systems used in the fly and in the mammal, because independent activation of the studied gene in the bloodstream consistently proceeds by ELC formation (Shiels et al submitted) (Fig. 6.5). Therefore, it appears that M-VSG genes are selected and expressed on their own telomeres in the fly by a mechanism which does not operate in normal bloodstream infection, but (at least one of) the same telomeres are not used as ES when activated in bloodstream infection. It is possible, however, that some M-VSG genes can be activated in situ and others by ELC production.

M-VSG telomeres, which are also ES in the fly, have a simple structure which contrasts markedly with the complex arrangement and high copy number of sequence in bloodstream ES (see Fig. 6.4). Most of the M-VSG telomere sequence is unique or of low copy number in the genome, being devoid of, or having very few, 70-bp repeats or ESAGs for up to 17 kbp upstream of the VSG gene (Son et al 1989, Shiels et al submitted). Preliminary analyses also suggest that transcription may begin very near the gene (Graham & Barry unpublished observations). This system looks radically different from what occurs in the bloodstream.

A current interpretation of these data is that, in the fly, the decision is made to initiate production of VSG, and transcription proceeds selectively, using at random the only set of genes available at that time: those contained at the telomeres of some of the large chromosomes. As there is no requirement for switching in the metacyclic population, the more complex bloodstream expression system is not yet active, and use of bloodstream ES may not be possible. Once the infection has run for several days in the mammal, the switching system is fully operational, and so the simple metacyclic telomeres may become incapable of activation.

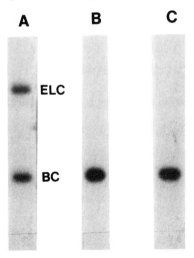

Figure 6.5 Activation of a metacyclic VSG gene. Southern blot of Hind III digested DNA from three trypanosome clones and probed with a 5' cDNA fragment of the ILTat 1.22 metacyclic VSG gene. Lane A, a bloodstream form trypanosome clone expressing the 1.22 VSG, demonstrating the basic copy (BC) and an extra expression-linked copy (ELC) of the gene; lane B, a metacyclic clone expressing another VSG, showing the silent BC; lane C, a metacyclic clone expressing the 1.22 gene, showing in situ activation and thus no extra gene copy

Why is the M-VSG repertoire predictable?

It is difficult to see any selective pressure for a set of *specific* VSGs being used in the fly (although it could be argued that only certain surface coats are compatible with existence in the tsetse fly). More significantly, there is probably a selective pressure for the presence of a *mixture* of VATs in this population (expressed as one VSG on each trypanosome), to enable a repeated re-infection of reservoir hosts. These hosts can cure infection by attaining immunity against the whole VSG repertoire (Barry 1986), but immunity wanes (Nantulya et al 1979). Should the metacyclic population express only one VAT, the chances of encountering an immune host are high; there is selection for a mixture in the metacyclic population. To achieve this mixture, the trypanosome must be capable of choosing at random from a pool of genes. The set of bloodstream telomeres does not allow such a degree of randomness, however, as they are dominated by one, or just a few, telomeres (Liu et al 1985, Delauw et al 1987, Myler et al 1988). One way of achieving a separate pool of genes is to maintain them in genomic locations which are potential ES in the fly but which do not participate in the conversion events which are so characteristic of bloodstream telomeres. This specification would be met by the existence of a set of telomeres composed mainly of unique sequence. More specifically, these would contain none of the recombinogenic 70-bp repeat sequence or so little that the telomere would act almost exclusively as a donor in gene conversion. When the non-switching gene expression system becomes active in the fly, exclusive use of these telomeres would result unavoidably in expression of the linked VSG genes. It is clear that the occasional loss of individual M-VSGs from the M-VSG repertoire (Barry et al 1983) is due to deletion of their genes (Cornelissen et al 1985, Barry unpublished observations), which would be the outcome of the predicted occasional use of the metacyclic telomere as a recipient in VSG gene conversion.

THE TRYPANOSOME DEVELOPMENTAL PROGRAMME

Basic studies on the developmental programme and growth control of trypanosomes may suggest novel approaches to control, in the form of receptor molecules which detect host factors. Such receptors may be present, but sufficiently sparse or exposed so transiently that they are not detectable by routine surface labelling techniques. Recent studies have indeed yielded findings of some promise, and at this stage it is worth considering how the trypanosome's developmental programme is organized, as this could indicate the level of dependence on host factors.

Developmental control in the trypanosome

As the trypanosome alters structurally and functionally during the life cycle, its gene expression is regulated stage-specifically. This is not achieved by the usual system of genes being subject individually to transcriptional control through individual promoters, and an increasingly convincing case can be made that much of this results from the need to respond rapidly to environmental change. The

110

trypanosome genome contains multigene transcription units (so far, no single-gene unit has been found) which appear to be expressed constitutively throughout the life cycle, producing long primary transcripts which are then processed by a trans-splicing mechanism to yield capped and polyadenylated gene-length transcripts (Borst 1986, Cornelissen et al 1986, Imboden et al 1987, Muhich & Boothroyd 1988, Tschudi & Ullu 1988). Differential control seems to be exerted pre-dominantly at the post-transcriptional level (Gibson et al 1988, Torri & Hajduk 1988). A most bizarre mechanism of post-transcriptional control occurs in the trypanosome mitochondrion, where some transcripts are nonsense until converted to sense by a very novel editing system which seems to be under developmental control (Benne et al 1986, Stuart 1989). Presumably by having genes already activated, or transcripts already present, the trypanosome can respond to environ-mental change rapidly, circumventing the time-consuming process of responding to a stimulus by selectively activating specific genes. The next areas for study are the molecular mechanisms for this post-transcriptional control and, returning to the question of dependence on host factors, the more complex question of what in turn controls these.

Triggering of a control system, leading to alteration in trypanosome growth (i.e. cell division) and development, can occur either as a result of intrinsic genetic programming or in direct response to external stimulus. It seems obvious that the trypanosome depends on both, as can be seen from the transitional life-cycle stages. Although the stumpy bloodstream and the metacyclic stages clearly are pre-adapted for survival and development in the next host, probably as a result of intrinsic programming, it would be lethally inappropriate for them to develop any further prior to encountering the new host. Hence, systems to detect external signals and to initiate appropriate responses are necessary. Very little is known as yet about what these signals may be or how they may be recognized, but the use of receptors seems a possibility. Simple changes in physical conditions such as temperature may be involved (Newport et al 1988).

Receptors do exist on trypanosomes. They are used for the uptake of the low-density lipoprotein–cholesterol complex, which is particulate, and the transferrin–iron complex (Coppens et al 1987). Receptors present a problem by being potentially exposed to the immune system although it is conceivable that restriction of such receptors to the plasma membrane of the flagellar pocket protects them, by an unknown mechanism. The complexes must either enter the pocket prior to binding or the receptors may make a transient appearance on the cell surface. Study of antigens of the flagellar pocket membrane has demonstrated that specific antibodies can actually bind to the surface of living trypanosomes at the region of emergence of the flagellum from the pocket and that these antigens can induce a degree of immunization (Olenick et al 1988). This raises interesting questions about parasite survival (Barry in press).

Evidence has now been obtained for a receptor used for growth control located all over the surface of bloodstream forms and procyclic forms of trypanosomes (Hide et al in press). The receptor is recognized by antibodies specific to the mam-malian epidermal growth factor (EGF) receptor and binds EGF; the trypanosome responding by undergoing division and biosynthesis. Why host growth factors may be involved with trypanosome multiplication is an interesting question;

perhaps those stages having the role of multiplying and establishing infection use a trigger. The distribution of this receptor contrasts with the flagellar pocket localization of other receptors, but this is not surprising, as EGF is a small protein which, unlike larger complexes, can presumably readily gain access to its receptor through the surface coat.

The tsetse–trypanosome interface
Environmental influence on trypanosome growth, and perhaps also on development, is apparent in the tsetse fly. Besides the presence of the growth factor

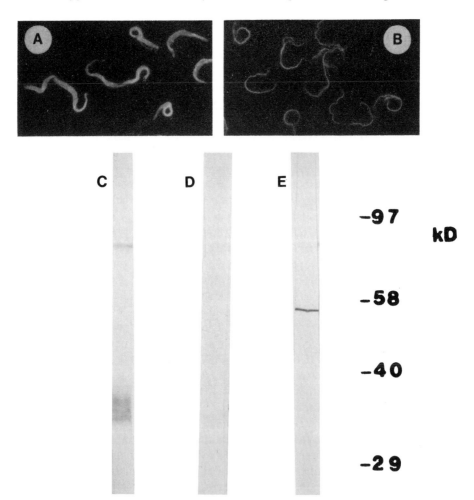

Figure 6.6 A surface antigen of procyclic *Trypanosoma congolense*. A, immunofluorescence pattern of acetone-fixed cells stained with monoclonal antibody GUGM 2.1, demonstrating a surface antigen. B, pattern with GUGM 4.8, demonstrating an intraflagellar antigen. Location of both antigens was confirmed by staining reaction with living procyclic cells. C, Western blot of procyclic cell lysate probed with GUGM 2.1, showing two antibody-reactive components, of which the lower separates as a diffuse, complex band. D, negative control Western, first antibody layer omitted. E, positive control Western, probed with GUGM 4.8, demonstrating a single antigen. The migration positions of molecular weight markers are shown (kD)

receptor on the procyclic form, there is evidence for tsetse factors influencing the parasite. Uptake of blood by the fly stimulates the appearance of two lectins, which bind, and are detrimental to, procyclic trypanosomes (Maudlin & Welburn 1988a). This may be a primitive form of defence against infection, which is circumvented for trypanosomes by a complex relationship between the fly and rickettsia-like organisms (Maudlin & Welburn 1988a). Investigation of the lectins in vivo is difficult, but indications are that, late in infection, the lectins may actually be required for development of the infection to the epimastigote and metacyclic stages (Maudlin & Welburn 1988b). Now that the lectins are being purified (Welburn & Maudlin personal communication), in vitro experiments may help to clarify this area and reveal whether novel growth factor receptors on the trypanosome should be sought.

Surface molecules on the procyclic trypanosome could be exploited for immunological control of parasite transmission. A series of monoclonal antibodies directed against a complex antigen on the surface of procyclic *T. congolense* (Fig. 6.6) have strong agglutinating activity against procyclic cells and, when incorporated into routine fly bloodmeals, one antibody markedly inhibited trypanosome transmission (Lainson et al submitted). Similar results have been obtained with an antibody against an uncharacterized antigen of *T. brucei* (Nantulya & Moloo 1988). The complex antigen of *T. congolense* shows a gel separation pattern and strong immunogenicity similar to those of procyclin, a surface protein of *T. brucei* procyclic cells (Richardson et al 1988). The function of this protein and its exploitation for control are areas worth further investigation.

ACKNOWLEDGEMENTS

I am grateful to P. Borst, I. Maudlin, E. Pays and A. Tait for communicating data prior to publication, to my colleagues in the laboratory (S. Graham, K. Matthews, P. Shiels and E. Kilbride), and to Christopher Barry for assistance with the figures. The author is a Wellcome Trust Senior Lecturer. Work quoted here is funded by the Wellcome Trust, the Medical Research Council and the Overseas Development Administration.

REFERENCES

Alexandre S, Guyaux M, Murphy N B, Coquelet H, Pays A, Steinert M, Pays E 1988 Putative genes of a variant-specific antigen gene transcription unit in *Trypanosoma brucei*. Mol Cell Biol 8: 2367–2378
Aline R F, MacDonald G, Brown E, Allison J, Myler P J, Rothwell V, Stuart K 1985 (TAA)n within sequences flanking several intrachromosomal variant surface glycoprotein genes in *Trypanosoma brucei*. Nucleic Acids Res 13: 3161–3177
Baltz T, Giroud C, Baltz D, Roth C, Raibaud A, Eisen H 1986 Stable expression of two variable surface glycoproteins by cloned *Trypanosoma equiperdum*. Nature 319: 602–604
Barry J D 1986 Antigenic variation during *Trypanosoma vivax* infections of different host species. Parasitology 92: 51–65
Barry J D 1989 African trypanosomiasis. In: Liew F Y (ed) Vaccination strategies of tropical diseases. CRC Press, Boca Raton (in press)

E

Barry J D, Crowe J S, Vickerman K 1983 Instability of the *Trypanosoma brucei rhodesiense* metacyclic variable antigen repertoire. Nature 306: 699–701

Barry J D, Crowe J S, Vickerman K 1985 Neutralization of individual variable antigen types in metacyclic populations of *Trypanosoma brucei* does not prevent their subsequent expression in mice. Parasitology 90: 79–88

Benne R, Van Den Burg J, Brakenhoff J, Sloof P, Van Boom J, Tromp M 1986 The major transcript of the frameshifted coxII gene from trypanosome mitochondria contains four nucleotides that are not encoded in the DNA. Cell 46: 819–826

Bernards A, De Lange T, Michels P A M, Liu A Y C, Huisman M J, Borst P 1984 Two modes of activation of single surface antigen gene of *Trypanosoma brucei*. Cell 36: 163–170

Borst P 1986 Discontinuous transcription and antigenic variation in trypanosomes. Annu Rev Biochem 55: 701–732

Capbern A, Giroud C, Baltz T, Mattern P 1977 *Trypanosoma equiperdum*: etude des variations antigeniques au cours de la trypanosomose experimentale du lapin. Exp Parasitol 42: 6–13

Coppens I, Opperdoes F R, Courtoy P J, Baudhin P 1987 Receptor-mediated endocytosis in the bloodstream form of *Trypanosoma brucei*. J Protozool 34: 465–472

Cornelissen A W C A, Bakkeren G A M, Barry J D, Michels P A M, Borst P 1985 Characteristics of trypanosome variant antigen genes active in the tsetse fly. Nucleic Acids Res 13: 4661–4676

Cornelissen A W C A, Verspieren M P, Toulme J J, Swinkels B W, Borst P 1986 The common 5' terminal sequence on trypanosome mRNAs: a target for anti-messenger oligodeoxynucleotides. Nucleic Acids Res 14: 5605–5614

Cross G A M 1975 Identification, purification and properties of clone-specific glycoprotein antigens constituting the surface coat of *Trypanosoma brucei*. Parasitology 71: 393–417

Crowe J S, Barry J D, Luckins A G, Ross C A, Vickerman K 1983 All metacyclic variable antigen types of *Trypanosoma congolense* identified using monoclonal antibodies. Nature 306: 389–391

Cully D F, Ip H S, Cross G A M 1985 Coordinate transcription of variant surface glycoprotein genes and an expression site associated gene family in *Trypanosoma brucei*. Cell 42: 173–182

Cully D F, Gibbs C P, Cross G A M 1986 Identification of proteins encoded by variant surface glycoprotein expression site-associated genes in *Trypanosoma brucei*. Mol Biochem Parasitol 21: 189–197

De Lange T, Kooter J M, Michels P A M, Borst P 1983 Telomere conversion in trypanosomes. Nucleic Acids Res 11: 8149–8165

Delauw M F, Laurent M, Paindavoine P, Aerts D, Pays E, Le Ray D, Steinert M 1987 Characterization of genes coding for two major metacyclic surface antigens in *Trypanosoma brucei*. Mol Biochem Parasitol 23: 9–17

Donelson J E 1988 Unsolved mysteries of trypanosome antigenic variation. In: Englund P T and Sher A (eds) The biology of parasitism: a molecular and immunological approach. Alan R. Liss, New York pp 371–400

Esser K M, Schoenbechler M J 1985 Expression of two variant surface glycoproteins on individual African trypanosomes during switching. Science 229: 190–193

Fincham J R S, Oliver P 1989 Initiation of recombination. Nature 338: 14–15

Gibson W C, Swinkels B W, Borst P 1988 Post-transcriptional control of the differential expression of phosphoglycerate kinase genes in *Trypanosoma brucei*. J Mol Biol 201: 315–325

Hajduk S L, Vickerman K 1981 Antigenic variation in cyclically transmitted *Trypanosoma brucei*. Variable antigen type composition of the first parasitaemia in mice bitten by trypanosome-infected *Glossina morsitans*. Parasitology 83: 609–621

Hajduk S L, Cameron C R, Barry J D, Vickerman K 1981 Antigenic variation in cyclically transmitted *Trypanosoma brucei*. Variable antigen type composition of metacyclic trypanosome populations from the salivary glands of *Glossina morsitans*. Parasitology 83: 595–607

Hide G, Gray A, Harrison C M, Tait A 1989 Identification of an epidermal growth factor receptor homologue in trypanosomes. Mol Biochem Parasitol, (in press)

Hoare C A 1972 The trypanosomes of mammals. Blackwell Sci Publi Oxford

Imboden M A, Laird P W, Affolter M, Seebeck T 1987 Transcription of the intergenic regions of the tubulin gene cluster of *Trypanosoma brucei*: evidence for a polycistronic transcription unit in a eukaryote. Nucleic Acids Res 15: 7357–7368

Johnson P J, Kooter J M, Borst P 1987 Inactivation of transcription by UV irradiation of *Trypanosoma brucei* provides evidence for a multicistronic transcription unit that includes a variant surface glycoprotein gene. Cell 51: 273–281

Kooter J M, Borst P 1984 Alpha-amanitin insensitive transcription of variant surface glycoprotein genes provides further evidence for discontinuous transcription in trypanosomes. Nucleic Acids Res 12: 9457–9472

Kooter J M, van der Spek H J, Wagter R, d'Oliveira C E, van der Hoeven F, Johnson P J, Borst P 1987 The anatomy and transcription of a telomeric expression site for variant-specific surface antigens in *Trypanosoma brucei*. Cell 51: 261–272

Lainson F A, Kilbride E, MacLennan C, Maudlin I, Barry J D 1989 Specific surface antigens of procyclic *Trypanosoma congolense* associated with transmission-blocking immunity. Mol Biochem Parasitol (submitted)

Lamont G S, Tucker R S, Cross G A M 1986 Analysis of antigen switching rates in *Trypanosoma brucei*. Parasitology 92: 355

Lenardo M J, Esser K M, Moon A M, Van der Ploeg L H T, Donelson J E 1986 Metacyclic variant surface glycoprotein genes of *Trypanosoma brucei* subsp. *rhodesiense* are activated in situ, and their expression is transcriptionally regulated. Mol Cell Biol 6: 1991–1997

Liu A Y C, Van der Ploeg L H T, Rijsewijk F A M, Borst P 1983 The transcription unit of variant surface glycoprotein gene 118 of *Trypanosoma brucei*. Presence of repeated elements at its border and absence of promoter-associated sequences. J Mol Biol 167: 57–75

Liu A Y C, Michels P A M, Bernards A, Borst P 1985 Trypanosome variant surface glycoprotein genes expressed early in infection. J Mol Biol 182: 383–392

Maudlin I, Welburn S C 1988a Tsetse immunity and the transmission of trypanosomiasis. Parasitol Today 4: 109–111

Maudlin I, Welburn S C 1988b The role of lectins and trypanosome genotype in the maturation of midgut infections in *Glossina morsitans*. Trop Med Parasit 39: 56–58

Michels P A M, Liu A Y C, Bernards A, Sloof P, Van der Bijl M M W, Schinkel A H, Menke H H, Borst P 1983 Activation of the genes for variant surface glycoproteins 117 and 118 in *Trypanosoma brucei*. J Mol Biol 166: 537–556

Miller E N, Turner M J 1981 Analysis of antigenic types appearing in first relapse populations of clones of *Trypanosoma brucei*. Parasitology 82: 63–80

Muhich M L, Boothroyd J 1988 Polycistronic transcripts in trypanosomes and their accumulation during heat shock: evidence for a precursor role in mRNA synthesis. Mol Cell Biol 8: 3837–3846

Myler P J, Allen A L, Agabian N, Stuart K 1985 Antigenic variation in clones of *Trypanosoma brucei* grown in immune-deficient mice. Infect Immun 47: 684–690

Myler P J, Aline R F, Scholler J K, Stuart K D 1988 Multiple events associated with antigenic switching in *Trypanosoma brucei*. Mol Biochem Parasitol 29: 227–241

Nantulya V M, Musoke A J, Barbet A F, Roelants G E 1979 Evidence for reappearance of *Trypanosoma brucei* variable antigen types in relapse populations. J Parasitol 65: 673–678

Nantulya V M, Moloo S K 1988 Suppression of cyclical development of *Trypanosoma brucei brucei* in *Glossina morsitans centralis* by an anti-procyclics monoclonal antibody. Acta Trop 45: 137–144

Newport G, Culpepper J, Agabian N 1988 Parasite heat-shock proteins. Parasitol Today 4: 306–312

Olenick J G, Wolff R, Nauman R K, McLaughlin J 1988 A flagellar pocket membrane fraction from *Trypanosoma rhodesiense*: immunogold localization and nonvariant immunoprotection. Infect Immun 56: 92–98

Pays E, Steinert M 1988 Control of antigen gene expression in African trypanosomes. Annu Rev Genet 22: 107–126

Pays E, Guyaux M, Aerts D, Van Meirvenne N, Steinert M 1985 Telomere reciprocal recombination as a mechanism for antigenic variation in trypanosomes. Nature 316: 562–564

Pays E, Tebabi P, Pays A, Coquelet H, Revelard P, Salmon D, Steinert M 1989 The genes and transcripts of an antigen gene expression site from *Trypanosoma brucei*. Cell 57: 835–845

Richardson J P, Beecroft R P, Tolson D L, Liu M K, Pearson T W 1988 Procyclin: an unusual immunodominant glycoprotein surface antigen from the procyclic stage of African trypanosomes. Mol Biochem Parasitol 31: 203–216

Shah J S, Young J R, Kimmel B E, Iams K P, Williams R O 1987 The 5' flanking sequence of a *Trypanosoma brucei* variable surface glycoprotein gene. Mol Biochem Parasitol 24: 163–174

Shea C, Lee M G-S, Van der Ploeg L H T 1987 VSG gene 118 is transcribed from a co-transposed pol-I like promoter. Cell 50: 603–612

Shiels P G, Matthews K R, Graham S G, Cowan C, Barry J D 1989 Structure and expression of a metacyclic variant surface glycoprotein gene in *Trypanosoma brucei*. (submitted)

Son H J, Cook G A, Hall T, Donelson J E 1989 Expression site associated genes of *Trypanosoma brucei rhodesiense*. Mol Biochem Parasitol 33: 59–66

Sternberg J, Tait A, Haley S, Wells J M, Le Page R W F, Schweizer J, Jenni L 1988 Gene exchange in African trypanosomes: characterisation of a new hybrid genotype. Mol Biochem Parasitol 27: 191–200

115

Stuart K 1989 RNA editing: new insights into the storage and expression of genetic information. Parasitol Today 5: 5–8

Tetley L, Turner C M R, Barry J D, Crowe J S, Vickerman K 1987 The onset of expression of the variant surface glycoproteins of *Trypanosoma brucei* in the tsetse fly studied using immunoelectron microscopy. J Cell Sci 87: 363–372

Torri A F, Hajduk S L 1988 Posttranscriptional regulation of cytochrome c expression during the developmental cycle of *Trypanosoma brucei*. Mol Cell Biol 8: 4625–4633

Tschudi C, Ullu E 1988 Polygene transcripts are precursors to calmodulin mRNAs in trypanosomes. EMBO J 7: 455–463

Turner M J 1985 The biochemistry of the surface antigens of the African trypanosomes. Br Med Bull 41: 137

Turner C M R, Barry J D 1989 High frequency of antigenic variation in *Trypanosoma brucei rhodesiense* infections. Parasitology (in press)

Turner C M R, Barry J D, Vickerman K 1986 Independent expression of the metacyclic and bloodstream variable antigen repertoires of *Trypanosoma brucei rhodesiense*. Parasitology 92: 67–74

Turner C M R, Barry J D, Maudlin I, Vickerman K 1988 An estimate of the size of the metacyclic variable antigen repertoire of *Trypanosoma brucei rhodesiense*. Parasitology 97: 269–276

Van der Ploeg L H T, Schwartz D C, Cantor C R, Borst P 1984a Antigenic variation in *Trypanosoma brucei* analysed by electrophoretic separation of chromosome-sized DNA molecules. Cell 37: 77–84

Van der Ploeg L H T, Cornelissen A W C A, Barry J D, Borst P 1984b Chromosomes of kinetoplastida. EMBO J 3: 3109–3115

Van Meirvenne N, Janssens P G, Magnus E 1975 Antigenic variation in syringe-passaged populations of *Trypanosoma* (Trypanozoon) *brucei*. I. Rationalization of the experimental approach. Ann Soc Belge Med Trop 55: 1–23

Vickerman K 1985 Developmental cycles and biology of pathogenic trypanosomes. Br Med Bull 41: 105–114

Vickerman K, Barry J D 1982 African trypanosomiasis. In: Cohen S, Warren K S (eds) Immunology of parasitic infections Blackwell Sci. Publ Oxford

Walter R D, Opperdoes F R 1982 Subcellular distribution of adenylate cyclase, cyclic-AMP phosphodiesterase, protein kinases and phosphoprotein phosphatase in *Trypanosoma brucei*. Mol Biochem Parasitol 6: 287–293

Discussion of paper presented by J. D. Barry

Introduced by G. Takle
Reported by L. Hudson

GENES, STRUCTURE AND SWITCHING FREQUENCY

The extraordinary degree of sequence diversity between variant surface glycoproteins (VSGs) accounts for the effective absence of immunological cross-reactivity between successive antigenic variants in trypanosome clones. Even so, each of these molecules with vastly different primary structures has been predicted to fold with a similar potential secondary and tertiary structure and form the characteristic closely packed coat of VSG dimers. Although similarities have been seen at the 3' end of the gene and the carboxy terminus of the protein, in each case these are hidden from the host's immune response.

There is a great deal of conservation of sequence between genes within each of the expression site associated gene (ESAG) families, and sequencing studies have confirmed that ESAG 1, which is nearest to the VSG gene, is well conserved. In one instance two different expression sites were compared from the same genome; all seven ESAGs were present at both sites and probably in the same order. Intriguingly, not all ESAGs are functional, some contain stop codons in the middle of the gene. Some ESAGs are probably present within chromosomes and so are not just features of telomeric sites. There is evidence that such internal ESAGs might be transcribed. It is interesting to speculate that a functional heterogeneity of ESAGs might contribute to specific differences seen between trypanosome populations, for example, division rates, virulence, etc.

The rate of switching between VSG genes is of crucial importance to trypanosome survival. If too many genes are turned on at once then the parasite could proliferate effectively without immune control and so kill its host before transmission had been effected. Conversely, too low a switching rate would allow immune depletion of the blood population and again lessen the chance of transmission. According to the new evidence presented by Barry, in a population of 10^9–10^{10} parasites typical of a parasitaemic peak, a VSG gene switch frequency of 10^{-2}–10^{-3} could result in every gene being expressed 100–1000 times at each generation (assuming a VSG gene repertoire of around 1000 genes per organism [Van der Ploeg et al 1984]) if expression occurred in an unregulated manner. Clearly, however, this is not a totally random process as there is considerable variation in the observed relative frequencies of particular switch combinations, for example a switch from VSG 1 to 4 might occur much more frequently than the switch of 1 to 7 or 3 to 4, and so on. These different frequencies of specific combinations of VSG switches may be related to sequences of flanking genes. The final spectrum of VSG represented on any population may also be subject to phenotypic selection, with the hybrid surface that formed during certain switches being lethal.

Recent work using inhibitors of ADP-ribosyl transferase (for example, 3-aminobenzamide) has shown inhibition of a specific VSG gene switch. If more potent inhibitors could be developed, then these compounds might offer a novel approach to the chemotherapy of trypanosomiasis in which at least some antigenic variation could be arrested, thus permitting effective immunological control of the infection.

THE FLAGELLAR POCKET – A VULNERABLE TARGET?

Membrane receptors for transferrin and low-density lipoprotein (LDL) are restricted to the flagellar pocket though an epidermal growth factor (EGF) receptor covers the whole cell surface.

Even though these receptors are fully immunogenic and probably can be recognized by the host's immune system, immune attack seems not to be deleterious to the parasite population. These receptors might represent a vulnerable immunological target. It will be interesting to see whether inhibition of receptor internalization by arsenical treatment renders the parasite susceptible to immune attack by anti-receptor antibodies.

CELL SURFACE PROTEINS OF T. cruzi

Although they both belong to the genus *Trypanosoma*, there is relatively little similarity between *T. cruzi*, the causative agent of South American trypanosomiasis, and *T. brucei*. *T. cruzi* shows no evidence of antigenic variation based on sequential VSG gene expression but instead survives as a result of its ability to invade cells and so evade the immune response by sequestering away in an immunologically privileged intracellular environment. Evidence is now emerging that many of the surface proteins of *T. cruzi* are encoded as multigene families (summarized in Fig. 6.7). Sequencing of different copies of these genes has shown that some copies possess regions of sequence variation at both the genomic DNA and mRNA level, suggesting that members of each family code for slightly different polypeptides. The *T. cruzi* stage-specific surface antigen gene family described by Manning & Peterson (1988) contains a nonapeptide repeat at the 3′ end of 3 gene copies and, intriguingly, the transcribed copy of one of the genes was located at a telomere; tantalizingly reminiscent of antigenic variation seen in *T. brucei*. Few research groups are working on the molecular biology of this important human pathogen and so relatively little is known about gene arrangement or the mechanisms of expression.

The procyclin gene of *T. brucei* is within a multigene family, different classes of which encode functionally different proteins; for example, one is associated with the cytoskeleton, whereas another is cell surface associated. This differs markedly from the highly polymorphic antigens of *Plasmodium* where each gene exists as a single copy.

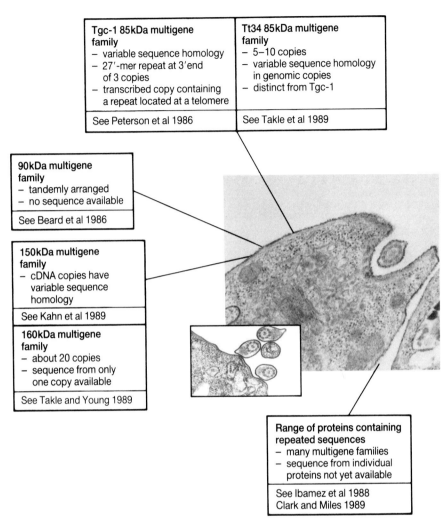

Tgc-1 85kDa multigene family – variable sequence homology – 27′-mer repeat at 3′end of 3 copies – transcribed copy containing a repeat located at a telomere	Tt34 85kDa multigene family – 5–10 copies – variable sequence homology in genomic copies – distinct from Tgc-1
See Peterson et al 1986	See Takle et al 1989

90kDa multigene family
– tandemly arranged
– no sequence available

See Beard et al 1986

150kDa multigene family
– cDNA copies have variable sequence homology

See Kahn et al 1989

160kDa multigene family
– about 20 copies
– sequence from only one copy available

See Takle and Young 1989

Range of proteins containing repeated sequences
– many multigene families
– sequence from individual proteins not yet available

See Ibamez et al 1988
Clark and Miles 1989

Figure 6.7 Multigene families of *Trypanosoma cruzi* cell surface proteins. Trypomastigotes of *T. cruzi* and *T. brucei* have profoundly different cell surface membranes; whereas the former has a typical eukaryotic cell surface membrane (large photograph; ×47 000), the latter has a thick surface coat of VSG molecules external to the phospholipid bilayer. (small inset). *T. cruzi* shows no evidence of antigenic variation via switching of VSG genes, but has an impressive array of multigene families which could confer antigenic diversity on important surface proteins. A major task for the future will be uncovering the means by which this mechanism contributes to trypomastigote survival in a hostile immune environment

REFERENCES

Beard C A, Wrightsman R A, Manning J E 1986 Stage and strain specific expression of the tandemly repeated 90kd surface antigen gene family in *Trypanosoma cruzi*. Mol Biochem Parasitol 28: 227–234
Clark J L, Miles M A 1989 Immunoselection of DNA clones encoding diagnostic antigens: a *Trypanosoma cruzi* specific antigen contains a 7 amino acid tandem repeat. J Cell Biochem (suppl) 13E: 100

Ibanez C F, Affranchino J L, Macina R A et al 1988 Multiple *Trypanosoma cruzi* antigens containing tandemly repeated amino acid sequence motifs. Mol Biochem Parasitol 30: 27–24

Kahn S J, Van Voorhis W, Eisen H A 1989 *Trypanosoma cruzi* mammalian stage specific transcripts reveal areas of sequence homology and diversity. J Cell Biochem (suppl) 13E: 107

Manning J E, Peterson D S 1988 Identification of the 85kDa surface antigen gene of *Trypanosoma cruzi* as a member of a multigene family. Current Communications in Molecular Biology. In: Turner M J, Arnot D (eds). Molecular genetics of parasitic protozoa. Cold Spring Harbor, pp 148–152

Peterson D S, Wrightsman R A, Manning J E 1986 Cloning of a major surface antigen gene of *Trypanosoma cruzi* and identification of a nonapeptide repeat. Nature 322: 566–568

Takle G B, Young A 1989 Characterisation of two trypomastigote-specific genes in *Trypanosoma cruzi*. J Cell Biochem (suppl) 13E: 123

Takle G B, Young A, Snary D, Hudson L, Nicholl S 1989 Cloning and expression of a trypomastigote-specific 85kDa surface antigen gene from *Trypanosoma cruzi*. Mol Biochem Parasitol (in press)

Van der Ploeg L H T, Schwartz D C, Cantor R C, Borst P 1984 Antigenic variation in *Trypanosoma brucei* analyzed by electrophoretic separation of chromosome-sized DNA molecules. Cell 37: 77–84

7. The membrane attachment of the variant surface glycoprotein coat of *Trypanosoma brucei*

M. A. J. Ferguson and S. W. Homans

INTRODUCTION

The trypanosome cell surface coat is an extraordinary structure. It is found on the bloodstream trypomastigote and insect-derived metacyclic trypomastigote forms of all species of African trypanosomes including *Trypanosoma brucei brucei, T. b. gambiense, T. b. rhodesiense, T. congolense, T. vivax* and *T. equiperdum*. The coat, which is absent from the non-infectious insect stages of the parasites, was first observed using electron microscopy, by Vickerman & Luckins (1969) as an electron-dense coat 12–15 nm thick which covers the entire plasma membrane and flagellar membrane of the trypanosome. The coat of an individual trypanosome is made of a single species of glycoprotein, a variant surface glycoprotein (VSG). The current model of the VSG coat is of a densely packed monolayer of VSG molecules, about 10^7 copies per cell, all of which are anchored in the plasma membrane by covalent linkage to a glycosyl phosphatidylinositol (GPI) membrane anchor. The coat serves as the primary defence mechanism of the parasite against both non-specific and specific host immunity. Firstly, the dense packing of the VSG molecules prevents host macromolecules from reaching the plasma membrane and so protects against non-specific attack by the alternative complement pathway. Secondly, a trypanosome population evades specific antibody-mediated immune attack through antigenic variation. The molecular basis of antigenic variation is the switching of discrete VSG genes encoding immunologically distinct VSG variants (see Ch. 6). In this paper we will consider only the structure, post-translational processing and membrane anchorage of trypanosome VSG.

THE VSG COAT AS A MACROMOLECULAR DIFFUSION BARRIER

The essence of VSG function is to prevent the approach of host macromolecules to the parasite's sensitive plasma membrane. The effective molecular weight 'cut-off' for access to the trypanosome plasma membrane is unknown but proteins as small as 50 kD are unable to penetrate the coat. Clearly, however, small nutrient molecules such as glucose and amino-acids have free access to the surface. There are several independent lines of evidence which demonstrate that the VSG coat is a macromolecular diffusion barrier:

(1) Bloodstream trypomastigote culture mutants of *T. congolense* which lack a VSG coat are rapidly lysed by the alternative complement pathway (ACP), whereas normal VSG-coated cells are resistant (Ferrante & Allison 1983).
(2) Antibodies to invariant surface antigens fail to bind to living trypanosomes, suggesting that these epitopes are hidden by the VSG coat (Rovis et al 1984).
(3) Concanavalin A lectin fails to bind to living trypanosomes prior to trypsinization (Cross & Johnson 1976).
(4) Bacterial phosphatidylinositol-specific phospholipase C (PI-PLC), an enzyme capable of cleaving the VSG GPI anchor in vitro, fails to release the coat from living trypanosomes (Low et al 1986).

Recently however, there have been reports of receptor-mediated endocytosis of macromolecules such as transferrin by *T. brucei* (Opperdoes et al 1987). These receptors are found only in the flagellar pocket; the exclusive site of exo- and endocytosis in trypanosomes. It is possible that such surface receptors might extend beyond the VSG coat or that the VSG coat is less densely packed in this specialized region of membrane. If the latter is true then mechanisms must exist either to exclude complement from the flagellar pocket or to render this membrane resistant to complement attack. The biochemistry of the flagellar pocket remains to be explored fully but might turn out to be the Achilles' heel of the African trypanosome.

The VSG coat with its high density of packing gives the trypanosome a peculiar property, namely the presentation of an entirely proteinaceous surface to its environment. With the possible exceptions of *Plasmodium* sporozoites and *Paramecium*, this is a unique phenomenon. All other eukaryotic cells display a rich polymorphous surface of phospholipid, protein and carbohydrate to their environment. The significance, if any, of this unusual surface chemistry is unclear.

ANATOMY OF THE VSG MOLECULE

The VSGs are a family of glycoproteins which have molecular weights around 55 kD, except for those of *T. vivax* which are somewhat smaller (46 kD) (Gardiner et al 1987). Each VSG is encoded by its own gene and the primary translation product undergoes extensive co- and post-translational processing before appearing at the cell surface as a coat component. A linear map of a representative mature VSG molecule is shown in Figure 7.1

VSG primary amino-acid sequence
The secret of antigenic variation lies in the disparity of the primary amino-acid sequence throughout the N-terminal two-thirds of the molecules. In these N-terminal domains there is no significant homology between VSG variants, unless conservative amino-acid substitutions are allowed (Olafson et al 1984). From monoclonal antibody mapping studies it seems that the majority of VSG epitopes reside in these N-terminal domains (Miller et al 1984, Masterson et al 1988), rather than in the more conserved C-terminal domains. Furthermore, only a small

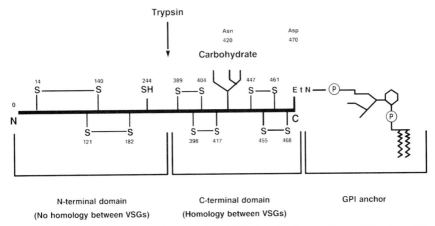

Figure 7.1 Linear map of mature mfVSG variant MITat1.4 showing positions of the disulphide bonds, aparagine glycosylation site, GPI anchor and the trypsin-sensitive hinge region between the N- and C-terminal domains

proportion of these variant-specific epitopes are available on living trypanosomes for antibody binding. The rest are presumably buried in the coat and inaccessible to antibody. This suggests that VSGs may be more immunologically distinct than is functionally required (Turner 1985). However, the unique immunological identity of each VSG may protect against antibody cross-reaction during any transient exposure of non-surface epitopes. After all, the surface of a cell is a highly dynamic environment and the VSG-coat molecules are known to display high lateral mobility (Bulow et al 1988).

The primary translation product of VSG contains both N- and C-terminal peptide extensions which are absent from the mature product (reviewed by Cross 1984, Boothroyd 1985, Turner 1985). The N-terminal peptide extension is a conventional 'signal sequence' involved in directing the translocation of nascent VSG polypeptide through the endoplasmic reticulum (ER) membrane and is co-translationally cleaved by a signal-peptidase (McConnell et al 1981). The C-terminal peptide represents another kind of signal sequence which is exchanged for a GPI membrane anchor (see below). During or immediately after completion of polypeptide synthesis, VSGs become *N*-glycosylated at one or more asparagine residues in the conventional Asn-Xaa-Ser/Thr glycosylation sequon. One would also predict that intramolecular disulphide bond formation would occur at this early stage of synthesis in the ER. Like other protein families the positions of several cysteine residues in the VSGs are strikingly conserved (Cross 1984). For one group 1 VSG (MITat1.4) the disulphide bridges have been determined (Allen & Gurnett 1983).

VSG subgroups

Significant homology between VSGs can be seen in their C-terminal domains. The homology becomes stronger towards the C-terminus of the mature protein and stronger still in the cleaved C-terminal GPI signalling sequence and beyond into the untranslated region of the mRNA (Rice-Ficht et al 1981, Boothroyd 1985).

Table 7.1 VSG subgroups based on COOH-terminal polypeptide homology

	Mature protein	Cleaved signal for GPI processing
Group 1		
MITat1.4	←DKCKGKLEDTCKKESNCKWENNACKD	SSILVTKKFALTVVSAAFVALLF
MITat1.6	←***************WEGETCKD	SSILVTKKFALTVVSAAFVALLF
ANTat1.1	←EKCTGKKKDDCKDG CKWEAETCKD	SSILLTKKFALSVVSAAFLALLF
ANTat1.8	←DKCKGKLEDTCKKESNCKWEGETCKD	SSILVNKQLALSVVSAAFAALLF
ILTat1.3	←*KCKDKKKDDCKSP DCKWEGETCKD	SSFILNKQFALSVVSAAFAALLF
Group 2		
MITat1.2	←KEEAKKVADETAKDGKTGNTNTTGSS	NSFVISKTPLWLAVLLF
MITat1.7	←*****************AETNTTG S	*****************
MITat1.1	←******************ANTTG S	NSFVIHKAPLLLAFLLF
ILTat1.1	←RVAEQAATNQETEGKDGKTTNTTG S	NSFVIHKAPLFLAFLLF
IOTat1.2	←EEAKKLEEKTEQNDSKTVTTNTTG S	HSFVINKTPPLLAFLLF
TXTat1	←*****EEAAENQEGKKEKTSNTTA S	NSFVINKAPLLLGFLLF
Group 3		
MITat1.5	←GKSADCGFRKGKDGETDEPDKEKCRN	GSFLTSKQFAFSVVSAAFVALLF

Data adapted from Cross (1984) and Boothroyd (1985)
*Denotes unknown amino-acid, gaps are present in some sequences to maximize homology matching

VSGs can be placed into three different subgroups based upon C-terminal homology (Table 7.1). One of these, group 3, has only one known member (VSG MITat1.5), whereas all other VSGs can be placed into either group 1 or group 2.

VSG N-glycosylation

All VSGs have one or more potential N-glycosylation site(s). Group 1 VSGs have a conserved glycosylation site about 50 amino-acid residues from the mature C-terminus which expresses a family of oligomannose structures; group 2 VSGs have a conserved glycosylation site 5 or 6 residues from the mature C-terminus which expresses a family of complex oligosaccharides (Holder 1985, Zamze et al in preparation). The location of other glycosylation sites in group 1 and 2 VSGs is variable but most often group 1 VSGs have only one oligomannose site whereas group 2 VSGs generally contain two glycosylation sites; the single group 3 variant contains at least three glycosylation sites. The role of VSG N-glycosylation is unclear but N-linked glycans are large structures and may play a role in overall coat architecture. Inhibition of N-glycosylation using tunicamycin renders the VSG molecules more sensitive to proteolysis (Reinwald 1985) and seems to affect their ability to dimerize (Strickler & Patton 1982).

VSG three-dimensional structure

VSGs appear to adopt a 2-domain structure linked by a short protease-sensitive 'hinge' region (Cross 1984). During the crystallization of two VSGs both molecules were found to be cleaved by trace amounts of protease in the samples. The crystals formed in both cases were of dimers of the N-terminal domains (Freymann et al 1984, Metcalf et al 1987). At the level of 0.6 nm resolution the N-terminal domains of MITat1.2 (a group 1 VSG) and ILTat1.24 (a group 2 VSG), with no primary sequence homology, adopt strikingly similar three-dimensional structures. The N-terminal domains account for about two-thirds of the VSG polypeptide and exist as elongated dimers containing fourfold α-helical bundles about 9 nm long. The tops of these α-helical cores are capped by non-helical regions which extend a further 2 nm with cross-sectional dimensions of about 3×5 nm (Freyman et al 1984, Metcalf et al 1987). The conservation of three-dimensional structure is surprising considering the disparity of primary sequences; however, similar shapes might be expected since all VSG molecules must be able to pack into similar arrays on the plasma membrane to form the protective cell surface coat.

THE GLYCOSYL PHOSPHATIDYLINOSITOL MEMBRANE ANCHOR

Historical perspective

The consensus that cell surface proteins could be anchored in the plasma membrane via covalent linkage to phospholipid was formed in 1985 through an amalgamation of data from several laboratories. Since the mid-1970s, data from the groups of Ikezawa & Low showed that the treatment of cells or membranes with bacterial phosphatidylinositol-specific phospholipase C (PI-PLC) resulted in the selective release of certain membrane proteins such as alkaline phosphatase, acetylcholinesterase (AChE) and 5′-nucleotidase (reviewed by Low 1987). In an extensive study Low showed that PI-PLC-released alkaline phosphatase could no longer re-bind to membranes and concluded that it was originally anchored through a tight, and probably covalent, linkage to phosphatidylinositol (PI) phospholipid (Low & Zilversmit 1980). However, in the absence of direct chemical evidence, this proposal was largely ignored. The first chemical evidence for covalent linkage of protein to phospholipid came from work on the rat Thy-1 antigen by Williams and colleagues (Campbell et al 1981) who found stoichiometric amounts of ethanolamine and fatty acid attached to C-terminal proteolysis fragments. Subsequently Holder showed that ethanolamine is in amide linkage with the C-terminal amino acid α-carboxyl group of VSG polypeptide and associated with a novel carbohydrate moiety (Holder & Cross 1981, Holder 1983). However the VSG, as conventionally isolated, was water soluble (sVSG) with no evidence of a hydrophobic membrane insertion site to account for its original stable association with the trypanosome plasma membrane. This paradox was explained by the elegant study of Cardoso de Almeida & Turner (1983) who isolated the amphiphilic membrane binding form of VSG (mfVSG) for the first time. They showed that trypanosomes contain a potent enzyme which rapidly converts mfVSG to sVSG unless specifically inhibited during VSG isolation. Together with Holder's data, it was concluded from this work that the membrane anchor of VSG was lipid in nature. Subsequent chemical analysis supported this view (Ferguson & Cross 1984, Ferguson et al 1985a) and a partial structure defining the term glycosyl phosphatidylinositol was elucidated (Ferguson et al 1985b). At the same time compositional analyses of *Torpedo* AChE (Futerman et al 1985), Thy-1 (Tse et al 1985) and erythrocyte AChE (Roberts & Rosenberry 1985) demonstrated the covalent association of GPI components with these proteins. Since then more than 40 examples of GPI-anchored eukaryotic proteins have been described (reviewed most recently by Ferguson & Williams 1988, Low 1989).

The VSG GPI anchor

The GPI anchor of the group 1 VSG MITatl.4 was the first to be structurally elucidated. Based on the known partial structure shown at the top of Figure 7.2 an analytical strategy was developed using proton nuclear magnetic resonance spectroscopy (^{1}H-n.m.r.), mass spectrometry and chemical and enzymatic modifications as principal tools (Ferguson et al 1988a). Of these techniques, n.m.r. provides the most information but requires reasonable quantities (> 50 nmol) of material in a suitable form, i.e. freely water soluble and fairly small (< 10 kD). Clearly mfVSG itself fails to meet either of these criteria. It was necessary therefore to remove the diacyl glycerol (DAG) portion (already known to be sn-1,2-dimyristyl glycerol [Ferguson et al 1985a, Schmitz et al 1986]) to produce sVSG and subsequently remove all the protein, except for the C-terminal amino-acid, by pronase digestion. The resulting fragment known as the soluble form C-terminal glycopeptide (sCt-gp, see Fig. 7.2) is ideal for n.m.r. analysis.

High-resolution Fourier transform n.m.r. using high-field (500 MHz) instruments has become an invaluable tool in the determination of complex carbohydrate structure. Many of the modern techniques were introduced to solve asparagine-linked glycoprotein oligosaccharides. Where previously solved structures are available, a one-dimensional n.m.r. spectrum 'fingerprint' can be compared with reference spectra to give rapid structural identification (Vliegenthart et al 1983). However, in cases such as GPI analysis no reference spectra are available and an 'ab initio' approach (Homans et al 1987) must be taken until sufficient spectra become available. The approach relies on two-dimensional n.m.r. techniques to extract the information available in the conventional one-dimensional spectrum (see Fig. 7.3 and legend).

Following non-destructive n.m.r. analysis the sCt-gp sample was chemically modified to remove all charged groups and to introduce a tritium radiolabel selectively into the molecule to aid subsequent fractionation (Fig. 7.2). This was achieved by nitrous acid deamination, which converts the glucosamine residue to 2,5-anhydromannose and simultaneously releases the inositol phosphate group, followed by sodium borotritiide reduction to yield labelled 2,5-anhydromannitol. This deaminated and reduced glycopeptide (dAR-gp) was further charge-neutralized by dephosphorylation with cold 50% aqueous HF to yield the neutral glycan (NG) fraction. This form of the GPI glycan is amenable to size-fractionation by a number of means including gel-filtration in Bio-Gel P4 columns (Fig. 7.4). This profile shows the heterogeneous nature of the GPI glycan from this single VSG derived from a cloned trypanosome cell line. Examination of each peak by n.m.r. and methylation analysis showed that they were identical in structure except for the presence and/or absence of the two terminal Gal residues depicted in Figure 7.5. This kind of peripheral microheterogeneity in oligosaccharide structures is common in all types of glycoconjugates and therefore not unexpected in GPI glycans. The precise location of the ethanolamine phosphate–protein bridge and the linkage position of the glucosamine residue to the inositol ring were solved using mannosidase

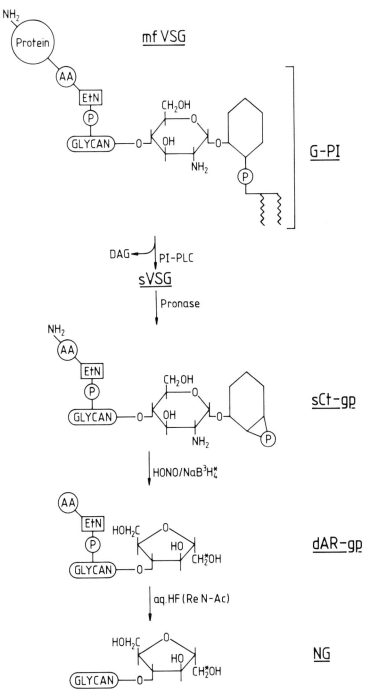

Figure 7.2 Fragmentation of VSG to produce GPI glycan fractions amenable to high resolution
^{1}H n.m.r. (the sCt-gp fraction) and size fractionation and methylation analysis (the NG fraction).
A tritium radiolabel is introduced selectively by nitrous acid deamination, sodium borotritiide
reduction which converts the glucosamine residue to [1-^{3}H]-2,5-anhydromannitol. Reproduced with
permission from Ferguson et al (1988a), copyright 1988 AAAS)

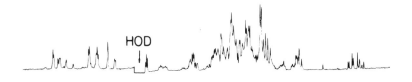

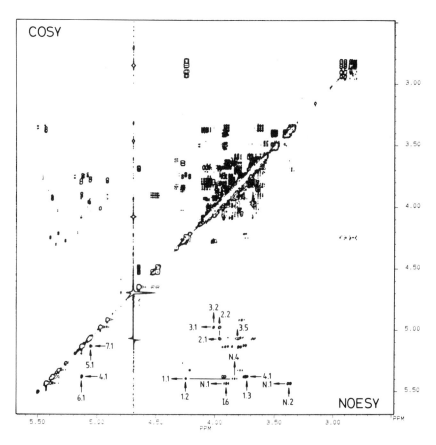

Figure 7.3 Combined contour plot derived from ¹H–¹H correlated n.m.r. spectroscopy (COSY) and ¹H–¹H nuclear Overhauser effect spectroscopy (NOESY) experiments upon the sCt-gp fraction of VSG GPI. The one-dimensional spectrum (top of figure) can be thought of as lying along the diagonal from lower left to upper right. Off-diagonal peaks (cross-peaks) correlate resonances derived from protons between which a through-bond (COSY) or through-space (NOESY) connectivity exists. Most of the resonances can be assigned to specific protons from the COSY experiment, by stepwise correlation from the resolved C-1 anomeric protons (between 4.8 and 5.5 ppm) of each monosaccharide residue. The primary sequence of the molecule is then derived by analysis of through-space connectivities across glycosidic linkages using the COSY assignments. Representative connectivities are labelled for the largest structure shown in Figure 7.5. Cross-peak labels correspond to the residue descriptor numbers:

```
3—2
7—5    1—N—I
    4
6
```

followed by the ring proton number. (Reproduced with permission from Ferguson et al (1988a), copyright 1988 AAAS)

128

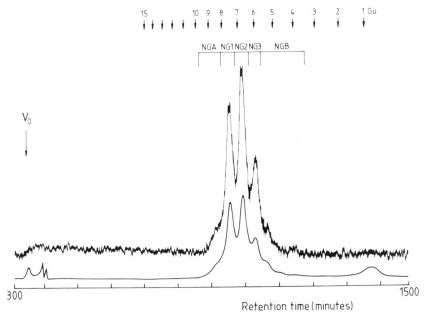

Figure 7.4 Bio-Gel P4 gel-filtration profile of the neutral glycan (NG) fraction showing the degree of microheterogeneity in the GPI glycan of VSG MITat1.4. The upper trace represents radioactivity introduced by deamination, reduction. The lower trace represents refractive index and demonstrates the fidelity of the radio-label. The numbers at the top represent the elution positions of dextran oligomers (number of glucose units). (Reproduced with permission from Ferguson et al (1988a), copyright 1988 AAAS)

digestions (before and after dephosphorylation) and periodate oxidation studies. The complete fine structure is shown in Figure 7.5.

Host–parasite structural comparison

All proteins which employ a GPI anchor are externally disposed plasma membrane proteins. However, they are functionally extremely varied and include protozoal coat proteins, hydrolases, lymphoid antigens, cell adhesion molecules and receptors. There is no clear correlation between protein function and the use of GPI anchors (Ferguson & Williams 1988). One interesting correlation that does exist with the data available so far is the distribution of GPI usage at different stages of eukaryotic evolution. In mammals, for example, it seems that a significant minority of cell surface proteins employ GPI whereas in the protozoa GPI appears to be the predominant form of anchorage. Indeed, in all cases where the mode of membrane anchorage has been studied directly in protozoons, GPI anchors have been found instead of single-pass transmembrane polypeptide domains. It is probable that multiple-pass transmembrane proteins exist in the protozoa in the form of nutrient and ion transporters.

This high frequency of GPI usage in the protozoa is also reflected in the expression of structurally related glycolipids which have no clearly defined analogues in higher eukaryotes. These novel glycolipid species include the lipophosphoglycans (LPG) and glyco-inositol phospholipids (GIPLs) of the

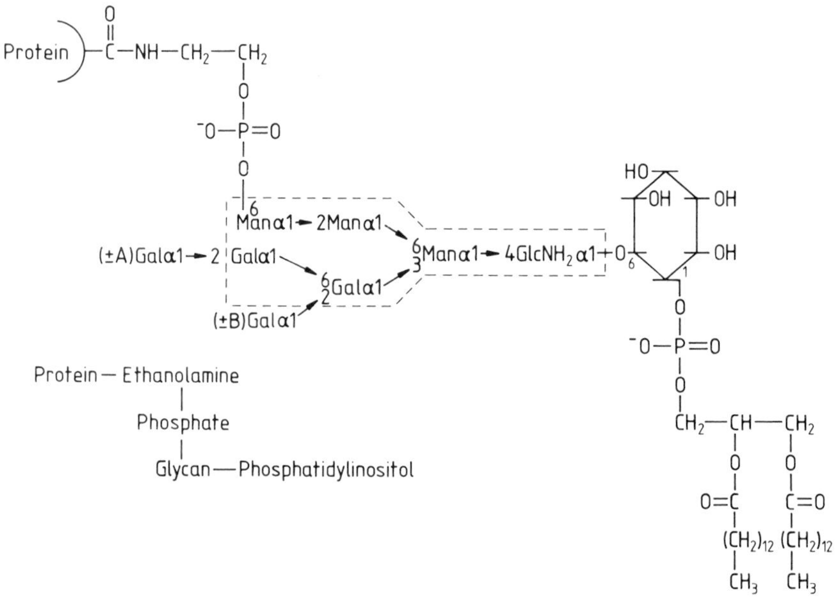

Figure 7.5 Complete primary structure of the GPI anchor of VSG MITat1.4. The size heterogeneity seen in Figure 7.4 is due to the two terminal Gal residues A and B which can be present or absent in all four combinations. (Reproduced with permission from Ferguson et al (1988a), copyright 1988 AAAS)

Leishmania (Turco et al 1989 McConville & Bacic 1989) and the lipopeptidophosphoglycan (LPPG) of *T. cruzi* (de Lederkremer 1989, Previato et al 1989). All of these molecules have the sub-structure $Man\alpha1–4GlcNH_2\alpha1–6myo$ inositol-1-PO_4 in common and may therefore share some biosynthetic enzymes in their formation.

In general, it would seem that the parasitic protozoa rely on GPI anchors and related molecules for their infectivity and survival (Ferguson & Homans 1988). If this evolutionary skew in GPI usage is to be understood, and possibly exploited, it is important to determine the full range of structures expressed by both parasite and host (mammalian) cells. So far only one other complete GPI structure has been reported, for rat brain Thy-1 antigen (Homans et al 1988), as well as a detailed partial structure for human erythrocyte AChE (Roberts et al 1989a). The VSG and Thy-1 structures are shown together in Figure 7.6. The data for human erythrocyte AChE are consistent with the Thy-1 structure except that the AChE GPI does not contain the GalNAc or $+/-$ Man residues. Comparing the two complete structures, it appears that the core structure which actually links the protein to the lipid (i.e. ethanolamine-PO_4–6Manα1–2Manα1–6Manα1–4GlcNH$_2\alpha$1–6myo inositol-1-PO_4-) is conserved between the protozoal and mammalian GPIs. While more examples are needed to draw convincing conclusions, the conservation of the core is striking and may suggest that the core region of GPI is conserved throughout the eukaryotes.

In contrast the side-chains attached to this core region are quite different. The VSG GPI contains a large and unusual alpha-galactose branched side-chain

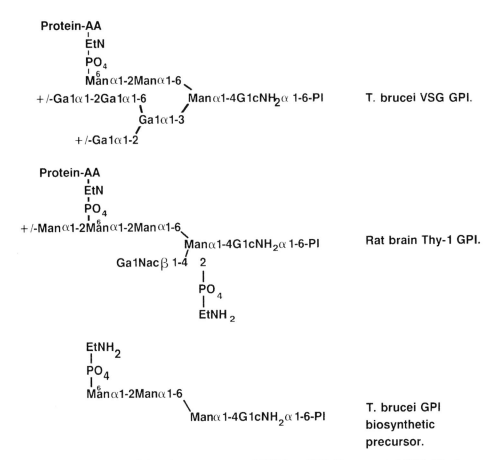

Figure 7.6 Comparison of the primary structures of GPI from VSG (Ferguson et al 1988), Thy-1 (Homans et al 1988) and the predicted structure of the GPI precursor from trypanosomes (Mayor et al in preparation)

linked α1–3 to the first Man residue whereas Thy-1 GPI contains a single *N*-acetyl galactosamine residue linked β1–4 to the equivalent Man residue. In addition, the Thy-1 structure can contain an extra Man residue at the end of the core region. Both Thy-1 and AChE bear a second ethanolamine phosphate group attached to the first Man residue. This extra ethanolamine phosphate, with a free amino group, appears to be common in mammalian GPIs (Ferguson & Williams 1988, and references therein) but its function is unknown. Thus there appear to be conserved and species-specific structures in GPI anchor carbohydrate.

Another notable difference between VSG GPI and those from other sources is in the lipid moiety. The VSGs from *T. brucei*, *T. congolense* and *T. equiperdum* all contain exclusively myristic acid (Ferguson & Cross 1984, Gurnett et al 1986, Lamont et al 1987, Ross et al 1987) as sn-1,2-dimyristyl glycerol (Ferguson et al 1985a, Schmitz et al 1986). In contrast GPIs of mammalian origin contain palmitic and stearic acids together with a variety of unsaturated fatty acids, probably in the form of 1-alkyl-2-acyl glycerols, as found for human erythrocyte AChE (Roberts et al 1989b).

BIOSYNTHESIS OF GPI

The addition of GPI to VSG polypeptide occurs extremely rapidly; within 1 min of the completion of protein synthesis (Bangs et al 1985, Ferguson et al 1986). The speed of addition led to the hypothesis that GPI was synthesized as an intact precursor and added to the VSG polypeptide *en bloc*, close to the site of protein synthesis in the endoplasmic reticulum (Fig. 7.7). This premise was supported by the isolation of glycolipid species from trypanosomes with physical and chemical properties consistent with being GPI precursors (Krakow et al 1986, Menon et al 1988a). The putative precursor contains glucosamine linked to dimyristyl-PI, mannose and ethanolamine bearing a free amino group. Recent structural analysis (Mayor et al in preparation) confirmed the lack of galactose in the precursor and showed that the tri-mannosyl glycan portion is identical to the core region of the mature anchor (i.e. Manα1–2Manα1–6Manα1–?GlcNH$_2$). A hypothetical structure for the biosynthetic precursor is shown in Figure 7.6.

The addition of GPI precusor to protein is controlled by two signals in the primary translation product. First, the protein moves through the rough endoplasmic reticulum membrane by virtue of a cleavable N-terminal signal sequence. Second, an enzyme or enzyme complex recognizes a C-terminal signal sequence which is cleaved and directly replaced by the GPI precursor to generate mfVSG. The nature of this transfer reaction is unknown although a transamidase activity has been suggested. The GPI addition C-terminal signal sequence shows considerable homology between VSG variants (see Table 7.1) but there is no correlation of the signals when other eukaryotic sequences are compared (Ferguson & Williams 1988). In general any C-terminal sequence which ends in a run of apolar amino acids, without any evidence of a polar cytoplasmic domain sequence following it, will serve as a GPI addition signal. The degeneracy in C-terminal GPI addition signals is similar to that found for N-terminal signal sequences.

Following the addition of GPI the VSG is transported through the Golgi apparatus and to the plasma membrane via the flagellar pocket (Duszenko et al 1988). The

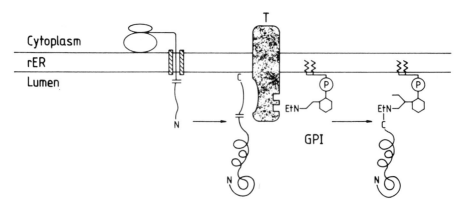

Figure 7.7 Model of GPI addition to protein. A cleavable N-terminal signal sequence directs the nascent polypeptide across the rough endoplasmic reticulum membrane. A C-terminal GPI addition signal peptide is recognized by an enzyme or enzyme complex (T) which cleaves off the peptide and adds the GPI precursor

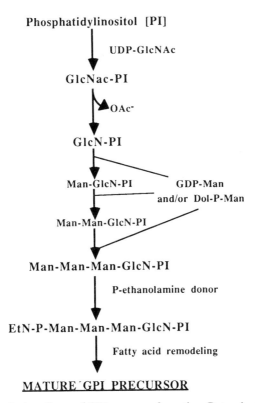

Figure 7.8 The biosynthetic pathway of GPI precursor formation. Data adapted from Masterson et al (1989), Doering et al (in press) and Schwartz et al (in press)

transport from endoplasmic reticulum to the plasma membrane is relatively rapid, with a t_{1M2} of 15 min (Bangs et al 1986). The addition of galactose to the GPI is believed to occur late in VSG processing in the Golgi stacks (Bangs et al 1988).

Considerable progress has been made recently in understanding the pathway of GPI precursor formation using cell-free membrane preparations (Menon et al 1988b, Masterson et al 1989). The pathway shown in Figure 7.8 is based on the work of Masterson et al (1989) and Doering et al (in press). In essence the pathway involves the sequential glycosylation of PI; GlcNAc is added from UDP-GlcNAc followed by de-N-acetylation to form GlcNH$_2$-PI. Subsequently three mannose residues are added from GDP-Man, at least one of which goes via a Dol-P-Man donor (Schwartz et al in press). Next, ethanolamine phosphate is added from an unknown donor and finally the fatty acids of the PI moiety are re-modelled to yield the dimyristyl-PI moiety of the mature GPI precursor.

THE GPI BIOSYNTHETIC PATHWAY AS A TARGET FOR CHEMOTHERAPY

The absolute dependence of the African trypanosomes on the integrity of their VSG surface coats for survival makes the coat an attractive target for the

133

development of chemotherapeutics. Any drug which interfered with GPI biosynthesis, and therefore VSG coat stability at the plasma membrane, should be trypanocidal in the presence of host serum components. Upon reviewing the current information on GPI structure and biosynthesis one can consider three areas of the biosynthetic pathway for possible intervention.

1. The common core region

Compounds which affect the formation of the ethanolamine-PO_4-6Manα1–2Manα1–6Manα1–4GlcNH$_2\alpha$1–6myo inositol core region of GPI, or the transfer of GPI precursor to protein, might be expected to affect the host as well as the parasite since it seems likely that the enzymes involved in synthesizing the core are conserved throughout the eukaryotes. However, despite this potential lack of parasite selectivity such drugs could be of some use when one considers the relative rates of GPI synthesis between parasite and host. African trypanosomes divide rapidly (about every 4–6 h) in the bloodstream by binary fission and must generate around 10^7 new copies of VSG GPI per cell division. Furthermore it may be only necessary to reduce the density of VSG packing at the cell surface by a small amount to render it permeable to complement. Thus, a drug which inhibited GPI synthesis or transfer by say 50% and with a serum half-life of around 2–4 h might be sufficient to clear bloodstream parasites without adversely affecting the host.

2. The dimyristyl glycerol moiety

The exclusive use of myristic acid in VSG GPI is unique to the African trypanosomes. The mechanism of myristic acid incorporation is unknown but appears to involve 'lipid re-modelling' during the terminal stages of GPI precursor synthesis (Masterson et al 1989). The reason why trypanosomes have chosen to use this non-abundant fatty acid for VSG GPI remains completely obscure. The enzymes involved in the remodelling process are unknown but are presumably trypanosome-specific phospholipases A and myristyl-CoA-dependent fatty acid transferases. These enzymes may be good targets for the development of parasite-specific inhibitors.

3. The alpha-galactose side-chain

The presence of galactose appears to be unique to the GPI of VSGs; compositional analyses show that galactose is absent from the GPIs of human, bovine, rat, hamster and squid proteins (reviewed in Ferguson et al 1988b). Furthermore the α-galactosyl linkages found in VSG GPI have not been described in mammalian glycoconjugates. It seems likely, therefore, that the galactosyl transferases involved in VSG GPI processing are trypanosome specific. In this respect the galactose side-chain fulfils the criterion of a potential parasite-specific target. However, at first sight the complex α-galactose side-chain of VSG GPI (see Fig. 7.6) seems to be a poor target since it is not directly involved in the linkage of VSG polypeptide to the membrane. In contrast the predicted three-dimensional structure of the VSG GPI presents a more promising picture.

The structure shown in Figure 7.9 is for a GPI containing four Gal residues and was deduced by computational chemistry and direct experimental measurements using nuclear Overhauser effect (n.O.e.) n.m.r. spectroscopy (Homans et al

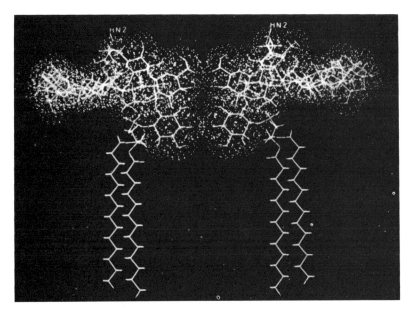

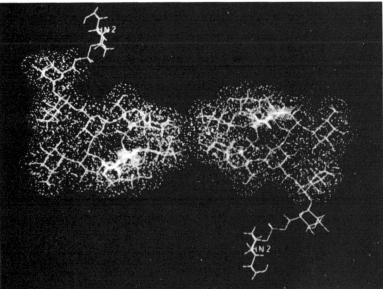

Figure 7.9 Predicted three-dimensional structure of the VSG GPI containing four Gal residues (data adapted from Homans et al 1989). Pairs of GPI structures are shown to reflect the dimeric nature of the VSG polypeptides to which they are attached. The relative orientation of the two GPIs is arbitrary. (Top) Side view showing the myristic acid chains which insert into the membrane lipid bilayer. (Bottom) Plan view showing the area of membrane covered by the GPI anchor glycan. NH_2 marks the amino group of the C-terminal aspartate of the VSG polypeptide

1989). The GPI carbohydrate appears to lie flat over the plasma membrane and, viewed from above, forms a plate-like structure with the galactose branch extending back towards the PI moiety. The dimensions of the GPI carbohydrate are quite surprising, the area of membrane covered by the GPI is around 60 nm². This is very similar to the estimated cross-sectional area of the N-terminal domain of a VSG monomer, as predicted by X-ray crystallography (Metcalf et al 1987). The GPI glycan may therefore make a significant contribution to the barrier characteristics of the VSG coat since it is both large and located right next to the membrane. The galactose branch contributes about 50% of the GPI area shown in Figure 7.9 and might be considered as space-filling material next to the membrane. Consistent with this notion there is an interesting correlation between the extent of GPI galactosylation and VSG subgroup (Holder 1985, Ferguson et al 1988b); group 1 VSGs (e.g. MITat1.4, MITat1.6 and ILTat1.3) contain an average of about 3–4 mol of Gal per mol GPI whereas group 2 VSGs (e.g. MITat1.2, MITat1.1 and MITat1.7) contain about 8 mol of Gal per mol GPI and the single known group 3 variant (MITat1.5) contains negligible amounts of galactose.

The extent of GPI galactosylation might depend on the differential expression of the relevant α-galactosyl transferases, regulated according to which VSG subgroup is being expressed. The coordinately transcribed expression site associated genes (ESAGs) (Cully et al 1985) would be good candidates to code for such enzymes. However this explanation seems unlikely since VSG variants MITat1.4 (group 1) and MITat1.5 (group 3) use the same expression site (Van de Ploeg et al 1982) yet differ dramatically in their GPI galactosylation state.

An alternative explanation is that the extent of GPI galactosylation is controlled by the structure of the VSG polypeptide itself (Ferguson et al 1988b, Homans et al 1989). This is certainly consistent with the fact that the GPI precursor appears to be free of galactose (Menon et al 1988a, Mayor et al in preparation) and that galactosylation appears to occur several minutes after the transfer of GPI precursor to VSG polypeptide (Bangs et al 1988). The galactosyl transferases might therefore be acting as spatial probes adding Gal residues until VSG intra- and intermolecular steric constraints prevent further addition of galactose. In this way VSG subgroup (and therefore C-terminal domain three-dimensional structure) would define the galactosylation pattern of a given VSG GPI.

CONCLUSION

Glycosyl phosphatidylinositol (GPI) membrane anchors are ubiquitous amongst the eukaryotes but are used most extensively by the protozoa. The GPI of *Trypanosoma brucei* variant surface glycoprotein (VSG) is the best studied in terms of its structure and biosynthesis and has become a paradigm in the field of GPI research. Comparative analysis of GPI anchors of higher eukaryotes suggests common and species-specific differences between host and parasite anchors which may have implications for the development of trypanocidal agents. The important steps in structure determination of novel molecules are summarized in Figure 7.10. The predicted three-dimensional structure of VSG GPI adds to the understanding of VSG surface coat architecture and points to a role for the GPI anchor in

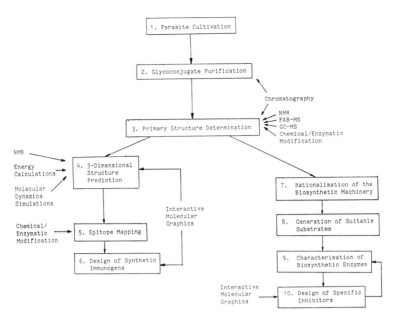

Figure 7.10 Steps in the determination of the structure of glycoconjugates.

maintaining the macromolecular diffusion barrier characteristics of this primary defence mechanism of the African trypanosome.

ACKNOWLEDGEMENTS

We are grateful to the Wellcome Trust for their continued support for our studies on GPI structure and biosynthesis. We would like to thank our colleagues for making data available to us prior to publication.

REFERENCES

Allen G, Gurnett L P 1983 Locations of the six disulphide bonds in a variant surface glycoprotein (VSG 117) from *Trypanosoma brucei*. Biochem J 209: 481–487
Bangs J D, Hereld D, Krakow J L, Hart G W, Englund P T 1985 Rapid processing of the carboxyl terminus of a trypanosome variant surface glycoprotein. Proc Natl Acad Sci USA 82: 3207–3211
Bangs J D, Andrews N W, Hart G W, Englund P T 1986 Post-translational modification and intracellular transport of a trypanosome variant surface glycoprotein. J Cell Biol 103: 255–263
Bangs J D, Doering T L, Englund P T, Hart G W 1988 Biosynthesis of a variant surface glycoprotein of *Trypanosoma brucei*. J Biol Chem 263: 17697–17705
Boothroyd J C 1985 Antigenic variation in African trypanosomes. Annu Rev Microbiol 39: 475–502
Bulow R, Overath P, Davoust J 1988 Rapid lateral diffusion of the variant surface glycoprotein in the coat of *Trypanosoma brucei*. Biochemistry 27: 2384–2388
Campbell D G, Gagnon J, Reid K B M, Williams A F 1981 Rat brain Thy-1 glycoprotein: the amino acid sequence, disulphide bonds and an unusual hydrophobic region. Biochem J 195: 15–30
Cardoso de Almeida M L, Turner M J 1983 The membrane form of variant surface glycoproteins of *Trypanosoma brucei*. Nature (Lond) 302: 349–352

Cross G A M 1984 Structure of the variant surface glycoproteins and surface coat of *Trypanosoma brucei*. Phil Trans R Soc Lond B 307: 3–12

Cross G A M, Johnson J G 1976 Structure and organisation of the variant-specific antigens of *Trypanosoma brucei*. In: Van den Bosche (ed) Biochemistry of parasites and host parasite relationships. Elsevier, Amsterdam, 413–420

Cully D F, Ip H S, Cross G A M 1985 Coordinate transcription of variant surface glycoprotein genes and an expression site associated gene family in *Trypanosoma brucei*. Cell 42: 173–182

de Lederkremer R M 1989 Data presented at the International Course and Workshop on Glycosyl-phosphatidylinositol Membrane Anchors, Angra dos Reis RJ, Brazil

Doering T L, Masterson W J, Englund P T, Hart G W 1989 Biosynthesis of the glycosyl-phosphatidylinositol membrane anchor of the trypanosome variant surface glycoprotein: origin of the non-acetylated glucosamine. J Biol Chem, (in press)

Duszenko M, Ivanov I E, Ferguson M A J, Plesken H, Cross G A M 1988 Intracellular transport of a variant surface glycoprotein in *Trypanosoma brucei*. J Cell Biol 106: 77–86

Ferguson M A J, Cross G A M 1984 Myristylation of the membrane form of *Trypanosoma brucei* variant surface glycoprotein. J Bio Chem 259: 3011–3015

Ferguson M A J, Homans S W 1988 Parasite glycoconjugates: towards the exploitation of their structure. Parasite Immunol 10: 465–479

Ferguson M A J, Williams A F 1988 Cell surface anchoring of proteins via glycosyl-phosphatidylinositol structures. Annu Rev Biochem 57: 285–320

Ferguson M A J, Haldar K, Cross G A M 1985a *Trypanosoma brucei* variant surface glycoprotein has a sn-1,2-dimyristyl glycerol membrane anchor at its COOH-terminus. J Biol Chem 260, 4963–4968

Ferguson M A J, Low M G, Cross G A M 1985b Glycosyl-sn-1,2-dimyristyl phosphatidylinositol is covalently linked to *Trypanosoma brucei* variant surface glycoprotein. J Biol Chem 260: 14547–14555

Ferguson M A J, Duszenko M, Lamont G, Overath P, Cross G A M 1986 Biosynthesis of *Trypanosoma brucei* variant surface glycoproteins. J Biol Chem 261: 356–362

Ferguson M A J, Homans S W, Dwek R A, Rademacher T W 1988a Glycosyl-phosphatidylinositol moiety that anchors *Trypanosoma brucei* variant surface glycoprotein to the membrane. Science 239: 753–759

Ferguson M A J, Homans S W, Dwek R A, Rademacher, T W 1988b The glycosyl-phosphatidylinositol membrane anchor of *Trypanosoma brucei* variant surface glycoprotein. Biochem Soc Trans 16: 265–268

Ferrante A, Allison A C 1983 Alternative pathway activiation of complement by African trypanosomes lacking a glycoprotein coat. Parasite Immunol 5: 491–498

Freymann D M, Metcalf P, Turner M, Wiley D C 1984 6A°- Resolution X-ray structure of a variable surface glycoprotein from *Trypanosoma brucei*. Nature (Lond) 311: 167–169

Futerman A H, Low M G, Ackerman K E, Sherman W R, Silman I 1985 Identification of covalently bound inositol in the hydrophobic membrane-anchoring domain of *Torpedo* acetylcholinesterase. Biochem Biophys Res Commun 129: 312–317

Gardiner P R, Pearson T W, Clarke M W, Mutharia L M 1987 Identification and isolation of a variant surface glycoprotein from *Trypanosoma vivax*. Science 235: 774–777

Gurnett A M, Raper J, Ward J, Turner M J 1986 Purification and characterisation of membrane form VSGs of *Trypanosoma brucei*. Mol Biochem Parasitol 20: 1–13

Holder A A 1983 Carbohydrate is linked through ethanolamine to the C-terminal amino acid of *Trypanosoma brucei* variant surface glycoprotein. Biochem J 209: 261–262

Holder A A 1985 Glycosylation of the variant surface antigens of *Trypanosoma brucei*. Curr Topics Microbiol Immunol 117: 57–74

Holder A A, Cross G A M 1981 Glycopeptides from variant surface glycoproteins of *Trypanosoma brucei*. C-terminal location of antigenically cross reacting carbohydrate moieties.Mol Biochem Parasitol 2: 135–150

Homans S W, Dwek R A, Rademacher T W 1987 Solution conformations of N-linked oligosaccharides. Biochemistry 26: 6571–6578

Homans S W, Ferguson M A J, Dwek R A, Rademacher T W, Anand R, Williams A F 1988 Complete structure of the glycosyl phosphatidylinositol membrane anchor of rat brain Thy-1 glycoprotein. Nature (Lond) 333: 269–272

Homans S W, Edge C J, Ferguson M A J, Dwek R A, Rademacher T W 1989 Solution structure of the glycosyl-phosphatidylinositol membrane anchor glycan of *Trypanosoma brucei* variant surface glycoprotein. Biochemistry 28: 2881–2887

Krakow J L, Hereld D, Bangs J D, Hart G W, Englund P T 1986 Identification of a glycolipid precursor of the *Trypanosoma brucei* variant surface glycoprotein. J Biol Chem 261: 12147–12153

Lamont G S, Fox J A, Cross G A M 1987 Glycosyl-sn-1,2-dimyristylphosphatidylinositol is the membrane anchor for *Trypanosoma equiperdum* and *T. (Nannomonas) congolense* variant surface glycoproteins. Mol Biochem Parasitol 24: 131–136

Low M G 1987 Biochemistry of the glycosyl-phosphatidylinositol membrane protein anchors. Biochem J 244: 1–13

Low M G 1989 Glycosyl-phosphatidylinositol: a versatile anchor for cell surface proteins. FASEB J 3: 1600–1608

Low M G, Zilversmit D B 1980 Role of phosphatidylinositol in attachment of alkaline phosphatase to membranes. Biochemistry 19: 3913–3918

Low M G, Ferguson M A J, Futerman A H, Silman I 1986 Covalently attached phosphatidylinositol as a hydrophobic anchor for membrane proteins. Trends Biochem Sci 11: 212–215

McConnell J, Cordingley J S, Turner M J 1981 Biosynthesis of *Trypanosoma brucei* variant surface glycoprotein. 1. Synthesis, size and processing of an N-terminal signal peptide. Mol Biochem Parasitol 4: 226–242

McConville M J, Bacic A 1989 A family of glycoinositol phospholipids from *Leishmania major*. J Biol Chem 264: 757–766

Masterson W J, Taylor D W, Turner M J 1988 Topological analysis of a variant surface glycoprotein of *Trypanosoma brucei*. J Immunol 140: 3194–3199

Masterson W J, Doering T L, Hart G W, Englund P T 1989 A novel pathway for glycan assembly: biosynthesis of the glycosyl-phosphatidylinositol anchor of the trypanosome variant surface glycoprotein. Cell 56: 793–800

Mayor S, Menon A K, Cross G A M, Ferguson M A J, Dwek R A, Rademacher T W 1989 (in preparation)

Menon A K, Mayor S, Ferguson M A J, Duszenko M, Cross G A M 1988a A candidate glycophospholipid precursor for the membrane anchor of *Trypanosoma brucei* VSG. J Biol Chem 263: 1970–1977

Menon A K, Schwartz R T, Mayor S, Cross G A M 1988b Glycolipid precursor of *Trypanosoma brucei* variant surface glycoproteins: incorporation of radiolabelled mannose and myristic acid in a cell free system. Biochem Soc Trans 16: 996–997

Metcalf P, Blum M, Freymann D, Turner M, Wiley D C 1987 Two variant surface glycoproteins of *Trypanosoma brucei* of different sequence class have similar 6A° resolution X-ray structures. Nature (Lond) 325: 84–86

Miller E N, Allan L M, Turner M J 1984 Relationship of antigenic determinants to structure within a variant surface glycoprotein of *Trypanosoma brucei*. Mol Biochem Parasitol 13: 309–322

Olafson R W, Clarke M W, Kielland S L, Pearson T W, Barbet A F, McGuire T C 1984 Amino terminal sequence homology among variant surface glycoproteins of African trypanosomes. Mol Biochem Parasitol 12: 287–298

Opperdoes F R, Coppens I, Baudhuin P 1987 Digestive enzymes, receptor-mediated endocytosis and their role in the bloodstream-form trypanosome. In: Chang K-P, Snary D (eds) Host–parasite cellular and molecular interactions. NATO ASI series H: Cell Biology, Vol 11, Springer-Verlag, Berlin

Previato J O, Gorin P A J, Xavier M T, Fournet B, Mendonca-Previato L 1989 Data presented at the International Course and Workshop on Glycosyl-phosphatidylinositol Membrane Anchors, Angra dos Reis RJ, Brazil

Reinwald E 1985 Role of carbohydrate within variant surface glycoprotein of *Trypanosoma congolense*. Europ J Biochem 151: 385–391

Rice-Ficht AC, Chen KK, Donelson J E 1981 Sequence homologies near the C-termini of the variable surface glycoproteins of *Trypanosoma brucei*. Nature (Lond) 294: 53–57

Roberts W L, Rosenberry T L 1985 Identification of covalently attached fatty acids in the hydrophobic membrane-binding domain of human erythrocyte acetylcholinesterase. Biochem Biophys Res Commun 133: 621–627

Roberts W L, Santikarn S, Reinhold V N, Rosenberry T L 1989a Structural characterization of the glycoinositol phospholipid membrane anchor of human erythrocyte acetylcholinesterase by fast atom bombardment mass spectrometry. J Biol Chem 263: 18776–18784

Roberts W L, Myher J J, Kuksis A, Low M G, Rosenberry T L 1989b Lipid analysis of the glycoinositol phospholipid membrane anchor of human erythrocyte acetylcholinesterase. J Biol Chem 263: 18766–18775

Ross C A, Cardoso de Almeida M L, Turner M J 1987 Variant surface glycoproteins of *Trypanosoma congolense* bloodstream and metacyclic forms are anchored by a glycolipid tail. Mol Biochem Parasitol 22: 153–158

Rovis L, Musoke A J, Moloo S K 1984 Failure of trypanosomal membrane antigens to induce protection against tsetse-transmitted *Trypanosoma vivax* or *T. brucei* in goats and rabbits. Acta Trop 41: 491–498

Schmitz B, Klein R A, Egge H, Peter-Katalinic J 1986 A study of the membrane attachment site of the membrane form variant surface glycoprotein from *Trypanosoma brucei* brucei using lipid vesicles as a model of the plasma membrane. Mol Biochem Parasitol 20: 191–197

Schwarz R T, Mayor S, Menon A K, Cross G A M 1989 Biosynthesis of the glycolipid membrane anchor of *Trypanosoma brucei* variant surface glycoproteins: involvement of Dol-P-Man. Biochem Soc Trans (in press)

Strickler J E, Patton C L 1982 *Trypanosoma brucei*: effect of inhibition of N-linked glycosylation on the nearest neighbor analysis of the major variable surface coat glycoprotein. Mol Biochem Parasitol 5: 117–131

Tse A G D, Barclay N, Watts A, Williams A F 1985 A glycophospholipid tail at the carboxyl terminus of the Thy-1 glycoprotein of neurons and thymocytes. Science 230: 1003–1008

Turco S J, Orlandi P A, Homans S W, Ferguson M A J, Dwek R A, Rademacher T W 1989 Structure of the phosphosaccharide-inositol core of the *Leishmania donovani* lipophosphoglycan. J Biol Chem 264: 6711–6715

Turner M J 1985 The biochemistry of the surface antigens of the African trypanosomes. Br Med Bull 41: 137–143

Van der Pleog L H T, Bernards A, Rijsewijk F A M, Borst P 1982 Characterization of the DNA duplication-transposition that controls the expression of two genes for variant surface glycoproteins in *Trypanosoma brucei*. Nucleic Acids Res 10: 593–609

Vickerman K, Luckins A G 1969 Localisation of variable antigens in the surface coat of *Trypanosoma brucei* using ferritin-conjugated anitbody. Nature (Lond) 224: 1125–1127

Vliegenthart J F G, Dorland L, van Halbeek H 1983 High resolution 1H NMR spectroscopy as a tool in the structural analysis of carbohydrates related to glycoproteins. Adv Carbohydr Chem Biochem 41: 209–374

Zamze S E, Wooten W, Ashford D A, Ferguson M A J, Dwek R A, Rademacher T W 1989 (in preparation)

Discussion of paper presented by M.A.J. Ferguson

Discussed by L. H. T. Van der Ploeg
Reported by L. Hudson

The sugar moieties on a typical cell surface glycoprotein occupy a considerable proportion of the total molecular volume when seen in a truly representative space-filling model; this is in striking contrast to their normal representation as 'merely a few sticks and balls'. A relatively small oligosaccharide composed, for example, of 2 sialic acid, 2 galactose, 4 N-acetyl glucosamine and 3 mannose residues occupies nearly as much space as a 20-kD globular protein. To put this into context, when the mouse glycoprotein Thy 1, which has a GPI anchor and three N-linked glycosylation sites, is modelled to the correct proportions it is seen as a protein core virtually completely enclosed within a sugar coat (Perkins et al 1988). Even so, the majority of antibodies raised against this antigen react with protein rather than sugar-based epitopes.

A similar picture emerges for the VSG molecules of African trypanosomes; the GPI glycan of each VSG covers the same (vast) area of the surface membrane as the protein, about 6 nm^2. Although there is considerable heterogeneity in patterns of asparagine glycosylation, these do not appear to contribute to the antigenic variety of the molecules; neither directly as epitopes nor by perturbation of the protein structure. The rich antigenic diversity of VSGs is derived purely from differences in primary amino-acid sequence. In any case the asparagine-linked carbohydrate tends to be sequestered away from the external environment as part of the VSG C-terminal domain and is composed mainly of the typical mammalian-type oligomannose and complex structures (SE Zamze, unpublished data) which are poorly immunogenic. However, the GPI is immunogenic and forms the cross-reacting determinant (CRD) common to all VSGs thus far examined. Significantly, however, the CRD epitope is only fully exposed for antibody binding once the dimyristylglycerol part of the molecule has been removed by phospholipase C (PLC) digestion and so it is not available for immune interaction in the intact trypanosome. Cleavage by endogenous trypanosome GPI-PLC is crucially dependent on the amino group of the glucosamine; once this is acetylated the GPI no longer acts as a substrate. In contrast, GPI-PLC cleavage is not affected by the α-galactose side-chain, as evidenced by the equal susceptibility of the lipid anchor of types 1, 2 and 3 VSG molecules to cleavage by bacterial and endogenous PLC.

In the gut of its tsetse fly host the trypomastigote transforms into the procyclic stage which loses its dense VSG surface and coat and acquires procyclin (Roditi et al 1989). Intriguingly, the relatively loose packing of the procyclin molecules might permit an interaction between the GPI α-glucosamine residues of the procyclin molecules and the glucosamine-specific lectin in the gut wall of the fly. This interaction might be crucially important for the parasite to retain or attain a preferred developmental site.

POTENTIAL DRUG TARGETS

Trypanosome-specific galactosyl transferases might have potential as chemotherapeutic targets as the galactose residues in the *T. brucei* GPI are unique among the GPIs analysed to date. Present studies are concentrating on the addition of galactose to de-galactosylated VSGs in a cell-free system to identify the enzymes involved. It is not yet clear, however, whether interference with this process will provide a lethal target as specific inhibitors of galactosylation are not yet available. In the one example of a VSG lacking the galactosyl side-chain, VSG 118, there are 3 N-linked glycosylation sites so that lack of GPI galactosylation might be compensated for by sugars elsewhere in the molecule.

Potential drug and immunological targets might also be found among the cell surface receptors now being described on these parasites. For example, insect and bloodstream forms of *T. brucei* and *T. equiperdum* express a cysteine-rich acidic repetitive integral membrane protein (CRAM) with the characteristics of a membrane receptor. (M G S Lee, B Bihain, R Deckelbaum, L H T Van der Ploeg unpublished observations). Immunofluorescence of insect form trypanosomes has shown that the molecule is located on the flagellum and the flagellar pocket. The flagellar pocket is believed to be a small domain where cellular immunity cannot affect cell viability, hence the expression of cell surface receptors. It is unclear, however, how the parasite prevents the action of antibody-stimulated complement-mediated cell lysis via the expression of flagellar pocket located, constitutively expressed, cell-surface proteins.

The CRAM has a predicted molecular weight of 130 kD and shares structural similarities with eukaryotic cell surface receptors, the homology being most striking when compared with four of the five significant domains of the human low-density lipoprotein (LDL) receptor (Brown & Goldstein 1986) and a single domain of the *Drosophila* epidermal growth factor (EGF) receptor (Livneh et al 1985, Scott 1989). CRAM contains a signal peptide, a 66-fold 12 amino-acid cysteine-rich acidic repeat with homology to the cysteine-rich human LDL receptor repeat, a 43-amino-acid extracellular stem, a 30-amino-acid transmembrane spanning domain and a 41-amino-acid cytoplasmic extension. The function of CRAM is not yet clear. However, based on the structural similarities of the CRAM protein and the LDL receptor it is possible that CRAM might serve as a protozoal LDL receptor and so provide a possible drug or antibody target.

It seems logical that these receptors should have a restricted surface distribution in view of the diffusional barrier provided by the VSG coat outside the flagellar pocket. Indeed the diffusional barrier itself might create an interesting environment immediately adjacent to the parasite's surface – a kind of periplasmic space in which molecules released through exocytosis could be trapped for salvage via say 5' nucleotidase or acetylcholine esterase.

African trypanosomes have evolved a life style that has bewildered immunologists, bemused biochemists and bewitched molecular biologists. It remains to be seen whether they will be overcome once the practitioners of these arts mount a concerted attack to understand and defeat the parasite. Fotunately, the current rate of progress gives cause for optimism.

REFERENCES

Brown M S, Goldstein J L 1986 A receptor-mediated pathway for cholesterol homeostasis. Science 232: 34–47
Livneh et al 1985 The *Drosophila* EGF receptor gene homologue; conservation of both hormone binding and kinase domains. Cell 40: 599–607
Perkins S J, Williams A F, Rademacher T W, Dwek R A 1988 The Thy-1 glycoprotein: a three dimensional model. Trends Biochem Sci 13: 302–303
Roditi I, Schwarz H, Pearson T W, Beechcroft R P, Liu M K, Richardson J P, Buhring H J, Pleiss J, Bulow R, Williams R D, Overath P 1989 Procyclin gene expression and loss of the variant surface glycoprotein during differentiation of *Trypanosoma brucei*. J Cell Biol 108: 137–246
Scott J 1989 Lipoprotein receptors: unravelling atherosclerosis. Nature 338: 118–119

Section III: Leishmaniasis

Chairman: S. Britton

Discussion for both papers on the immunology of Leishmaniasis is on page 173–75.

F

8. CD4+ T cell subsets in murine leishmaniasis

R. M. Locksley   M. D. Sadick   B. J. Holaday
M. S. Bernstein   R. T. Pu   R. S. Dawkins and
F. P. Heinzel

INTRODUCTION

Leishmaniasis affects approximately 20 million people on all continents except Antarctica and Australia. The organisms are transmitted from a reservoir of infected mammals to humans by the bite of phlebotomine sandflies. Control of the natural reservoir is clearly unachievable, and resistance to currently available drugs has been problematic when prolonged, parenteral administration is not observed. Based on the immunology of the disease, vaccines would seem to offer the best chance for realistic control of *Leishmania* infection. A successful vaccine strategy, however, must take into consideration the many aspects of the immune response in a heterogeneous population.

The potential spectrum of the disease is perhaps best represented by visceral leishmaniasis, or kala-azar (Fig. 8.1). People with infection, usually children, have fever and prominent hepatosplenomegaly. Marked hypergammaglobulinaemia and anaemia are typical, and patients die with profound cachexia if untreated. A high titre antibody response to the intramacrophage parasite is present, but there is no skin test reactivity to *Leishmania* antigens. Most interesting, however, are studies demonstrating that humans with overt leishmaniasis constitute only a

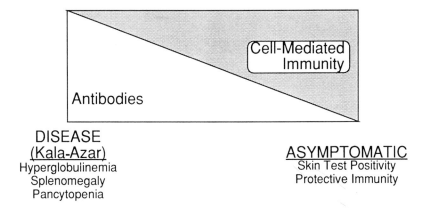

Fig. 8.1   The spectrum of leishmaniasis

portion of those infected with the protozoa; 6–8 cases of asymptomatic or subclinical disease probably occur for every recognized case (Badaro et al 1986). These patients demonstrate skin test reactivity to *Leishmania* antigens and low titres of antibodies. Among patients with disease, the cellular defect that underlies the failure to respond to *Leishmania* antigens is, in cases of visceral (Carvalho et al 1985, Sacks et al 1987) and some cutaneous (Murray et al 1984, Akuffo et al 1988) syndromes, restored following successful drug therapy. Thus, failure to control infection is not an irreversible phenotype. Such studies suggest that successful vaccination can be accomplished even in susceptible genotypes if the proper choice of antigens or route of vaccination can be established.

EXPERIMENTAL MURINE LEISHMANIASIS

Major insights into the spectral nature of leishmaniasis have derived from animal studies, primarily using inbred mouse strains. Infection with *Leishmania major* results in infection that mimics human visceral leishmaniasis in most aspects. Susceptible mice, such as the BALB/c strain, develop localized swelling and infection at the site of inoculation and, over a period of weeks, suffer visceralization with hepatosplenomegaly and, if untreated, progressive cachexia and death. Marked hypergammaglobulinaemia and anaemia are consistent findings. In contrast, genetically resistant mice, such as the C57BL/6 strain, develop localized infection followed shortly by control of disease, eradication of parasites, and the development of immunity to re-infection. The genetics of susceptibility have not been defined precisely, although it is clear that the lesion is not linked to major histocompatibility complex (MHC). The course of disease can be conveniently followed by measuring the size of the local lesion in the footpad, a measurement that correlates well with the presence of viable parasites (Fig. 8.2).

As in the human cases, the BALB/c strain is not susceptible due to a genetic deletion of the requisite T-cell repertoire. A variety of manipulations – thymectomy (Howard et al 1980), sublethal irradiation (Howard et al 1981), anti-μ-mediated B-cell depletion (Sacks et al 1984), and anti-CD4-mediated T-cell depletion (Sadick et al 1987, Titus et al 1985) have been shown to confer either a delay in expression of the disease or even cure on subsequently infected BALB/c mice (Table 8.1). Despite their differences, when tested each has been shown to establish protective immunity that can be transferred into naive mice using $CD4^+$ T cells. Since disease in susceptible mice is associated with expansion of $CD4^+$ T

Table 8.1 Immunological manipulations affecting the susceptible phenotype of BALB/c mice to *Leishmania major*

Manipulation	Approximate cure rate	Immunity re-infection	Immunity transferred by $CD4^+$ cells
Thymectomy	Disease slowed	–	–
Irradiation	50–60%	Yes	Yes
B-cell depletion	Transient	–	Yes
Transient CD4 depletion	65–90%	Yes	Yes

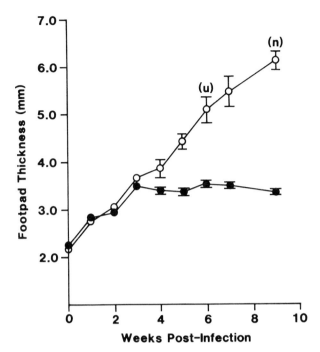

Fig. 8.2 Footpad thickness of BALB/c (open circles) or C57BL/6 (closed circles) mice infected with *Leishmania major* in the hind footpads. Times of ulceration (u) and necrosis (n) are marked. (Adapted from Heinzel et al 1988)

cells that abrogate protection in transfer experiments (Liew et al 1982, Mitchell 1983), these various interventions must share the capacity either to inhibit activation of an 'infection-promoting' $CD4^+$ T cell or to preferentially activate an 'immunoprotective' $CD4^+$ T cell. The ability of anti-CD4 antibody itself to confer a protective phenotype on BALB/c mice infected with *L. major* suggests that these interventions directly affect T-cell responses, since the CD4 molecule is not expressed on murine macrophages (Crocker et al 1987).

MACROPHAGE ACTIVATION AND RESOLUTION OF INFECTION

Leishmania are exclusively intramacrophage parasites in their mammalian hosts, and macrophage activation is required for elimination of the organisms in vitro. In experiments designed to test whether the appearance of T cells producing macrophage activating factors (MAFs) correlated with the resolution of infection (Sadick et al 1986, Sadick et al 1987), mononuclear cells from the draining lymph nodes or spleen were collected from infected BALB/c or C57BL/6 mice, stimulated in vitro with *Leishmania* antigens, and the supernatants assayed for macrophage activating activity (Table 8.2). Coincident with resolution of infection, C57BL/6 lymphocytes produced MAF for the destruction of *Leishmania* and MHC class II antigen induction, as well as classic anti-viral interferon activity. All of these activities could be removed using a neutralizing anti-IFN-γ antibody. In contrast,

Table 8.2 Generation of macrophage activating factors by lymph node cells and spleen after 8 weeks of *Leishmania major* infection

Mouse	Pre-treatment	Mφ activation to kill *Leishmania*	IFN-γ
C57BL/6	None	Yes	Yes
BALB/c	None	No	No
BALB/c	Irradiation	Yes	Yes
BALB/c	Anti-CD4 antibody	Yes	Yes

(Adapted from Sadick et al 1986, 1987)

BALB/c mice produced almost no measurable macrophage activating activity or IFN-γ. If BALB/c mice were treated with sublethal irradiation or anti-CD4 monoclonal antibody prior to infection, however, the animals healed and the isolated mononuclear cells produced readily measurable IFN-γ. These data suggested that resolution of *Leishmania* infection was related to the establishment in the host of cells that produced IFN-γ in response to *Leishmania* antigens.

CD4+ T-CELL SUBSETS

The inability of the infected BALB/c mice to respond to antigen stimulation with IFN-γ production was not due to a failure of CD4+ T cells to expand. At the time that these assays were performed, infected BALB/c mice had comparable or even greater numbers of CD4+ T lymphocytes in the lymph nodes as did healer C57BL/6 or immunologically manipulated BALB/c mice (Milon et al 1986, Sadick et al 1987). This perplexing situation of disparate CD4 cell populations awaited the discovery that murine CD4+ T-cell clones could be consistently divided into two subsets (Cherwinski et al 1987) (Fig. 8.3). The first, designated Th 1, generated IFN-γ, IL-2 and lymphotoxin following mitogen or antigen stimulation, while the second, designated Th 2, released IL-4, IL-5 and IL-6. Other lymphokines, including TNF, GM-CSF and IL-3, were less clearly segregated between the subsets. Th-2 cells required IL-1 as a co-factor for IL-4-mediated proliferation (Kurt-Jones et al 1987). Experiments in naive and immunized mice established that counterparts for these clones were present in normal animals (Finkelman et al 1986, Powers et al 1988), although it is apparent that additional subsets, including mixed secretors and unresponsive, null secretors, may also be present (Hayakawa & Hardy 1988).

In order to test whether differential CD4+ T-cell subset activation might account for the disparate outcomes in murine leishmaniasis, mRNA was extracted immediately from harvested lymph nodes or spleen from infected healer and non-healer mice and hybridized with specific lymphokine probes (Heinzel et al 1989). Northern analysis was used in order to avoid manipulation of cells in vitro that might change cytokine expression. The lymphokine genes are largely transcriptionally controlled and short-lived (Shaw & Kamen 1986), thus mRNA detected in vivo correlates with secretion of mature protein product. Remarkably, expression of mRNA for IFN-γ and IL-4 was reciprocal, consistent with differential

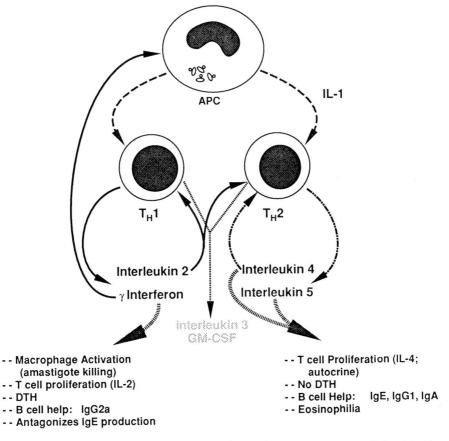

- - Macrophage Activation
   (amastigote killing)
- - T cell proliferation (IL-2)
- - DTH
- - B cell help: IgG2a
- - Antagonizes IgE production

- - T cell Proliferation (IL-4;
   autocrine)
- - No DTH
- - B cell Help: IgE, IgG1, IgA
- - Eosinophilia

Fig. 8.3 The two distinct subsets of murine L3T4$^+$ (CD4$^+$) T-cell clones can be distinguished by their lymphokine profiles following stimulation by appropriate antigen-presenting cells (APC)

CD4$^+$ T-cell subset activation in healing or progressive disease (Fig. 8.4). Although IFN-γ was consistently seen in the healer C57BL/6 but not in the BALB/c, IL-4 was present in the non-healer BALB/c but not in the C57BL/6. IL-1, a co-factor for activation of Th-2 but not Th-1 cells, was also preferentially expressed in the non-healer mice. IL-2 less consistently segregated between healer and non-healer mice, although expression was 2- to 3-fold greater in healer animals. Similar experiments established that this differential cytokine expression was not related to differences in mouse strains, since anti-CD4-pretreated BALB/c develop a healer phenotype and express mRNA for IFN-γ but not IL-4 in both spleen and lymph nodes (Fig. 8.5). The presence of IL-4 mRNA correlated directly with levels of IgE in the serum (Table 8.3), consistent with the known role of IL-4 as an IgE switch factor (Snapper & Paul 1987).

Taken together, these data suggested that the outcome of *Leishmania* infection is predicated on the bias in CD4$^+$ subset expansion during the disease. Several important questions remain, however. Although prior experiments by numerous investigators had demonstrated that CD4$^+$ cells could mediate both protection and exacerbation, confirmation that the message for these cytokines is contained

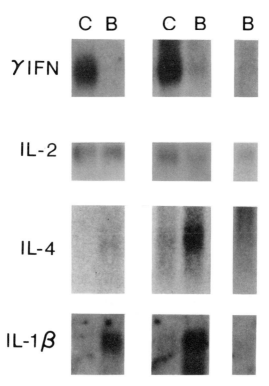

Fig. 8.4 Cytokine mRNA in infected spleen (left two columns) and lymph node (third, fourth columns) during leishmaniasis in healer C57BL/6 (C) or non-healer BALB/c (B) at 8 weeks of infection. Levels in uninfected BALB/c mice are shown in the right column. (Adapted from Heinzel et al 1989)

Table 8.3 Serum IgE levels in mice infected with *Leishmania major* for 8 weeks

Mouse	Pre-treatment	Serum IgE
C57BL/6	None	<0.10
BALB/c	None	28.5 ± 7.4
BALB/c	Anti-CD4	1.2 ± 1.7

(Adapted from Heinzel et al 1989)

in CD4$^+$ T cells is required. The ability of cloned, parasite-specific CD4$^+$ T cells to function in transfer experiments is important. The mechanisms by which the Th subsets interact in genetically susceptible mice is of fundamental importance to the understanding of the genetic predisposition to disease. In particular, are there ways to interfere preferentially with expansion of one or the other Th subsets and thus alter the outcome of infection? Finally, the identification of parasite antigens that stimulate the respective clones is critical in the rational development of vaccine candidate antigens. Answers to at least some of these questions are being addressed in several laboratories.

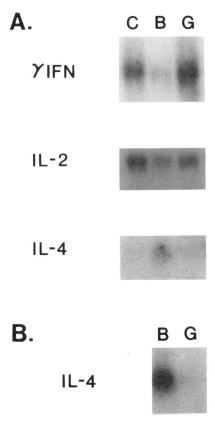

Fig. 8.5 Lymphokine mRNA in infected spleens from healer C57BL/6 (C), non-healer BALB/c (B) or healer anti-CD4 pretreated BALB/c (G) after 8 weeks of *Leishmania major* infection. (A) Levels of IFN-γ, IL-2 and IL-4 mRNA in spleen. (B) Levels of IL-4 mRNA in lymph nodes. (Adapted from Heinzel et al 1989)

CYTOKINES FROM CD4⁺ T-CELL SUBSETS

Identification of the cellular origin of the lymphokine messages was achieved following isolation of CD4⁺ cells using anti-CD4-coated iron microspheres that could be separated in a magnetic field. Using separation at 4°C to inhibit decay of mRNA, it was clear that mRNA for IFN-γ was only in CD4⁺ T cells in healing C57BL/6 mice, whereas small amounts were contained in non-CD4⁺ cells in non-healing BALB/c (Table 8.4). In contrast, IL-4 mRNA was present only in the CD4⁺ cell population isolated from the non-healing BALB/c. These data demonstrate directly that CD4⁺ T cells isolated from infected mice contain either IFN-γ or IL-4 depending on the status of disease. Experiments to extend this observation to the syngeneic healer models of BALB/c mice will be necessary to confirm the general nature of this observation.

Experiments by Scott and colleagues have extended these studies to the clonal level (Scott et al 1988). Using T-cell lines derived from mice immunized with soluble *Leishmania* antigens, these investigators were able to show that two

Table 8.4 Lymphokine mRNA in CD4$^+$ T cells in mice infected with *Leishmania major* for 8 weeks

Mouse	IFNγ mRNA		IL-4 mRNA	
	CD4$^+$	CD4$^-$	CD4$^+$	CD4$^-$
C57BL/6	+ + +	–	–	–
BALB/c	–	+	+ +	–

CD4$^+$ lines were separable by their abilities to transfer either resistance or exacerbation of disease to subsequently infected BALB/c mice. The line that transferred resistance generated IFN-γ and IL-2 following stimulation with antigens, whereas the line that exacerbated infection released IL-4 and IL-5. These findings are consistent with distinct roles for Th 1 and Th 2 in disease, and support the prior findings using mRNA isolated directly from infected animals. Importantly, using two-dimensional T-cell blots, these investigators demonstrated that the lines responded to distinct antigen fractions from the parasite. Thus, the Th-1 and Th-2 cells seem to respond to distinct antigens, a critical observation in terms of vaccine development.

Another method for demonstrating causality rather than association is to interfere with expansion of specific subsets in vivo during infection in order to assess their role in outcome. Several investigators have shown that sustained depletion of CD4$^+$ cells renders animals unable to control infection (Louis et al 1986). IL-4 is a specific autocrine growth factor for Th-2 cells; blockade of IL-4 completely abolishes Th-2 expansion (Harel-Bellan et al 1988). Using a neutraliz-

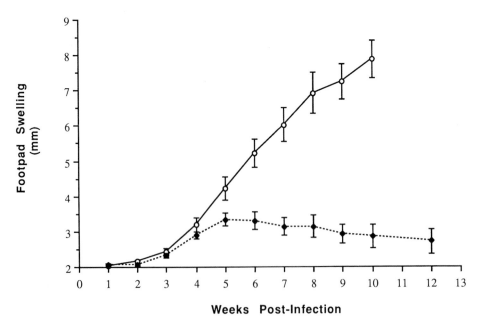

Fig. 8.6 Course of footpad swelling in susceptible BALB/c mice infected with *Leishmania major* and treated for 6 weeks with intraperitoneal neutralizing anti-IL-4 monoclonal antibody (closed symbols) or isotype control (open symbols)

ing anti-IL-4 monoclonal antibody, it is possible to assess the contribution of Th-2 cells to progression of disease in susceptible BALB/c by inhibiting their expansion. Consistent with their association with progressive disease, blockade of these cells attenuated subsequent infection in all mice, and, when stopped after 6 weeks of therapy, resulted in sustained cure in 15 of 23 mice (Fig. 8.6). These data, together with those of Scott et al (1988) utilizing T-cell clones, suggest that parasite-specific Th-2 cells can directly mediate the failure of genetically susceptible mice to generate a protective immunological response.

CONCLUSION

Although a thorough understanding of the immunology remains incomplete at present, the following hypothesis is consistent with our current understanding. Infection or intravenous immunization using *Leishmania* antigens of susceptible BALB/c mice results in the preferential activation and/or maturation of $CD4^+$ T cells into effector $CD4^+$ T lymphocytes expressing the Th-2 phenotype. Preliminary evidence suggests that both Th-1 and Th-2 cells arise from a common precursor memory cell that initially responds to antigen stimulation with IL-2-dependent clonal expansion (Swain et al 1988, Street et al 1989). Maturation to the Th-1 or Th-2 phenotype may occur via an intermediate that secretes some combination of lymphokines that are segregated in the final effector phenotype. Commitment to the Th-1 or Th-2 pathways may be a function of how antigen is presented by the antigen-presenting cell (APC), an hypothesis consistent with the ability of B cells but not macrophages to present concanavalin A to Th-2-like cells (Hayakawa & Hardy 1988), and with the IL-1 co-requirement for IL-4-dependent Th-2 cells (Kurt-Jones et al 1987). The dependence of certain APCs for the generation of Th-2 cells may explain the observation that deletion of B cells prior to infection could ameliorate the disease in BALB/c mice (Sacks et al 1984). By this hypothesis, sublethal irradiation or transient depletion of $CD4^+$ T cells must interfere with activation requirements of Th-2 cells but not Th-1 cells. Once Th-2 cells have expanded, soluble factors are released that interfere with the expansion of antigen-specific Th-1 cells (Mosmann et al 1989), and disease progresses inexorably. In genetically resistant mice, APCs present antigen in such a manner that $CD4^+$ precursors are activated to mature to effector Th-1 cells, the soluble products of Th-1 cells interfere with Th2 cell expansion (Gajewski & Fitch 1988), and successful activation of macrophages and resolution of infection occur. Although much work remains, the availability of recombinant cytokines and neutralizing antibodies, the ability to clone and transfer T cells from both subsets, and the identification of antibodies that distinguish among the subsets (Hayakawa & Hardy 1988) should allow rapid progress into the previously complicated immunology of leishmaniasis.

ACKNOWLEDGEMENT

This work was supported by AI-26918 and AI-27461 from the National Institutes of Health and a grant from the MacArthur Foundation.

REFERENCES

Akuffo H O, Fehniger T E, Britton S 1988 Differential recognition of *Leishmania aethiopica* antigens by lymphocytes from patients with local and diffuse cutaneous leishmaniasis. Evidence for antigen-induced immune suppression. J Immunol 141: 2461–2466

Badaro R, Jones T C, Lorenco R et al 1986 A prospective study of visceral leishmaniasis in an endemic area of Brazil. J Infect Dis 154: 639–649

Carvalho E M, Badaro R, Reed S G, Jones T C, Johnson W D Jr 1985 Absence of gamma-interferon and interleukin-2 production during active visceral leishmaniasis. J Clin Invest 76: 2066–2069

Cherwinski H M, Schumacher J H, Brown K D, Mosmann T R 1987 Two types of mouse helper T cell clone. III. Further differences in lymphokine synthesis between Th1 and Th2 clones revealed by RNA hybridization, functionally monospecific bioassays, and monoclonal antibodies. J Exp Med 166: 1229–1244

Crocker P R, Jefferies W A, Clark S J, Chung L P, Gordon S 1987 Species heterogeneity in macrophage expression of the CD4 antigen. J Exp Med 166: 613–618

Finkelman F D, Ohara J, Goroff D K et al 1986 Production of BSF-1 during an in vivo, T-dependent immune response. J Immunol 137: 2878–2885

Gajewski T R, Fitch F W 1988 Anti-proliferative effect of IFN-γ in immune regulation. I. IFN-γ inhibits the proliferation of Th2 but not Th1 murine helper T lymphocyte clones. J Immunol 140: 4245–4252

Harel-Bellan A, Durum S, Muegge D, Abbas A K, Farrar W L 1988 Specific inhibition of lymphokine biosynthesis and autocrine growth using antisense oligonucleotides in Th1 and Th2 helper T cell clones. J Exp Med 168: 2309–2318

Hayakawa K, Hardy R R 1988 Murine CD4$^+$ T cell subsets defined. J Exp Med 168: 1825–1838

Heinzel F P, Sadick M D, Locksley R M 1988. *Leishmania major*: analysis of lymphocyte and macrophage cellular phenotypes during infection of susceptible and resistant mice. Exp Parasitol 65: 258–268

Heinzel F P, Sadick M D, Holaday B J, Coffman R L, Locksley R M 1989 Reciprocal expression of interferon γ or interleukin 4 during the resolution or progression of murine leishmaniasis. Evidence for expansion of distinct helper T cell subsets. J Exp Med 169: 59–72

Howard J G, Hale C, Liew F Y 1980 Immunological regulation of experimental cutaneous leishmaniasis. III. Nature and significance of specific suppression of cell-mediated immunity in mice highly susceptible to *Leishmania tropica*. J Exp Med 152: 594–607

Howard J G, Hale C, Liew F Y 1981 Immunological regulation of experimental cutaneous leishmaniasis. IV. Prophylactic effect of sublethal irradiation as a result of abrogation of suppressor T cell generation in mice genetically susceptible to *Leishmania tropica*. J Exp Med 153: 557–568

Kurt-Jones E A, Hamberg S, Ohara J, Paul W E, Abbas A K 1987 Heterogeneity of helper/inducer T lymphocytes. I. Lymphokine production and lymphokine responsiveness. J Exp Med 166: 1774–1787

Liew F Y, Hale C, Howard J G 1982 Immunologic regulation of experimental cutaneous leishmaniasis. V. Characterization of effector and specific suppressor T cells. J Immunol 128: 1917–1922

Louis J A, Mendonca S, Titus R G et al 1986 The role of specific T cell subpopulations in murine cutaneous leishmaniasis. In: Progress in Immunology VI, Academic Press, New York, 762–769

Milon G, Titus R G, Cerottini J-C, Marchal G, Louis J A 1986 Higher frequency of *Leishmania major*-specific L3T4$^+$ T cells in susceptible BALB/c as compared with resistant CBA mice. J Immunol 136: 1467–1471

Mitchell G F 1983 Murine cutaneous leishmaniasis: resistance in reconstituted nude mice and several F_1 hybrids infected with *Leishmania tropica major*. J Immunogenet 10: 395–412

Mosmann T R, Fiorentino D F, Bond M W 1989 Inhibition of Th1 proliferation and IFN-γ secretion by activities in Th2 supernatants. FASEB J 3: 6058 (abstract)

Murray H W, Rubin B Y, Carriero S, Acosta A M 1984. Reversible defect in antigen-induced lymphokine and γ-interferon generation in cutaneous leishmaniasis. J Immunol 133: 2250–2254

Powers G D, Abbas A K, Miller R A 1988 Frequencies of IL-2- and IL-4-secreting T cells in naive and antigen-stimulated lymphocyte populations. J Immunol 140: 3352–3357

Sacks D L, Scott P A, Asofsky R, Sher F A 1984 Cutaneous leishmaniasis in anti-IgM-treated mice: enhanced resistance due to functional depletion of a B cell-dependent T cell involved in the suppressor pathway. J Immunol 132: 2072–2077

Sacks D L, Lal S L, Shrivastava S N, Blackwell J, Neva F A 1987 An analysis of T cell responsiveness in Indian kala-azar. J Immunol 138: 908–913

Sadick M D, Locksley R M, Tubbs C, Raff H V 1986 Murine cutaneous leishmaniasis: resistance correlates with the capacity to generate interferon-γ in response to *Leishmania* antigens in vitro. J Immunol 136: 655–661

Sadick M D, Heinzel F P, Shigekane V M, Fisher W L, Locksley R M 1987 Cellular and humoral immunity to *Leishmania major* in genetically susceptible mice after in vivo depletion of L3T4[+] T cells. J Immunol 139: 1303–1309

Scott P, Natovitz P, Coffman R L, Pearce E, Sher A 1988 Immunoregulation of cutaneous leishmaniasis. T cell lines that transfer protective immunity or exacerbation belong to different T helper subsets and respond to distinct parasite antigens. J Exp Med 168: 1675–1684

Shaw G, Kamen R 1986 A conserved AU sequence from the 3′ untranslated region of GM–CSF mRNA mediates selective mRNA degradation. Cell 46: 659–667

Snapper C M, Paul W E 1987 Interferon-γ and B cell stimulatory factor-1 reciprocally regulate Ig isotype production. Science 236: 944–947

Street N E, Bass H, Fiorentino D et al 1989 Influence of immune status on commitment to Th1 and Th2 phenotypes. FASEB J 3: 6081 (abstract)

Swain S L, McKenzie D T, Weinberg A D, Hancock W 1988 Characterization of T helper 1 and 2 cell subsets in normal mice. Helper T cells responsible for IL-4 and IL-5 production are present as precursors that require priming before they develop into lymphokine-secreting cells. J Immunol 141: 3445–3455

Titus R G, Ceredig R, Cerottini J-C, Louis J A 1985 Therapeutic effect of anti-L3T4 monoclonal antibody GK1.5 on cutaneous leishmaniasis in genetically-susceptible BALB/c mice. J Immunol 135: 2108–2114

9. T-cell responses in resistance and susceptibility to experimental infection with *Leishmania major*

I. Müller   R. Titus   I. Caldumbide and J. A. Louis

INTRODUCTION

Leishmaniases are infectious diseases of protozoan origin that have only recently been recognized to represent an important public health problem worldwide (Modabber 1987). The organisms responsible for these diseases are trypanosoma-tid protozoans of the genus *Leishmania* which are transmitted to their mammalian hosts by the bite of infected female phlebotomine sandflies. In their vertebrate hosts, the flagellate promastigotes penetrate mononuclear phagocytes where they transform into the amastigote forms. It is important to mention that there are indications that these diseases affect an increasing number of immunocompromised patients and, indeed, leishmaniasis has been reported to develop as an opportunistic infection in AIDS patients several years after time spent in areas where transmission by insects does occur (Fuzibet et al 1988)

The spectrum of clinical manifestations seen in humans infected with *Leishmania* ranges from the localized cutaneous form (oriental sore) to the visceral form (kala-azar). The features of the disease appear to be the consequence of the characteristics of the species of *Leishmania* involved and of the immune response of the host.

Numerous observations showing that the resolution of natural infection often leads to the development of a state of immunity to re-infection strongly suggest that prophylactic immunization (i.e. vaccination) would be an important tool by which to effectively control leishmaniasis. It is clear that the rational design of a vac-cine against leishmaniasis will depend upon the precise understanding of the im-mune mechanisms involved in resistance to infection together with the identification of the molecules from the parasites which are the target of protective responses.

The different clinical manifestations observed in human leishmaniasis can be reproduced in mice according to their genetic background. This availability of inbred strains of mice that are either resistant (e.g. CBA, C57BL/6) or susceptible (BALB/c) to infection with *Leishmania major* has greatly facilitated the analysis of the immune mechanisms involved either in resistance or susceptibility. In this experimental model of infection, no clear evidence exists that specific anti-*Leishmania* antibodies, detectable as early as 2 weeks after experimental infection, play an important role in the resolution of an established infection (Mitchell 1984, Liew 1986). However, recent results have demonstrated that antibodies specific for

158

molecules of the parasites' surface, responsible for binding to receptors at the surface of macrophages, may passively protect mice against infection. Indeed, monoclonal antibodies specific for the glycolipid of the surface of *L. major* have been demonstrated to inhibit the binding of these parasites to murine macrophages (Handmann & Goding 1985). Furthermore, it has been demonstrated that not only the passive transfer of antibody specific for a 46-kD membrane glycoprotein (M-2) of *Leishmania amazonensis* protected mice against infection with this parasite (Anderson et al 1983) but also that immunization with M-2 in adjuvant elicited a protective response which was reflected by an increased antibody response (Champsi & McMahon-Pratt 1988). Therefore, it is possible that antibodies might have some protective function by hampering the binding of *Leishmania* promastigotes to their obligate host cell and thereby interfering with their entry and survival in macrophages.

In their mammalian hosts, *Leishmania* live and multiply obligatorily in mononuclear phagocytes; the functions of these cells are relevant to the expression of diseases induced by these parasites. The central role of macrophages in infection with intracellular pathogens is not surprising since these cells are involved in all aspects of immune responses, i.e. the induction as well as the effector phase. In this vein, it has been recognized for some time that the activation of macrophages harbouring *Leishmania* amastigotes is an important mechanism for the destruction of intracellular parasites. Observations which have documented a dramatic increase in the number of precursor cells of the macrophage–granulocyte lineage, presumably phagocytic but refractory to activating lymphokines, in the spleen of infected susceptible mice, support the notion of the importance of macrophages in leishmanial infections (Mirkovich et al 1986). Parasite survival and multiplication inside macrophages have also been related to an ability of these organisms to impair some non-vital functions of their host cells such as the expression of major histocompatibility complex (MHC) class I and II gene products (Reiner et al 1987, Reiner et al 1988).

Available information clearly indicates that T-cell-mediated immunity, rather than humoral response, is instrumental in the acquisition of resistance to infection with *Leishmania*. In addition, it is also becoming evident that the activity of specific T-cell responses triggered during experimental infection may favour parasite multiplication in vivo and therefore play a role in determining the susceptibility of the host to infection. Although it is now generally agreed that resolution of lesions and promotion of parasite growth are the result, at least in part, of distinct parasite-specific T cells, it has proved difficult to delineate the mechanisms by which T cells mediate these two opposite effects on the disease process in vivo.

In this paper, we summarize the results of several research groups, including our own, pertaining to the role of specific T cells triggered during experimental infection on the course of disease.

RESISTANCE TO INFECTION WITH *L. major*: ROLE OF T CELLS

Early work of the group of Mitchell in Australia has clearly shown that T cells were involved in resistance to infection with *L. major* by demonstrating (a) that nu/nu athymic mice belonging to both susceptible and resistant strains were extremely susceptible to *L. major* infection, and (b) that this exquisite susceptibility was abrogated after adoptive transfer of relatively small numbers of T cells from non-infected syngeneic mice (Mitchell 1984).

CD4$^+$ T cells

The results of adoptive cell transfer experiments, performed by several laboratories have shown that protective immunity in resistant strains was dependent upon the activity of CD8$^-$ (Lyt2$^-$) T cells (Mitchell 1984, Liew 1986). The role of CD4$^+$ T cells in resistance to infection with *L.major* was directly evaluated in vivo by studying the course of infection in mice in which CD4$^+$ cells had been eliminated (>95%) by intensive treatment with anti-CD4 monoclonal antibodies GK-1.5 (Titus et al 1987) during the entire course of infection. Results have shown that, in the absence of CD4$^+$ T cells, even mice from resistant strains developed severe lesions. Thus, there is now a general consensus that CD4$^+$ T cells are essential for the development of protective immunity.

CD8$^+$ cells

Although the role of CD8$^+$ cells in the immunological control of infection by *L.major* is still controversial (Titus et al 1987, Moll et al 1988), results recently obtained in our laboratory indicate that specific CD8$^+$ cells participate, to some extent, in the healing of *L. major*-induced lesions. Indeed, depletion of CD8$^+$ T cells in vivo by administration of anti-Lyt2 mAb (mAb H–35–17.2) during the course of infection led to the development of more severe lesions in mice from both resistant and susceptible strains (Titus et al 1987). It is, however, noteworthy that resistant mice depleted of CD8$^+$ cells eventually resolved their lesions. It is also of interest that, compared with susceptible BALB/c mice, the number of CD8$^+$ T cells, in lymph node cells draining the lesions, capable of transferring specific delayed-type hypersensitivity (DTH) reactions into normal mice was three times higher in CBA mice at a time when lesions start to heal in these resistant mice (Titus et al 1987). Taken together these results could suggest that, even though CD8$^+$ T cells are not the main protective cells against *L. major* infection, they play some role in the resolution of primary lesions.

Evidence indicates that CD8$^+$ T cells could play a more important role in controlling the lesions that developed in immunized mice. Indeed, it has recently been shown that in vivo depletion of CD8$^+$ cells, effectively prevented the induction of resistance that can be seen following i.v. immunization with 1×10^7 killed promastigotes (Liew et al 1984) suggesting that CD8$^+$ T cells may be a critical component of this immune response (Farrell et al 1989). Furthermore, the small lesions that developed upon infectious challenge of resistant mice, 2 weeks after resolution of primary infection, were substantially enhanced after depletion of either CD4$^+$ or CD8$^+$ T cells with the corresponding monoclonal antibodies (Fig. 9.1). Interestingly, resistant mice depleted of either CD4$^+$ or CD8$^+$ T cells were eventually able to control their secondary infection. In contrasts, secondary lesions in resistant animals severely depleted of both CD4$^+$ and CD8$^+$ T cells progressed inexorably without tendency to heal (Fig. 9.1, panel D). Collectively these results might indicate that, although CD4$^+$ T cells are mainly responsible for the resolution of lesions resulting from a first infection with *L. major*, both CD8$^+$

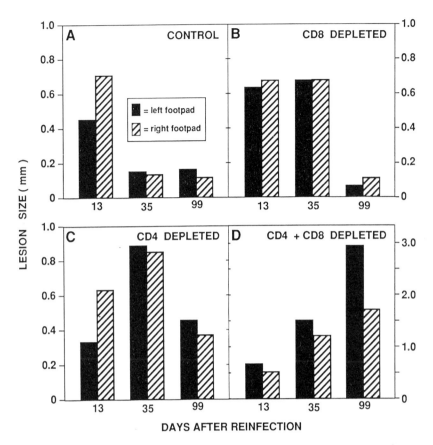

Figure 9.1 Contribution of CD4$^+$ and CD8$^+$ T-cell subpopulations to the resolution of cutaneous lesions that develop in resistant animals re-infected with *L. major*. CBA-mice were infected s.c. in one hind footpad with 2×10^6 virulent *L. major* parasites. Twelve weeks later, when the primary lesions were completely resolved, all animals were re-infected in the contralateral footpad with 2×10^6 *L. major* parasites (5–8 mice per group). The figure depicts the size of the lesions developing at the site of rechallenge (right footpad) and the size of lesions at the primary site of infection (left footpad) which was 0 at the time of re-infection. Panel A = control group; panel B = mice depleted of CD8$^+$ positive T cells during the entire course of re-infection by administration of 200 μg H35 MAb twice a week starting at day 3 before re-infection; panel C = mice depleted of CD4$^+$ positive T cells during the entire course of re-infection by administration of 300 μg GK 1.5 MAb twice a week starting at day 3 before re-infection; panel D = depleted of both T-cell subpopulations during the entire course of re-infection by injection of both mAB twice a week

and CD4$^+$ cells are implicated in the healing of lesions developing in immune mice. Evidence for a role of CD8$^+$ T cells in the elimination of intracellular parasites and/or bacteria by infected hosts has also been obtained in murine models of infection with *L. donovani, Listeria monocytogenes* and *Mycobacterium tuberculosis* (De Libero & Kaufmann 1986, Kaufmann et al 1986a, 1986b, Kaye et al 1987, Müller et al 1987).

Lymphokines
Since the activation of macrophages harbouring *Leishmania* probably represents the major mechanism by which these intracellular organisms are eliminated from

the hosts, the importance of macrophages activating lymphokines released by specific T cells in the healing process has long been recognized. Indeed, interferon γ (IFN-γ) has been shown to be important for macrophage activation in vitro which leads to the destruction of intracellular *Leishmania* amastigotes (Nathan et al 1983, Ralph et al 1983, Titus et al 1984). The crucial role of IFN-γ in the resolution of *Leishmania*-induced lesions in vivo has been documented by several observations. First, the capacity of genetically resistant mice to resolve spontaneously their cutaneous lesions has been found to be directly related to the ability of their draining lymph node T cells to release IFN-γ after stimulation with parasite antigens in vitro (Sadick et al 1986). Second, compared with susceptible mice, the lymph node and spleen cells of resistant mice contained greater amounts of IFN-γ mRNA a few weeks after infection (Locksley et al 1987, Heinzel et al 1989). Third, the administration of neutralizing anti-IFN-γ mAb during the course of infection of resistant mice interferred with the spontaneous resolution of lesions normally seen in these mice (Müller et al 1989, P. Scott and A. Sher personal communication).

Specific T-cell lines and clones
Using a panel of murine T-cell clones specific for a given antigen, it has been shown recently that the murine CD4$^+$ T-cell population comprises two functionally distinct subsets, designated Th-1 and Th-2 which differ in the pattern of lymphokines produced after stimulation with antigens or mitogens (Mosmann et al 1986, Mosmann & Coffman 1987). Th-1 clones were shown to produce IFN-γ and interleukin 2 (IL-2) whereas Th-2 clones produced interleukin 4 (IL-4) and interleukin 5 without producing IFN-γ and IL-2. Therefore, lines and clones of *Leishmania*-specific T lymphocytes represent important tools to dissect the characteristics of T cells which mediate resolution of lesions induced by *L. major*.

Studies by Scott et al (1987) had previously shown that immunization with two distinct fractions separated from a preparation of soluble extract of *L. major* parasites (soluble leishmanial antigens, SLA), which both elicited strong T-cell responses, was capable of either protecting BALB/c mice against challenge with virulent parasites or enhancing the infection. These authors derived a T-cell line recognizing the protective fraction and correlated defined immunological functions with protective capacity. The adoptive transfer of a CD4$^+$ T-cell line, recognizing the fraction of SLA capable of vaccinating BALB/c mice, to either 2 Gy irradiated or normal mice was shown to protect them against this normally fatal infection. After antigenic or mitogenic stimulation in vitro, this protective T-cell line was found to produce IFN-γ and IL-2, a lymphokine profile corresponding to the Th-1 subset (Scott et al 1988).

Recently, we have derived two *L. major*-specific cloned T-cell lines which were capable of significantly protecting normal recipient BALB/c mice against challenge with virulent *L. major* promastigotes (Müller & Louis 1989). This protective effect was reflected by an important reduction of the size of cutaneous lesions and a dramatic reduction of the number of parasites found in lesions of mice adoptively transferred with the cloned T cells (Fig. 9.2). The protective CD4$^+$ T-cell clones were derived from the spleen of BALB/c mice infected intravenously with live stationary phase promastigotes. Clones were derived in the presence of live

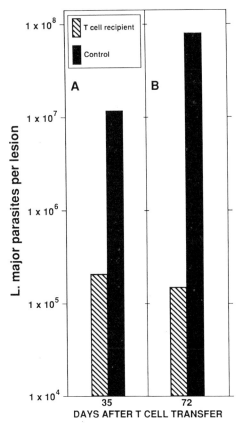

Figure 9.2 Estimation of the number of viable *L. major* parasites in lesions of susceptible BALB/c mice protected by the adoptive transfer of *L. major*-specific T-cell clones. One day after the i.v. transfer of 3.8×10^6 BS3.H5 cloned T cells or 3.4×10^6 BS3.G9 cloned T cells animals were infected with 2×10^6 live *L. major* promastigotes in one hind footpad. The frequencies of viable parasites in the infected footpad were determined by limiting dilution analysis (Titus et al 1985) and the number of viable parasites per lesion was calculated by multiplying the footpad weight (g) with the frequency of parasites/g. Panel A = number of parasites in the lesions of BS3.H5 T cell recipients 35 days after T-cell transfer, compared with control infected BALB/c mice. Panel B = number of parasites in the lesions of BS3.G9 T-cell recipients 72 days after T-cell transfer, compared with control infected BALB/c mice

L. major promastigotes as antigen and expressed the CD4$^+$ cell surface phenotype since blocking of the CD4 surface molecule by specific mAb interferred with their specific activation (Fig. 9.3). They were shown to produce IFN-γ and IL-2 after specific stimulation in vitro, indicating that they also belong to the recently described Th-1 subset. Observations which have shown that treatment of protected recipient mice with anti-IFN-γ neutralizing mAb abolished the protection conferred by the transferred cloned T cells strongly suggest that IFN-γ is involved in this effect (Müller & Louis 1989). A remarkable characteristic of these two protective CD4$^+$ T-cell clones is that they appear to recognize antigens associated only with live *L. major* parasites. Activation of these T-cell clones in vitro was only seen after stimulation with either live *L.major* promastigotes, parasites inactivated by a short exposure to u.v. radiation or promastigotes incubated overnight at 37°C

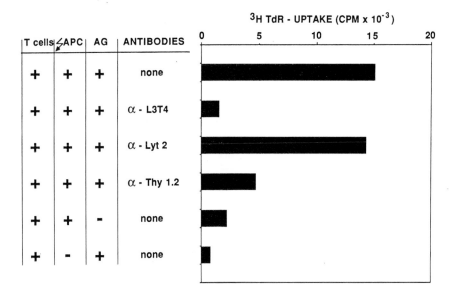

Figure 9.3 Inhibition of IL-2 secretion by cloned T cells using anti-CD4 monoclonal antibodies. Protective cloned T cells (1×10^5) were incubated with syngeneic irradiated antigen-presenting cells (2×10^5) and live *L. major* parasites as antigen (5×10^5) in the presence of 10% of either anti-L3T4, anti-Lyt 2⁻ or anti-Thy 1.2 MAb. Twenty-four hours later 100 µl of culture supernatants were removed and IL-2 activity was determined using an IL-2 dependent CTLL line

prior to addition to lymphocyte cultures. In contrast, no activation was observed when either glutaraldehyde-fixed *L. major* promastigotes or lysates of *L. major* promastigotes (obtained by repeated freezing and thawing of the parasites) were used as a source of antigen in vitro. It is also noteworthy that these protective T-cell clones recognized neither antigen present in the fraction of the soluble extract of *L. major* promastigotes (SLA) which has been shown to induce protective immunity in susceptible BALB/c mice (Scott et al 1987) nor the major surface protein of *Leishmania* promastigotes (PSP) which has been shown to vaccinate mice against infection with *L. mexicana* (Russel & Alexander 1988). The results depicted in Fig. 9.4 summarize the antigen-reactivity pattern of these two protective clones.

The results summarized in this section strongly indicate that (i) the anti-*Leishmania* effector function of CD4⁺ T cells is performed by cells belonging to the Th-1 subset and is related to their ability to release IFN-γ, (ii) some protective T cells could exhibit a unique specificity, i.e. recognize antigens associated with live parasites (Müller & Louis 1989). Observations are accumulating, suggesting that CD8⁺ T cells could also play a role in the immunological control of experimentally induced cutaneous leishmaniasis.

SUSCEPTIBILITY TO INFECTION WITH *L. major*: ROLE OF T CELLS

In addition to their predominant role in the resolution of *L. major*-induced lesions, it is now established that CD4⁺ T cells are also important in determining

164

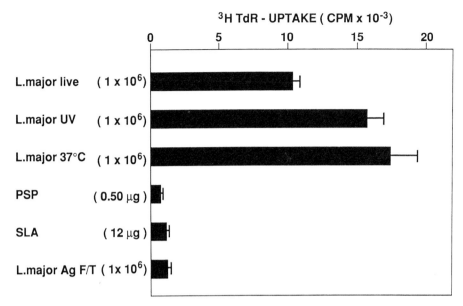

Figure 9.4 Antigen-reactivity pattern of protective *L. major*-specific cloned T cells. Cloned protective T cells (1×10^4) were stimulated with different preparations of *L. major* major parasites in the presence of syngeneic irradiated spleen cells. As antigen, untreated live parasites, 5 min u.v.-inactivated parasites, promastigotes incubated overnight at 37°C, the amphiphilic form of PSP, soluble extracts of *L. major* promastigotes (SLA) or the soluble fraction of 5x frozen and thawed (F/T) parasites were used. Proliferation was determined after 3 days of culture

susceptibility to infection with *L. major*. This contention was already supported by early observations which have shown that (a) in contrast to what was observed after the injection of small numbers of CD4$^+$ (Lyt 1$^+$2$^-$) T cells from normal susceptible BALB/c mice, the adoptive transfer of high numbers of these CD4$^+$ (Lyt 1$^+$2$^-$) T cells into syngeneic nu/nu mice failed to confer resistance (Mitchell et al 1980), (b) nu/nu mice receiving CD4$^+$ (Lyt 1$^+$2$^-$) T cells from chronically infected BALB/c mice were more susceptible to infection and could no longer be rendered resistant as a result of the administration of small numbers of normal syngeneic T cells (Mitchell et al 1987). Furthermore, it has been known for several years that s.c. immunization of resistant and susceptible mice with crude preparations of *Leishmania* antigens emulsified or not in complete Freund's adjuvant prior to infection with virulent parasites enhanced the course of infection (Titus et al 1984, Liew et al 1985a), an effect which has been attributed to the activity of CD4$^+$ T cells expanding after immunization (Liew et al 1985b).

A role for CD4$^+$ T cells in susceptibility to infection with *L. major* was strongly supported by the demonstration that the specific immune response generated in susceptible mice during infection was characterized by the expansion of large numbers of parasite-specific CD4$^+$ T cells. Indeed, comparison of the numbers of specific CD4$^+$ T cells triggered in susceptible and resistant mice, as a result of experimental infection, revealed that the frequency of CD4$^+$ T cells capable of mediating specific DTH reactions was 10–50 times higher in lymphoid tissues of susceptible mice (Milon et al 1986). Furthermore, treatment of susceptible mice with anti-CD4 mAb, using a regimen which did not result in the complete and permanent elimination of CD4$^+$ T cells from lymphoid tissues, has been demonstrated to render these mice resistant to infection with *L. major* (Titus et al 1985). Similarly, administration of cyclosporin A has also been shown to render genetically susceptible mice resistant to infection with *L. major* and this effect was attributed to the ability of cyclosporin A to modulate T-cell responses and to increase the destruction of intracellular *Leishmania* by macrophages (Solbach et al 1986, Bogdan et al 1989). Although these observations taken together confirmed the paradox that CD4$^+$ T cells favour the growth of parasites in vivo although they are required for resolution of lesions, they did not permit us to ascribe 'disease-promotion' and 'resolution of lesion' to the activity of distinct parasite-specific CD4$^+$ T cells.

Evidence has been obtained recently which clearly shows that CD4$^+$ T cells which confer resistance are different from those which mediate susceptibility. The existence of functionally distinct parasite-specific CD4$^+$ T cells triggered during experimental infection has been suggested by observations showing that immunological manipulation of the immune system, such as the transient depletion of CD4$^+$ T cells at the beginning of infection, not only allowed highly susceptible mice to resolve their *L. major*-induced lesions, but also modulated various functions ascribed to parasite-specific CD4$^+$ T cells (Sadick et al 1987, Müller et al 1989). Elegant studies by Heinzel et al (1989) have shown that resistance to infection resulting from prior treatment of normally susceptible mice with anti-CD4 MAb was associated with the appearance of mRNA for IFN-γ and with the disappearance of mRNA for IL-4 in their lymph node cells. Furthermore, compared to susceptible mice the lymph node cells of resistant mice contained 50–100-fold more IFN-γ mRNA and up to 50-fold less IL-4 mRNA 8 weeks after infection (Heinzel et al 1989). Taken together, these observations lend strong support to the hypothesis that healing of *L. major*-induced lesions results from the activity of Th-1 CD4$^+$ T cells and that severe disease in susceptible mice could result from the expansion of Th 2 CD4$^+$ T cells. However, the demonstration of increased numbers of CD4$^+$ cells, capable of transferring specific DTH reactions into normal mice, in lymphoid tissues of infected susceptible mice (Milon et al 1986) would also indicate that some CD4$^+$ cells expressing certain characteristics of the Th-1 cells might also play a role in the exacerbated disease that occurs in mice of this strain.

Specific T-cell lines and clones

T-cell lines recognizing antigen(s) present in a fraction of SLA (see above) which failed to trigger protective immunity in BALB/c mice (Scott et al 1987) were shown recently to exacerbate the course of infection after adoptive transfer to syngeneic BALB/c recipients (Scott et al 1988). These T-cell lines had the functional properties of the Th-2 subset since, after antigenic or mitogenic stimulation in vitro, they produce IL-4 and IL-5 but no IFN-γ or IL-2. Therefore, these results combined with those described above showing that a T-cell line recognizing antigen(s) in the protective fraction from SLA expressed the Th-1 functional phenotype and could protect BALB/c mice against fatal infection support the concept that 'protective' and 'exacerbating' T cells belong to the Th-1 and Th-2 subset respectively. In this context, it would therefore be of great interest to determine whether or not the protective or exacerbating properties of parasite antigens are determined solely by their ability to preferentially stimulate one population of CD4$^+$ T cells. Several years ago, we derived parasite-specific CD4$^+$ T-cell lines from the lymph nodes of mice which had been infected with *L. major* or immunized by the s.c. injection of a crude lysate of promastigotes emulsified in adjuvant. These T-cell lines were always selected in vitro in the presence of a lysate of *L. major* promastigotes as a source of antigen and were found to exacerbate the course of disease after adoptive transfer to syngeneic recipients (Titus et al 1984). These specific T-cell lines were able to transfer strong DTH reactions to syngeneic recipients and to release substantial amounts of MAF/IFN-γ, interleukin 3 (IL-3) and granulocyte–macrophage colony-stimulating factors (GM-CSF) after specific activation in vitro (Titus et al 1984, Feng et al 1988). To exclude the possibility that these cell lines contained a mixture of T cells with different functional properties, cloned T-cell lines were derived from these homogeneous populations and their effect on the disease process and functional properties studied. Results of a representative experiment depicted in Figure 9.5, show that such T-cell clones led to exacerbation of cutaneous lesions after adoptive transfer to normal BALB/c mice (Titus et al in preparation). These T-cell clones expressed the CD4$^+$ T-cell surface phenotype and released IFN-γ after specific stimulation in vitro (Fig. 9.6). Taken together, these results indicate that some parasite-specific T cells exhibiting functional characteristics of Th-1 cells can promote disease progression. In contrast to these exacerbating T cells, a remarkable characteristic of the protective T-cell clones described above is that they appear to recognize antigen(s) associated only with live *L. major* parasites. It could be hypothesized that the capacity of

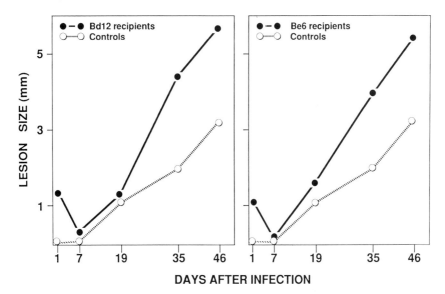

Figure 9.5 Exacerbation of cutaneous leishmaniasis by adoptive transfer of *L. major*-specific T cell clones. The size of lesion was monitored in groups of BALB/c mice injected with 1×10^7 *L. major* promastigotes ($\bigcirc$ - - - - $\bigcirc$) or with 1×10^7 *L. major* promastigotes and 2×10^6 of either (left) Bd 12 or (right) Be 6 cloned T cells ($\bullet$ – $\bullet$)

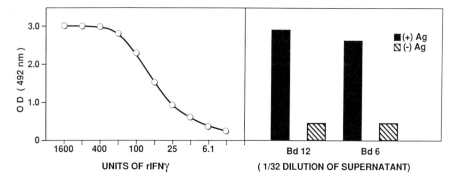

Figure 9.6 Interferon-γ secretion of 'exacerbating' *L. major*-specific T cell clones. Two exacerbating L3T4[+] T-cell clones (Bd6 2×10^4; Bd12 5×10^4) were incubated with syngeneic irradiated spleen cells (5×10^5) in the presence or absence of *L. major* promastigotes lysates (1×10^6), as a source of antigen, for 24 h. Afterwards, culture supernatants were removed and tested for IFN-γ content using a specific ELISA assay. In left panel: standard curve with r-IFN-γ

TH-1 parasite-specific T cells to protect mice against *L. major* infection also depends upon their fine specificity. It is tempting to speculate that the antigens recognized by protective CD4[+] T cells are preferentially expressed at the surface of infected macrophages containing multiplying microorganisms. It is possible that the failure of some T cells recognizing antigens present in a lysate of *L. major* promastigotes contributes to the resolution of lesions, is the consequence of the lack of presentation of these antigens by macrophages containing multiplying *L. major* amastigotes. Accordingly, these T cells would not be able to focus the IFN-γ that they release after activation, at the surface of parasitized macrophages. The inability of macrophages harbouring living amastigotes to present antigens in an extract of *L. major* promastigotes could result from a competition between peptides derived from proteins synthesized only by the intracellular amastigote form of *Leishmania* and other parasite antigens for binding to MHC class II molecules which are reduced at the surface of infected macrophages from susceptible mice (Handmann et al 1979, Reiner et al 1988). It is also possible that the capacity of macrophages to process and present antigen is modified by the presence of living intracellular organisms. Inasmuch as the majority of living *L. major* promastigotes are destroyed extremely rapidly after their s.c. injection into mice (Table 9.1), it is likely that the majority of parasite antigens presented at the start of infection derive from these degraded parasites and preliminary evidence exists which indicate that they might trigger T-cell responses detrimental to the host (Müller et al 1989).

Lymphokines
After specific activation in vitro, the CD4[+] T-cell lines capable of exacerbating cutaneous leishmaniasis were found to release, in addition to IFN-γ, substantial amounts of IL-3 and GM-CSF. In an attempt to assess whether or not such molecules, promoting the growth and differentiation of cells of the haemopoietic lineage including granulocytes and macrophages, were related to the capacity of these CD4[+] T cells to enhance the development of lesions, the effect of the administration of both recombinant IL-3 and GM-CSF on the course of

Table 9.1 Number of viable parasites in the lesion of mice infected with 5×10^6 _L. major_ promastigotes[a]

Time after injection (h)	Number of viable parasites per lesion ($\times 10^{-5}$)[b]	
	BALB/c	CBA
0	0.68	0.27
1.5	0.30	0.19
3	0.86	0.57
6	0.79	1.10
12	0.94	1.11
48	0.82	1.74
672	1750	5.14

[a]Stationary phase _L. major_ parasites (5×10^6) were injected s.c. into one hind footpad
[b]The numbers of viable parasites were determined by limiting dilution analysis and the frequency of viable parasites per nanogram of tissue was calculated according to Poisson statistics. The number of viable parasites per lesion was calculated by multiplying the number of parasites/g of footpad tissue by the average weight (g) of the footpad (Titus et al 1985)

cutaneous leishmaniasis was studied. The administration of both IL-3 (Feng et al 1988) and GM-CSF (Greil et al 1988) led to a significant enhancement of the size of lesions in genetically susceptible mice infected with _L. major_. This effect has been related to the capacity of these lymphokines to increase the pool of circulating mononuclear cells, the host cells in which _Leishmania_ multiply. It is therefore possible that exacerbation of cutaneous leishmaniasis by the $CD4^+$ T-cell lines described above results from their capacity to release molecules capable of increasing the pool of circulating mononuclear cells, the host cells in which _Leishmania_ multiply. Furthermore, it has been shown that this deleterious effect of $CD4^+$ T cells depended upon the continuous recruitment, to the site of infection, of blood-derived mononuclear phagocytes, in which parasites grow (Louis et al 1986). In addition, it has been reported recently that IL-3 completely abolished the activation of macrophages by IFN-γ by a mechanism still unknown (Liew 1989). Inasmuch as IL-3 has been shown to be released by both subsets of $CD4^+$ T cells (i.e. Th-1 and Th-2), this finding suggests that anti-Leishmania effector T cells belong to another category of $CD4^+$ T cells not secreting IL-3.

The severe disease that develops in susceptible BALB/c mice has been related to the expansion of Th-2 $CD4^+$ T cells preferentially secreting IL-4 after stimulation. Recent results indicate that this lymphokine plays a role in disease progression since the administration of anti-IL4 mAb to BALB/c mice significantly reduced the progression of lesions (Heinzel et al 1989). The mechanism(s) by which IL-4 favours the development of lesions and the growth of parasite in vivo is unclear since on the one hand it has been suggested that IL-4 also hampers the activation of macrophages by IFN-γ (Liew 1989) and, on the other hand, it has been shown that the capacity of macrophages to resist infection with amastigotes of _L. major_ in vitro required IFN-γ in combination with other lymphokines, including IL-4 (Belosevic et al 1988). In this context, IL-4 has been shown to increase the uptake and the killing by macrophages of another protozoan parasite, namely _Trypanosoma cruzi_ (Wirth et al 1989).

CONCLUSION

The course of disease after inoculation of mice with *L. major* appears to be greatly influenced by the specific T-cell responses triggered as a result of infection.

There is a consensus that healing of lesion and exacerbation of disease are, at least in part, the consequence of the activity of different parasite-specific CD4[+] T cells and the lymphokines they release. Results from several studies strongly suggest that CD4[+] cells belonging to the Th-1 subpopulation (i.e. secreting IFN-γ) are the protective cells which are preferentially induced during infection in genetically resistant mice. Recent observations indicate that parasite-specific Th-2 cells are expanding preferentially in susceptible animals and play a causal role in the severe disease seen in these mice.

Delineating the precise mechanism by which parasite-specific Th-2 cells promote susceptibility to this infection becomes very important and might reveal fundamental mechanisms operating in several infectious diseases. Analysis of the parameters accounting for the preferential expansion of cells from the Th-2 subset in susceptible mice and determining whether or not some leishmanial antigens selectively trigger Th-1 or Th-2 cells are areas of investigation extremely relevant for the design of a molecularly defined vaccine.

Evidence also exists that some T cells mediating protection and susceptibility belong to the Th-1 subset (i.e. release IFN-γ) but display different antigenic specificity. It is tempting to speculate that the ability of T cells to recognize antigens expressed by macrophages harbouring living parasites determines their protective capacity. T cells recognizing parasite antigens presented only by non-parasitized macrophages might not be able to concentrate the IFN-γ, that they release, on infected macrophages. This finding imposes an important requirement for *Leishmania*-specific Th-1 T cells in order to be protective.

Finally, it appears that CD8[+] T cells play a role in the immunological control of infection with *L. major* and it becomes important to study the parameters of their induction as well as the precise mechanism(s) by which they contribute to resolution of lesions.

ACKNOWLEDGEMENTS

Experimental work was supported by grants from the Swiss National Science Foundation, the UDNP/World Bank/WHO Special Programme for Research and Training in Tropical Diseases, the Roche Research Foundation and the Deutsche Forschungsgemeinschaft.

REFERENCES

Anderson S, David J R, McMahon-Pratt D 1983 In vivo protection against *Leishmania mexicana* mediated by monoclonal antibodies. J Immunol 131: 1616–1618
Belosevic M, Davis C E, Meltzer M, Nacy C A 1988 Regulation of activated macrophage antimicrobial activities. Identification of lymphokines that cooperate with IFN-γ for induction of resistance to infection. J Immunol 141: 890–896

Bogdan C, Streck H, Röllinghoff M, Solbach W 1989 Cyclosporin A enhances elimination of intracellular *L. major* parasites by murine macrophages. Clin Exp Immunol 75: 141–146

Champsi J, McMahon-Pratt D 1988 Membrane glycoprotein M-2 protects against *Leishmania amazonensis* infection. Infect Immun 56: 3272–3279

De Libero G, Kaufmann S H E 1986 Antigen-specific Lyt-2$^+$ cytolytic T lymphocytes from mice infected with the intracellular bacterium *Listeria monocytogenes.* J Immunol 137: 2688–2694

Farrell J, Müller I, Louis J A 1989 A role for Lyt-2$^+$ T cells in resistance to cutaneous leishmaniasis in immunized mice. J Immunol 142: 2052–2056

Feng Z, Louis J, Kindler V, Pedrazzini T, Eliason J, Behin R, Vassalli P 1988 Aggravation of experimental cutaneous leishmaniasis in mice by administration of interleukin 3. Eur J Immunol 18: 1245–1251

Fuzibet J G, Marty P, Taillan B, Bertrand F, Pras P, Pesce A, Le Fichoux Y, Dujarin P 1988 Is *Leishmania infantum* an opportunistic parasite in patients with anti-human immunodeficiency virus antibodies? Arch Intern Med 148: 1228

Greil J, Bodendorfer B, Röllinghoff M, Solbach W 1988 Application of recombinant granulocyte-macrophage colony-stimulating factor has a detrimental effect in experimental murine leishmaniasis. Eur J Immunol 18: 1527–1533

Handmann E, Ceredig R, Mitchell G F 1979 Murine cutaneous leishmaniasis: disease patterns in intact and nude mice of various genotypes and examinations of some differences between normal and infected macrophages. Aust J Exp Biol Med Sci 57: 9–30

Handmann E, Goding J W 1985 The *Leishmania* receptor for macrophages is a lipid-containing glycoconjugate. EMBO J 4: 329–396

Heinzel F P, Sadick M D, Holaday B J, Coffman R L, Locksley R M 1989 Reciprocal expression of interferon-γ or interleukin 4 during the resolution or progression of murine leishmaniasis. J Exp Med 169: 59–72

Kaufmann S H E, Hug E, De Libero G 1986a *Listeria monocytogenes*-reactive T lymphocyte clones with cytolytic activity against infected target cells. J Exp Med 164: 363–368

Kaufmann S H E, Chiplunkar S, Flesh I, De Libero G 1986b Possible role of helper and cytotoxic T cells in mycobacterial infections. Lepr Rev 57: (suppl. 2) 101–106

Kaye P M, Roberts M B, Blackwell J M 1987 Analysing the immune response to *L. donovani* infection. Ann Inst Pasteur/Immunol 138: 762–768

Liew F Y 1986 Cell-mediated immunity in experimental cutaneous leishmaniasis. Parasitol Today 2: 264–270

Liew F Y 1989 Functional heterogeneity of CD4$^+$ T cells in leishmaniasis. Immunol Today 10: 40–45

Liew F Y, Howard J G, Hale C 1984 Prophylactic immunization against experimental leishmaniasis. III. Protection against fatal *Leishmania tropica* infection induced by irradiated promastigotes involves Lyt 1$^+$2$^-$ T cells that do not mediate DTH. J Immunol 132: 456–461

Liew F Y, Hale C, Howard J G 1985a Prophylactic immunization against experimental leishmaniasis. IV. Subcutaneous immunization prevents the induction of protective immunity against fatal *Leishmania major* infection. J Immunol 135: 2095–2101

Liew F Y, Singleton A, Cillari E, Howard J G 1985b Prophylactic immunization against experimental leishmaniasis. V. Mechanism of the anti-protective blocking effect induced by subcutaneous immunization against *Leishmania major*. J Immunol 135: 2101–2107

Locksley R M, Heinzel F P, Sadick M D, Holaday B J, Gardner K D 1987 Murine cutaneous leishmaniasis: susceptibility correlates with differential expansion of helper T cell subsets. Ann Inst Pasteur/Immunol 138: 744–749

Louis J A, Mendonça S, Titus R G et al 1986 The role of specific T cell subpopulations in murine cutaneous leishmaniasis. In: Cinader B, Miller R G (eds) Progress in immunology, VI. Academic Press, New York, pp 762–769

Milon G, Titus R G, Cerottini J C, Marchal G, Louis J A 1986 Higher frequency of *Leishmania major* specific L3T4$^+$ T cells in susceptible BALB/c mice than in resistant CBA-mice. J Immunol 136: 1467–1471

Mirkovich A M, Galelli A, Allison A C, Modabber F Z 1986 Increased myelopoiesis during *L. major* infection in mice: generation of 'safe targets', a possible way to evade the effector immune mechanism. Clin Exp Immunol 64: 1–7

Mitchell G F 1984 Host-protective immunity and its suppression in a parasitic disease: murine cutaneous leishmaniasis. Immunol Today 5: 224–226

Mitchell G F, Curtis J M, Handmann E, McKenzie I F C 1980 Cutaneous leishmaniasis in mice: disease pattern in reconstituted nude mice of several genotypes infected with *Leishmania tropica*. Aust J Exp Biol Med Sci 58: 521–532

Mitchell G F, Handmann E, Moll H, McConville M J, Spithill T W, Kidane G Z, Samaras N, Elhay M J 1987 Resistance and susceptibility of mice to *Leishmania major*. A view from Melbourne. Ann Inst Pasteur/Immunol 138: 738–743

Modabber F 1987 The leishmaniasis. In: Maurice J, Pearce A M (eds) Tropical disease research. A global partnership, 8th Programme Report of the UNDP/World Bank/WHO special programme for research and training in tropical diseases. WHO, Geneva, pp 99–112

Moll H, Scollay R, Mitchell 1988 Resistance to cutaneous leishmaniasis in nude mice injected with L3T4+ T cells but not with Lyt 2+ T cells. Immunol Cell Biol 66: 57–61

Mossmann I R, Cherwinski I I, Bond M W, Giedlin M A, Coffman R L 1986 Two types of murine helper T cell clone. I. Definition according to profiles of lymphokine activities and secreted proteins. J Immunol 136: 2348–2357

Mossman T R, Coffman R L 1987 Two types of mouse helper T cell clone. Implications for immune regulation. Immunol Today 8: 223–227

Müller I, Louis J A 1989 Immunity to experimental infection with *Leishmania major*: Generation of protective L3T4+ T cell clones recognizing antigen(s) associated with live parasites. Eur J Immunol 19: 865–871

Müller I, Cobbold S P, Waldmann H, Kaufmann S H E 1987 Impaired resistance to *Mycobacterium tuberculosis* infection after selective in vivo depletion of L3T4+ and Lyt 2+ T cells. Infect Immun 55: 2037–2041

Müller I, Pedrazzini Th, Farrell J P, Louis J A 1989 T cell responses and immunity to experimental infection with *Leishmania major*. Annu Rev Immunol 7: 561–578

Nathan C F, Murray H W, Wiebe M E, Rubin B Y 1983 Identification of interferon-γ as the lymphokine that activates human macrophages oxidative metabolism and antimicrobial activity. J Exp Med 158: 670–689

Ralph P, Nacy C A, Meltzer M S, Williams N, Nakoinz I, Leonard E J 1983 Colony-stimulating factors and regulation of macrophage tumoricidal and microbicidal activities. Cell Immunol 76: 10–21

Reiner N E, Ng W, McMaster W R 1987 Parasite-accessory cell interactions in murine leishmaniasis. II *Leishmania donovani* suppresses macrophages expression of class I and class II major histocompatibility complex gene products. J Immunol 138: 1926–1932

Reiner N E, Ng W, Ma T, McMaster W R 1988 Kinetics of interferon binding and induction of major histocompatibility complex class II mRNA in *Leishmania*-infected macrophages. Proc Natl Acad Sci USA 85: 4330–4334

Russel D G, Alexander J 1988 Effective immunization against cutaneous leishmaniasis with defined membrane antigens reconstituted into liposomes. J Immunol 140: 1274–1279

Sadick M D, Locksley R M, Tubbs C, Raff H V 1986 Murine cutaneous leishmaniasis: Resistance correlates with the capacity to generate interferon-γ in response to *Leishmania* antigens in vitro. J Immunol 136: 655–661

Sadick M D, Heinzel F P, Shigekane V N, Fisher W L, Locksley R M 1987 Cellular and humoral immunity to *Leishmania major* in genetically susceptible mice following in vivo depletion of L3T4+ cells. J Immunol 139: 1303–1309

Scott P, Pearce E, Natovitz P, Sher A 1987 Vaccination against cutaneous leishmaniasis in a murine model. II. Immunologic properties of protective and non-protective subfractions of a soluble promastigote extract. J Immunol 139: 3118–3125

Scott P, Natovitz P, Coffman R L, Pearce E, Sher A 1988 Immunoregulation of cutaneous leishmaniasis: T cell lines that transfer protective immunity or exacerbation belong to different T helper subsets and respond to distinct parasite antigens. J Exp Med 168: 1675–1684

Solbach W, Forberg K, Kammerer E, Bogdan C, Röllinghoff M 1986 Suppressive effect of cyclosporin A on the development of *Leishmania tropica* induced lesions in genetically susceptible BALB/c mice. J Immunol 137: 702–707

Titus R G, Lima G C, Engers H D, Louis J A 1984 Exacerbation of murine cutaneous leishmaniasis by adoptive transfer of parasite-specific helper T cell populations capable of mediating *Leishmania major*-specific delayed type hypersensitivity. J Immunol 133: 1594–1600

Titus R G, Kelso A, Louis J A 1984 Intracellular destruction of *Leishmania tropica* by macrophages activated with macrophage activating factor/interferon. Clin Exp Immunol 55: 157–165

Titus R G, Marchand M, Boon T, Louis J A 1985 A limiting dilution assay for quantifying *Leishmania major* in tissue of infected mice. Parasite Immunol 7: 545–555

Titus R G, Ceredig R, Cerottini J C, Louis J A 1985 Therapeutic effect of anti-L3T4 monoclonal antibody GK1.5 on cutaneous leishmaniasis in genetically susceptible BALB/c mice. J Immunol 135: 2108–2114

Titus R G, Milon G, Marchal G, Vassalli P, Cerottini J C, Louis J A 1987 Involvement of specific Lyt 2+ T cells in the immunological control of experimentally induced murine cutaneous leishmaniasis. Eur J Immunol 17: 1429–1433

Wirth J J, Kierszenbaum F, Zlotnik A 1989 Effects of IL-4 on macrophage functions: increased uptake and killing of a protozoan parasite (*Trypanosoma cruzi*). Immunology 66: 296–301

172

Discussion of papers presented by R. M. Locksley and J. A. Louis

Discussed by J. M. Blackwell and R. Lane
Reported by S. Britton

Both papers in this section have made clear that, in response to a *Leishmania major* challenge, mice can mount a CD4$^+$ T-cell response of two functional types: (1) genetically resistant mice (C57BL and CBA background) preferentially generate a Th-1 response, i.e. CD4$^+$ cells which respond with gamma-interferon secretion when challenged with *Leishmania* antigen; (2) susceptible mice (BALBc background) preferentially produce a Th-2 response, which is characterized by IL-4 production. There was little variation in data between the two papers on this point except in Louis's paper where Th-1 cells secreted gamma-interferon in response to antigen, and were disease promoting. It should be noted that cells were selected in vitro. Whether they are activated in vivo is unknown. Thus, there might be discernible subgroups of Th-1 cells – some being protective, others not. It was pointed out that the form of antigen presentation was very important for the outcome of the Th-1 response. Soluble promastigote antigens tended to stimulate a disease-promoting Th-1 response, whereas live promastigotes, particularly if grown at 37°C for some time, gave rise to a protective Th-1 response. Presumably, these experiments indicate that the protective response is generated through the intracellular amastigote form of the parasite.

ARE THERE FUNCTIONALLY DIFFERENT CD4$^+$ SUBSETS IN MAN?

The first issue addressed during the discussion was whether this functional subdivision of CD4$^+$ cells had any counterpart in man and, indeed, in human leishmaniasis. It was reported that lymphocytes from kala-azar patients with progressive disease exposed to *Leishmania* antigens show no gamma-interferon response. However, after successful treatment for leishmaniasis, lymphocytes from those same patients showed a very substantial gamma-interferon response to the same antigen preparation. Thus, looking positively, there seems to be an analogous situation in man. There were no reports about a preferential secreted IL-4 response from antigen-exposed CD4$^+$ T cells of heavily parasitized men. Using the PCR technique, however, the IL-4 response could be detected and very preliminary data seemed to indicate that it was quantitatively correlated with disease progression. The high prevalence of concomitant helminthic infections would complicate the interpretation of elevated IL-4 concentrations.

CD4$^+$ SUBSETS AND VACCINE DEVELOPMENT

Clearly, if we have disease-promoting and disease-inhibiting CD4$^+$ T cells, it must be mandatory to test any vaccine candidate – be it of parasitic or any other origin – for the type of response it will elicit. From the ongoing vaccine trials with killed *Leishmania* promastigotes in Venezuela it was reported that vaccinees converted their skin reactivity to a larger extent than they changed their reactivity in a lymphocyte transformation assay. This fits with data from various mouse models where DTH reactive cells can be clearly dissociated from protective cells. A possible method of testing vaccine antigens for CMI stimulatory capacity was reported where SDS-PAGE separated promastigote antigens had been attached to a nitrocellulose filter in a two-dimensional system and, following elution, the various antigen preparations had been exposed to lymphocytes from patients naturally exposed to *Leishmania*. It was shown that several of these antigen preparations produced a gamma-interferon response, measurable in 2×10^5 effector cells.

A promising murine model now seems likely since, apparently for the first time, it is possible to show protection in a mouse model using *L. donovani* as the pathogen. At the Department of Parasitology, London School of Hygiene and Tropical Medicine, preparations of *Leishmania donovani* amastigotes prepared essentially as above, i.e. eluted from SDS-separated antigens on nitrocellulose filters, have been used to immunize mice before a challenge with live parasites. Several of these nitrocellulose particulated antigen preparations made the mice counteract the infection much faster than normal mice.

Thus there seems to be a murine model in which antigen preparations for the most relevant human *Leishmania* pathogen can be tested in vivo. These protection data can then be correlated with data on the cytokine and proliferative responses of antigen-exposed lymphocytes.

Certainly, any vaccine candidate in the future has to be tested in a functional T-cell assay where parameters such as proliferation, secretion of gamma-interferon, IL-2, IL-4 and other cytokines can be measured. Prior selection of antigens by antibodies, as with the Western blot system, may not be adequate as it is by no means clear that protective T cells recognize the same antigen epitopes.

A word of caution was added about extrapolating mouse models to man. As an example of this, a limited vaccine trial in humans was cited where non-pathogenic *Leishmania* promastigotes failed to protect against an injection of live *L. major* promastigotes although lymphocytes from these recipients showed a very good proliferative response to *L. major* antigens as a result of the previous exposure to the non-pathogenic *Leishmania*. It was agreed, however, that this was an expected outcome in light of the very low cross-protective capacity of different *Leishmania* strains. It also shows that antigen-specific lymphocyte proliferation does not always equate with protection but needs to be complemented by, for example, cytokine production.

MECHANISM OF SELECTION OF Th-1 VERSUS Th-2 RESPONSES

Leishmania-resistant mice produce preferentially an inhibiting Th-1 response, whereas susceptible mice produce a disease-promoting Th-2 response. Data so far seem to indicate that the division point is at the T cell level as this can be modulated by anti $CD4^+$ antibodies which in the mouse are not represented on monocytes and macrophages as they are in man. So far, this question must be left unanswered as in most other responder/non-responder systems the site of action is at the macrophage level. Indirect evidence that antigen presentation is of importance came from the reported data where soluble *Leishmania* promastigote antigens selectively stimulated disease-promoting Th-1 cells. Indeed, if animals were made tolerant to these antigens such disease-promoting response was no longer generated. Thus, an important remaining component in these studies is to determine whether *Leishmania* antigens may preferentially induce one or the other T cell response before or after macrophage processing. Clearly, both types of T cells can be generated in both susceptible and resistant mice and thus there must be a genetically non-H-2-linked process determining how to select each type of response. Until proved to the contrary, a macrophage-linked difference in antigen processing must be one possibility.

There has been virtually no work done on the antigen-binding specificity of the Th-1 versus the Th-2 cells nor is there any information on their respective degree of antigen restriction in cell-mediated effector assays.

GENERAL ASPECTS ON CONTROL OF *Leishmania* INFECTION

There was no agreement as to whether promastigote or amastigote antigens would be preferentially used as protective antigens. Most work so far has been on promastigotes as these are more easily available. From an entomologist's perspective it was pointed out that promastigotes are injected into humans from the sandfly, in a metacyclic form; this is a stationary phase showing a distinct profile with regard to lipophosphoglycan and glycoprotein surface molecules. These change considerably in promastigotes in an active growth phase which thus may represent an immunologically irrelevant form of the promastigote.

The number of promastigotes injected by each infected sandfly appears to be very small per bite, i.e. from 20 to 200. However, the sandfly saliva contains growth-promoting substances which appear essential for a successful infection. Work is going on to isolate the material in the sandfly saliva that is the promoter of promastigote survival. This substance appears to be similar in the many subspecies of sandflies which serve as vectors for *Leishmania* parasites. If such a substance is immunogenic in man it could actually be tried as an immunogen which would prevent promastigotes reaching their target cells.

Finally, it was pointed out that control of leishmaniasis in its visceral or cutaneous forms must be individualized as the epidemiology appears to differ in different parts of the world. For example, in China very successful eradication programmes had been reported where the approach had been mainly the elimination of the primary host (dogs), insecticides (DDT) and intensive chemotherapy of infected individuals. Clearly, such approaches cannot be taken in all parts of the world but they do indicate that this human disease can be stopped successfully with specifically targeted action.

Section IV: Schistosomiasis

Chairman: M. Capron

10. Idiotype networks in schistosomiasis

D. G. Colley   M. A. Montesano
S. M. Eloi-Santos   M. R. Powell   J. C. Parra
A. Goes B. L. Doughty   R. Correa-Oliveira
R. S. Rocha and G. Gazzinelli

INTRODUCTION

Recent studies in experimental and clinical schistosomiasis have demonstrated idiotypic/anti-idiotypic (Id/anti-Id) interactions, some of which correlate with the presence or absence of immunoregulatory events, clinical morbidity and/or resistance. The development of prominent Id/anti-Id interactions has been predicted, based on two epidemiological characteristics of schistosomiasis. First, age-prevalence curves show that schistosomal infections have their highest prevalence during the early child-bearing years. Thus, infections must occur in many pregnant women in endemic areas. This leads to intra-uterine and neonatal opportunities for schistosome antigens and idiotypes, related to a mother's antischistosome immune responses, to influence her child's developing immune repertoire. Second, the chronicity of schistosomiasis leads to long-term, continuous stimulation of antischistosomal immune responses. This provides increased opportunities for anti-Id responses against the chronically expressed idiotypes of the receptors and combining sites on these specific cellular and humoral reactants. This paper will present evidence that Id/anti-Id interactions develop in the maternal/neonatal setting, and occur during the chronic stages of infection. During chronic infection, they can be involved in the regulation of potential immunopathological processes. Furthermore, the occurrence of certain Ids correlates with the absence of severe disease. We hypothesize that the presence and nature of the Id/anti-Id responses during schistosomiasis, which may be determined by perinatal exposure to Ids, influence the clinical outcome of the infection.

INVOLVEMENT OF REGULATORY IDIOTYPIC RESPONSES IN EXPERIMENTAL MODEL SYSTEMS

The immunopathogenesis of experimental schistosomiasis mansoni is largely attributed to cellular immune reactivities against soluble schistosome egg antigens (SEA) (Warren 1982), and the control of these responses has been shown to be primarily mediated by cellular immunoregulation (Colley 1981, Phillips & Lammie 1986). A link between this regulation and Id/anti-Id interactions was found when it was shown that a T-suppressor factor activity capable of modulating schisto-some egg-induced granuloma formation possessed anti-Id characteristics (Abe & Colley 1984).

Furthermore, anti-Id plaque-forming cells (PFC) which make auto-anti-Id antibodies specific for Ids expressed on anti-SEA antibodies can be detected in the spleens of *S. mansoni*-infected mice (Powell & Colley 1985). A strong inverse relationship ($p < 0.001$) exists between the presence of anti-SEA antibodies in the sera and anti-anti-SEA PFC in the spleens of individual mice (Fig. 10.1). This inverse correlation was observed by plotting the number of splenic reverse PFCs in the spleens of individual CBA/J mice infected for 8–16 weeks vs the anti-SEA ELISA values obtained using the serum from each spleen donor. The reverse PFCs were developed using immunoaffinity-purified anti-SEA antibodies from the sera of CBA/J mice with *S. mansoni* infections of ≥ 16 weeks' duration, after subtrac-tion of the number of PFCs in the PBS control (Powell & Colley 1985). The data indicate that a mouse that exhibits a high level of anti-SEA antibodies in its serum has reciprocally fewer anti-Id PFCs against anti-SEA antibodies in its spleen. Auto-anti-Id T cells are also demonstrable in the lymph nodes of *S. mansoni*-infected mice (Powell & Colley 1987, see below).

Anti-SEA antibodies from mice infected with *S. japonicum* have been shown to express a major cross-reactive Id (CRI). An anti-Id mAb (monoclonal antibody)

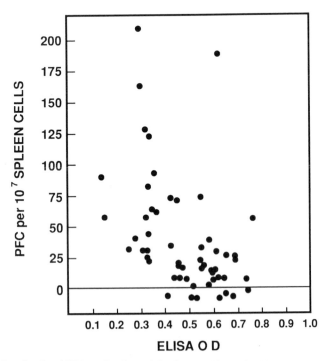

Figure 10.1 Levels of anti-SEA antibodies (Id) in the sera (determined by ELISA) vs the number of anti-Id PFC per 1×10^7 spleen cells (minus the number of control PFC in PBS) from mice infected with *S. mansoni* for 8–16 weeks. The *p* value of the inverse correlation of the parameters is < 0.001

against this Id can mediate strong regulation of granuloma formation (Olds & Kresina 1985). The expression of this Id by the antibodies from infected mice is greatest 6 weeks after infection and decreases beyond this time. Splenic B lymphocytes express this Id during acute infection (5–10 weeks). However, the CRI can be detected on the surface membranes of some thymocytes until 15 weeks after infection (Kresina & Olds 1986).

Other investigators have described Id/anti-Id involvement in immune-mediated resistance to schistosome infection. Both immunization by an anti-Id vaccine (Grzych et al 1985) and resistance-regulating Id/anti-Id interactions (Phillips et al 1986, Percy & Harn 1988, Phillips et al 1988) have been demonstrated. Thus, Id/anti-Id interactions develop during experimental schistosomiasis, and participate in phenomena which may impinge on, or contribute to, both protective responses and pathogenesis.

THE RESPONSE OF AUTO-ANTI-IDIOTYPIC T LYMPHOCYTES FROM PATIENTS TO PATIENTS' ANTI-SEA ANTIBODIES

We have reported an experimental approach which demonstrates the anti-Id responsiveness of anti-Id T lymphocytes in the peripheral blood mononuclear cells (PBMC) of patients with schistosomiasis (Lima et al 1986). All studies of human subjects were preceded by appropriate discussions with the patients and were done only if informed consent was obtained from the patients or their guardians. The manipulations of patients' PBMCs and sera, on which the system is based, are systematically presented in Figure 10.2. In this anti-Id T cell system, anti-SEA antibodies are immunoaffinity-purified from the sera of patients with schistosomiasis on antigen (Ag) columns. Patients' PBMCs are then cultured in the presence of these antibodies, and if there are T cells in the culture which are specific for specificities expressed on the antibodies (considered to be the Ids of those antibodies), proliferative (Blast) responses result. Monoclonal anti-SEA Abs are from mouse or human hybridomas. The Ids (anti-SEA Abs or mAbs) are also used to stimulate rabbit anti-Ids (rendered Id-specific by absorptions on normal human immunoglobulins (NIg)) and/or mouse anti-Id mAbs, which are used in competitive ELISAs. Not all anti-SEA preparations stimulate in this system, and not all patients have PBMCs which are stimulated by all stimulatory anti-SEA preparations (Table 10.1). It is possible to stimulate anti-Id T cells by culturing them with some anti-SEA human mAbs (Table 10.1) (Colley et al 1987), and even some mouse anti-SEA mAbs (Colley et al 1989). The production of hybridomas which have yielded these human mAbs has been described previously (Doughty et al 1987).

PBMCs from individuals who do not have, and never have had, schistosomiasis are not stimulated by anti-SEA antibodies, and normal human immunoglobulin preparations do not stimulate PBMCs from either schistosomiasis patients or uninfected individuals (Lima et al 1986). The specificity of the requirement for anti-SEA antibodies has been demonstrated by observing that anti-epimastigote antibodies, immunoaffinity-purified from the sera of patients with Chagas' disease, do not stimulate PBMC from patients with schistosomiasis, unless they also have Chagas' disease. The reverse is also true (Gazzinelli et al 1988).

Table 10.1 Responses of PBMC from patients with schistosomiasis mansoni, or former patients, upon exposure to *S. mansoni* soluble egg antigen (SEA), pooled anti-SEA antibodies from patients with schistosomiasis (anti-SEA Ids), or human anti-SEA monoclonal antibodies (anti-SEA Hu mAb)

Patient number	SEA	anti-SEA Ids	anti-SEA Hu mAb		
			E5	A7	F3
B1	26 506	17 945	43 167	485	713
B2	5 884	12 053	645	135	161
B3	16 121	19 488	5 106	9 554	9 365
B4	2 678	8 892	<C	<C	281
B5	1 859	36 049	110	152	65
B6	23 714	44 108	100 910	<C	<C
B7	1 374	28 513	–	–	–
B8	4 430	13 358	–	–	–
B9	48 535	6 328	–	–	–

Experimental minus control (E-C) values in counts/min. Mean C counts/min $\pm$ s.e.m.: 1164 ± 351

Examination of the mode of stimulation of anti-Id T cells by anti-SEA preparations shows that these molecules stimulate T cells in the presence of chloroquine (i.e. without 'antigen processing') and in the absence of HLA antigens. However, proliferation does require a source of IL-1 (Parra et al 1988).

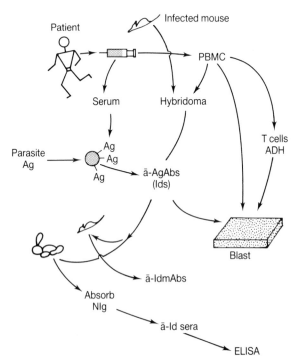

Figure 10.2 Diagram to illustrate the preparation and use of anti-SEA Abs (Ids) from patients and mice, the demonstration of patients' anti-Id T cells (Blast), and the production of anti-Id reagents

EVIDENCE FOR MATERNAL/NEONATAL IDIOTYPIC INFLUENCES IN HUMAN SCHISTOSOMIASIS

During gestation and breast feeding, children born to and/or fed by infected mothers are potentially exposed to circulating schistosome antigens (Carlier et al 1975, Santoro et al 1977, Nash & Deelder 1985, Feldmeier et al 1986) and their mothers' antischistosomal IgG antibodies. Prenatal sensitization and/or the induction of unresponsiveness has been demonstrated in experimental and clinical schistosomiasis (Lewert & Mandlowitz 1969, Hang et al 1974, Camus et al 1976, Tachon & Borojevic 1978) and another chronic, endemic helminthic disease, filariasis (Haque & Capron 1982, Weil et al 1983). High levels of the mothers' antischistosome antibodies have been documented in neonates born of *S. mansoni*-infected mothers (Lees & Jordan 1968, Hillyer et al 1970). However, these antibodies usually disappear from the newborn's circulation prior to the time of initial exposure of the child to infectious cercariae and infection. Therefore, the maternal antibodies appear not to offer any direct assistance to the child in regard to antibody-mediated resistance mechanisms against schistosome infections. Instead, the Ids expressed by these antibodies may exert their effects by having influenced the immune status of the child during gestation and development. Certainly in experimental studies of idiotypic interactions, such a situation is known to have profound influences on the immunological repertoire subsequently expressed by the offspring (Bona 1981, Kohler et al 1984, Stein & Soderstrom 1984, Takemori & Rajewsky 1984, Kearney & Vakil 1986, Freitas et al 1988).

We have now found that cord blood mononuclear cells (CBMC) from neonates born of mothers with schistosomiasis respond to purified anti-SEA antibodies (Table 10.2). It thus appears that anti-Id T cells develop in children prenatally, if the mother has an active schistosome infection. Anti-SEA antibodies which are stimulatory for CBMC from neonates born of infected mothers can be derived from their own mothers, or from serum pools from suitable patients (Eloi-Santos et al in press). For reasons which are not yet known, anti-SEA antibodies purified from the sera of the mothers collected during the latter half of the pregnancy usually do not stimulate neonatal CBMC, at least not under the conditions used to date (Eloi-Santos et al in press). Anti-SEA antibodies from sera obtained during a

Table 10.2 Responses of CBMC from neonates born of mothers with schistosomiasis or uninfected, upon exposure to an anti-SEA antibody pool or other immunoglobulin preparations

Stimulant	Mothers' condition			
	Schistosomiasis			Uninfected
	A	B	C	D
Anti-SEA	52 108	9 037	13 010	2 960
Ig Preps	92	208	4 186	1 908

Data given as E-C values in counts/min. Mean C value = 1669 ± 1031 s.d.
Ig Preps indicates that the immunoglobulins added were either antibodies purified from infected, gravid women late in their pregnancies or normal human immunoglobulin (Sigma). All antibody or Ig preparations were added to cultures at comparable concentrations (i.e. a final concentration of 40–60 μg/ml of protein/culture). A, B, C or D indicate CBMC responses of individual neonates

mother's first trimester of pregnancy are almost always stimulatory for the CMBC of her child at parturition (data not shown).

The actual consequences, if any, of having been born of a mother with active schistosomiasis, and having developed anti-Id T cells prior to birth, against the mother's idiotypes, are not yet known. However, the opportunity for these inter-actions to have long-range influences on the responsiveness and repertoire of the immune system are considerable. When a child born of an infected mother later becomes infected (which most often occurs several years later) (Jordan 1985), these altered responses may be anamnestically revived. This could result in consequences upon infection which differ from those generated by persons from outside endemic areas (who are usually not born of infected mothers).

IDIOTYPIC CORRELATIONS WITH CLINICAL FORMS OF HUMAN *SCHISTOSOMA MANSONI* INFECTION

Anti-SEA antibodies purified from patients' sera, pooled according to the clinical form of the donor patients, differ idiotypically as judged by both their abilities to stimulate PBMC proliferation and their recognition by anti-Id rabbit sera (Montesano et al 1989). As seen in Figure 10.3, anti-SEA antibodies prepared from patients with either the asymptomatic (Intestinal, INT) form (AM1, AM5) or the hepatointestinal (HI) form (AM7) of the infection, are stimulatory to PBMC of patients with either INT, HI or hepatosplenic (HS) infections. If, however, anti-SEA antibodies of comparable SEA-binding ability are prepared

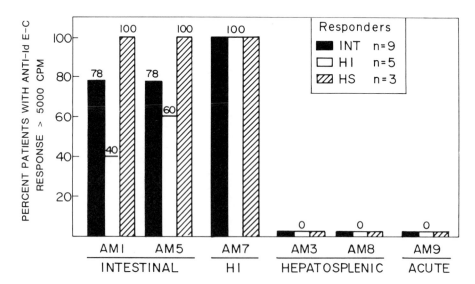

Figure 10.3 Percentage of patients with either asymptomatic, intestinal (INT, ■), hepatointestinal (HI, □) or hepatosplenic (HS, ▨) schistosomiasis mansoni who responded well (E-C counts/min > 5000) to anti-SEA antibodies from pooled sera from patients with INT (AM1, AM5), HI (AM7), HS (AM3, AM8) or acute (AM9) schistosomiasis mansoni. This figure is derived from data presented in Montesano et al 1989

from either HS patients (AM3, AM8) or those with acute (2–4 month) infections (AM9), these do not stimulate PBMC from INT, HI or HS patients.

Comparisons of anti-SEA antibodies from two different groups of INT patients have led to a disparate finding. Table 10.3 demonstrates that two different anti-SEA antibodies preparations, AM4 and AM-α from children (≤ 13 years of age) with chronic INT infections, fail to stimulate PBMCs from either children or adults with the INT form. However, the PBMCs of such children are stimulated by exposure to anti-SEA antibodies from adult chronic INT patients (AM1, AM5). Use of increased concentrations of AM4 or AM-α failed to alter their inability to stimulate (data not shown). The patients in both groups (adults and children) had been infected for years, albeit (based on epidemiological data from most endemic areas; Jordan 1985) the chronic infections of the children were probably of shorter duration than most of those of the adults. Such a distinct difference in the abilities of their anti-SEA antibodies to stimulate anti-Id PBMCs cells seems to indicate that younger patients lack antibodies which express stimulatory Ids. Yet, the detection of PBMCs in their circulation which mount a detectable response when cultured with appropriate stimulatory anti-SEA antibodies indicates the presence of suitable, expanded clones of anti-Id T cells. It is possible that these clones are the result of the earlier, intra-uterine expansion/sensitization phenomena discussed above.

Rabbits exposed to the anti-SEA preparations AM1, AM5 or AM8, respond by production of antibodies which, after appropriate absorption on normal human IgG columns, discern between AM1 and AM8, and AM5 and AM8, but not AM1 and AM5 (Montesano et al 1989) (Figure 10.2). Competitive ELISA systems using these antibodies and the specific antisera against them show that AM1 and AM5 (both from INT patients) share almost identical pools of cross-reactive Ids (CRI). The Ids expressed on the anti-SEA antibodies which comprise AM7 (from HI patients) are partially shared with AM1 and AM5. AM3 and AM8 (from HS patients) share some Ids with AM1 and AM5, but do so to a much lesser extent. AM9 (from acute patients) does not compete at all with AM1, AM5 or AM8, in

Table 10.3 PBMC responses of adults and children with chronic, intestinal schistosomiasis to pooled anti-SEA antibodies prepared from sera of adults or children with chronic, intestinal schistosomiasis

Patients		Source of Anti-SEA preparations			
		Adults		Children	
		AM1	AM5	AM4	AM-α
Adults	A	23 109	24 559	574	–
	B	20 243	23 096	< C	< C
	C	15 405	26 678	673	1 065
	D	16 541	9 906	199	–
Children	A	25 075	–	108	1 198
	B	25 748	–	< C	< C
	C	42 199	–	438	905
	D	15 237	–	49	35

E-C values in counts/min. Children ≤ 13 years of age

their respective competitive ELISAs. Only AM3 competes to any degree in the AM8/anti-AM8 competitive ELISA. AM3 and AM8 were each prepared from totally separate pools of sera from different HS patients.

The human anti-SEA mAb E5 (Table 10.1) has also been tested in these competitive ELISAs, and is seen to compete to approximately 20–25% with the AM1/anti-AM1 and AM5/anti-AM5 systems (data not shown). E5 is completely non-competitive in the AM8/anti-AM8 (HS patients) ELISA. These data should be considered with those in Table 10.1 that demonstrate that E5 can be stimulatory from PBMC, and earlier data that show E5 stimulates immunoregulation of anti-SEA responses (Doughty et al 1987, see next section). Together, these results indicate that E5 expresses CRI identical to a sizeable proportion of the anti-SEA-related Ids in chronic, adult INT patients' sera. The converse is that the E5 CRI are not represented in HS patients' sera.

HUMAN ANTI-ID RESPONSES AS IMMUNOREGULATORY MECHANISMS

Exposure of PBMCs or T cells to anti-SEA antibodies from adult INT patients, and some anti-SEA mAbs, leads to proliferation (Lima et al 1986, Parra et al 1988, Table 10.1). When the responding cells are from INT patients, one consequence of this stimulation is an ability to suppress in vitro granuloma formation against SEA-coated beads by autologous PBMC (Table 10.4; Colley et al 1989, Sher & Colley in press) or T cells (Doughty et al 1987). Several points about this Id-stimulated induction of immunoregulatory function can be seen in Table 10.4. The induction of this anti-Id suppressor function is dependent on the concentration of

Table 10.4 Anti-SEA Id induction of granuloma modulation of PBMC from intestinal (asymptomatic) or former patients, but not PBMC from hepatosplenic patients

Patient	Anti-SEA	[conc.]	Granuloma index
A (FP)	–		3.5 ± 0.1
	Id-A	150 µg	1.5 ± 0.1
	E5 (mAb)	150 µg	1.3 ± 0.1
B (INT)	–		3.5 ± 0.2
	Id-A	25 µg	3.2 ± 0.2
	Id-A	75 µg	2.6 ± 0.2
	Id-A	150 µg	2.2 ± 0.2
C (HS)	–		4.5 ± 0.4
	Id-A	25 µg	4.8 ± 0.2
	Id-A	75 µg	4.7 ± 0.2
	Id-A	150 µg	4.5 ± 0.1
D (HS)	–		2.6 ± 0.4
	Id-B	250 µg	2.6 ± 0.2
	Id-C	250 µg	2.7 ± 0.5

Data given as mean granuloma index $\pm$ s.d. (Doughty et al 1987).
Patient A, former INT case; Patient B, chronic INT case; Patients C and D, decompensated HS cases. PBMC were pre-incubated 24 h alone (–) or with anti-SEA antibodies (Id-A, Id-B and Id-C: from three different pools of adult INT patient sera or E5: human anti-SEA mAb) at the concentrations indicated, then washed and co-cultured with autologous PBMC and SEA-coated beads for granuloma formation

anti-SEA antibodies used during the 24-h pre-incubation, and it can be stimulated by anti-SEA mAbs (Table 10.4, Patient A; mAb E5). This anti-Id suppression is the characteristic response of cells from both former INT patients and chronic INT patients, but cells from decompensated HS patients do not react by mounting this regulatory response. As seen in Figure 10.3, HS patients' PBMCs proliferate when exposed to these Id preparations, but it appears that their response does not lead to functional suppression of an anti-SEA response.

EXPRESSION OF CROSS-REACTIVE, SHARED IDIOTYPES OF ANTI-SEA ANTIBODIES FROM HUMANS AND MICE WITH SCHISTOSOMIASIS

We have reported preliminary data which show that some mouse anti-SEA mAbs can stimulate PBMC from patients (Colley et al 1989), and are therefore hypothesized to express CRI. Using E5-specific rabbit antisera in an E5/anti-E5 competitive ELISA (Figure 10.2), we have screened sera from normal or *S. mansoni*-infected mice at different times after infection. The ability of sera from infected mice (8 and 16 weeks after infection) to compete with E5 in this system (Table 10.5) indicates that some of the antibodies in the sera from infected mice bear CRI which compete with those expressed on E5, and are recognized by the absorbed antisera from an E5-immunized rabbit. Remembering that E5 shares CRI with a reasonable proportion of the anti-SEA antibodies from INT patients, these preliminary competitive ELISA data imply that some mouse anti-SEA related Ids are the same as some INT patients' anti-SEA Ids. In fact, mouse sera and immunoaffinity-purified mouse anti-SEA antibodies do compete in the AM1/anti-AM1 and AM5/anti-AM5 ELISAs (data not shown). Furthermore, AM1 and AM5 can stimulate proliferation of spleen cells and lymph node cells from mice infected for 8 and 16 weeks (data not shown).

In our earlier demonstration of auto-anti-Id T cells in infected mice (Powell & Colley 1987), we observed that anti-SEA antibodies from mice with chronic infections (≥ 16 weeks) stimulated lymph node cells from mice with 8-week infections more (and more consistently) than those from mice infected for either 12

Table 10.5 Competitive inhibition of E5/anti-E5 ELISA by sera from mice infected with *S. mansoni*

Serum dilution	Weeks of infection				
	0	8	16	20–30	30–40
1/64	0.467	0.467	0.466	0.465	0.466
1/32	0.466	0.466	0.466	0.467	0.465
1/16	0.465	0.463	0.465	0.466	0.466
1/8	0.466	**0.453**	0.466	0.464	0.466
1/4	0.466	**0.439**	**0.457**	0.465	0.466
1/2	0.463	**0.423**	**0.444**	**0.460**	0.463

Data given as OD at 405 nM
Values which differ from normal mouse serum values, at any given dilution, are underlined

or 16 weeks. Based on anti-SEA Id expression, as evaluated by Id/anti-Id competitive ELISA, it seems that mice also express more Ids comparable to the human stimulatory Ids at the earlier times (Table 10.5). Further studies concerning the expression of CRI on anti-SEA antibodies from infected mice and men will need to carefully address the kinetics of Id expression during murine infection (Kresina & Olds 1986).

DISCUSSION AND CONCLUSIONS

We and others have predicted the occurrence of auto-Id/anti-Id interactions in schistosomiasis, and other chronic, endemic infections. It is now clear that these internal humoral and cellular immunological responses do develop. Perinatal exposure to maternal schistosome-related Ids, as well as schistosomal antigens, occurs, and impacts on the immune responsiveness of neonates born to mothers who harbour the infection at the time of their pregnancy. It seems likely that, due to these alterations during early development, children born to infected mothers, in an endemic environment, may well respond differently upon subsequent exposure and infection, than if they had been born to uninfected mothers. In schistosomiasis, host immune responses are directly involved in both resistance and pathogenesis, and these perinatal immune interactions could, therefore, manifest themselves in regard to either or both phenomena. It is known, for example, that most individuals who develop severe morbidity with acute schistosomal infection are visitors to endemic areas from non-endemic areas (von Lichtenberg 1987), and would most probably have been born to uninfected mothers. The pathogenesis of acute morbidity is often ascribed to the expression of a transient hypersensitivity state (Colley 1981, Colley 1987, von Lichtenberg 1987), which is then self-regulated. While cause and effect have not been studied (and certainly not proven), it seems possible that children born to infected mothers may either express less hypersensitivity, or down-regulate their reactivity more quickly, upon initial infection, than individuals in whom initial infection is also their initial immunological exposure to schistosome immunogens and antischistosome-related idiotypes.

We have observed a correlation between the expression of some Ids by anti-SEA antibodies and asymptomatic INT infections. Anti-SEA antibodies from HS patients express different Ids. Furthermore, PBMCs from HS patients fail to respond to Id exposure by regulation of in vitro anti-SEA granuloma formation. These findings are consistent with a hypothesis that some patients are unable (or lose the capacity) to produce anti-SEA-related Ids which induce regulation of anti-SEA responses, and that their cells are (or become) unable to respond to the regulatory stimuli induced by such Ids.

Our recent data indicate the presence of shared, immunoregulatory, cross-reactive Ids on anti-SEA antibodies from mice and men with S. mansoni infections. The ability to study these Id/anti-Id phenomena using anti-SEA mAbs which express these CRI should assist in the unravelling of the multiple effector and regulatory interactions which occur in this infection, and appear to be mediated through Id/anti-Id mechanisms.

ACKNOWLEDGEMENTS

We thank Iramaya Veira and Judith O'Connell for their assistance, and the UNDP/World Bank/WHO Special Programme for Research and Training in Tropical Diseases, the CNPq (Brazil), the Veterans Administration and NIAID, NIH (USA), for the funding of these studies.

REFERENCES

Abe T, Colley D G 1984 Modulation of *Schistosoma mansoni* egg-induced granuloma formation. III. Evidence for an anti-idiotypic, I-J-positive, I-J-restricted, soluble T suppressor factor. J Immunol 132: 2084–2088
Bona C A 1981 Idiotypes and lymphocytes. Academic Press, New York
Camus D, Carlier Y, Bina J C, Borojevic R, Prata A, Capron A 1976 Sensitization to *Schistosoma mansoni* antigen in uninfected children born to infected mothers. J Infect Dis 134: 405–408
Carlier Y, Bout D, Bina J C, Camus D, Figueiredo J F M, Capron A 1975 Immunological studies in human schistosomiasis. I. Parasitic antigen in urine. Am J Trop Med Hyg 24: 949–954
Colley D G 1981 Immune responses and immunoregulation in experimental and clinical schistosomiasis. In: Mansfield J M (ed) Parasitic diseases, Volume 1 The Immunology, Marcel Dekker, New York, pp 1–83
Colley D G 1987 Dynamics of the human immune response to schistosomes. In: Mahmoud A A F (ed) Clinics in tropical medicine and communicable diseases, W B Saunders, London, pp 315–332
Colley D G, Parra J C, Montesano M A et al 1987 Immunoregulation in human schistosomiasis by idiotypic interactions and lymphokine-mediated mechanisms. Memorias do Instituto Oswaldo Cruz, Rio de Janeiro 82 (suppl): 105–109
Colley, D G, Goes A M, Doughty B L et al 1989 Antiidiotypic T cells and factors in murine and human schistosomiasis. In: Kaplan J G, Green D R, Bleackley R C (eds) The cellular basis of immune modulation, Alan R Liss, Philadelphia, pp 367–378
Doughty B L, Goes A M, Parra J C et al 1987 Granulomatous hypersensitivity to *Schistosoma mansoni* egg antigens in human schistosomiasis. I. Granuloma formation and modulation around polyacrylamide antigen-conjugated beads. Memorias do Instituto Oswaldo Cruz, Rio de Janeiro 82 (suppl): 47–54
Eloi-Santos S M, Novato-Silva E, Maselli V M, Gazzinelli G, Colley D G, Correa-Oliveira R In utero idiotypic sensitization in human schistosomiasis and Chagas' disease. J Clin Invest (in press)
Feldmeier H, Nogueira-Queiroz J A, Peixoto-Queiroz M A et al 1986 Detection and quantification of circulating antigen in schistosomiasis by monoclonal antibody. II. The quantification of circulating antigens in human schistosomiasis mansoni and haematobium: relationship to intensity of infection and disease status. Clin Exp Immunol 65: 232–243
Freitas A A, Burlen O, Coutinho A 1988 Selection of antibody repertoires by anti-idiotypes can occur at multiple steps of B cell differentiation. J Immunol 140: 4097–4102
Gazzinelli R T, Parra J F C, Correa-Oliveira R et al 1988 Idiotypic/anti-idiotypic interactions in schistosomiasis and/or Chagas' disease. Am J Trop Med Hyg 39: 288–294
Grzych J P, Capron M, Lambert P H, Dissous C, Torres S, Capron A 1985 An anti-idiotype vaccine against experimental schistosomiasis. Nature 316: 74–76
Hang L M, Boros D L, Warren K S 1974 Induction of immunological hyporesponsiveness to granulomatous hypersensitivity in *Schistosoma mansoni* infection. J Infect Dis 130: 515–522
Haque A, Capron A 1982 Transplacental transfer of rodent microfilariae induces antigen-specific tolerance in rats. Nature 299: 361–363
Hillyer G V, Menendez-Corrada R, Lluberes R, Hernandez-Morales F 1970 Evidence of transplacental passage of specific antibody in schistosomiasis mansoni in man. Am J Trop Med Hyg 19: 289–291
Jordan P 1985 Schistosomiasis, The St Lucia project. Cambridge University Press, Cambridge
Kearney, J F, Vakil, M 1986 Idiotype-directed interactions during ontogeny play a major role in the establishment of the adult B cell repertoire. Immunol Rev 94: 39–50
Kohler H, Urbain J, Cazenave P A 1984 Idiotypy in biology and medicine. Academic Press, New York
Kresina T F, Olds G R 1986 Concomitant cellular and humoral expression of a regulatory cross-reactive idiotype in acute *Schistosoma japonicum* infection. Infect Immun 53: 90–94

189

Lees R E M, Jordan P 1968 Transplacental transfer of antibodies to *Schistosoma mansoni* and their persistence in infants. Trans R Soc Trop Med Hyg 62: 630–631

Lewert R M, Mandlowitz S 1969 Schistosomiasis: prenatal induction of tolerance to antigens. Nature 224: 1029–1030

Lima M S, Gazzinelli G, Nacimento E et al 1986 Immune responses during human schistosomiasis mansoni: evidence for antiidiotypic T lymphocyte responsiveness. J Clin Invest 78: 983–988

Montesano M A, Lima M S, Correa-Oliveira R, Gazzinelli G, Colley D G 1989 Immune responses during human schistosomiasis mansoni. XVI. Idiotypic differences in antibody preparations from patients with different clinical forms of infection. J Immunol 142: 2501–2506

Nash T E, Deelder A M 1985 Comparison of four schistosome excretory-secretory antigens: phenol sulfuric test active peak, cathodic circulating antigen, gut-associated proteoglycan, and circulating anodic antigen. Am J Trop Med Hyg 34: 236–241

Olds G R, Kresina T F 1985 Network interactions in *Schistosoma japonicum* infection. Identification and characterization of serologically distinct immunoregulatory auto-antiidiotypic antibody population. J Clin Invest 76: 2338–2347

Parra J C, Lima M S, Gazzinelli G, Colley D G 1988 Immune responses during human schistosomiasis mansoni. XV. Anti-idiotypic T cells can recognize and respond to anti-SEA idiotypes directly. J Immunol 140: 2401–2405

Percy A J, Harn D A 1988 Monoclonal anti-idiotypic and auto-anti-idiotypic antibodies from mice immunized with a protective monoclonal antibody against *Schistosoma mansoni*. J Immunol 140: 2760–2762

Phillips S M, Lammie P J 1986 Immunopathology of granuloma formation and fibrosis in schistosomiasis. Parasitol Today 2: 296–302

Phillips S M, Fox E G, Fathelbab N G, Walker D 1986 Epitopic and paratopically directed anti-idiotypic factors in the regulation of resistance to murine schistosomiasis mansoni. J Immunol 137: 2339–2347

Phillips S M, Perrin P J, Walker D J, Fathelbab N G, Linette G P, Idris M A 1988 The regulation of resistance to *Schistosoma mansoni* by auto-anti-idiotypic immunity. J Immunol 141: 1728–1733

Powell M R, Colley D G 1985 Demonstration of splenic auto-anti-idiotypic plaque-forming cells in mice infected with *Schistosoma mansoni*. J Immunol 134: 4140–4145

Powell M R, Colley D G 1987 Anti-idiotypic T lymphocyte responsiveness in murine schistosomiasis mansoni. Cell Immunol 104: 377–385

Santoro F, Carlier Y, Borojevic R, Bout D, Tachon P, Capron A 1977 Parasite 'M' antigen in milk from mothers infected with *Schistosoma mansoni* (preliminary report). Ann Trop Med Parasitol 71: 121–122

Sher A, Colley D G Immunoparasitology, Chapter 35. In: Paul W E (ed) Fundamental Immunology, 2nd Edition, Raven Press, New York (in press)

Stein K E, Soderstrom T 1984 Neonatal administration of idiotype or antiidiotype primes for protection against *Escherichia coli* K13 infection in mice. J Exp Med 160: 1001–1011

Tachon P, Borojevic R 1978 Mother–child relation in human schistosomiasis mansoni: skin test and cord blood reactivity to schistosomal antigens. Trans R Soc Trop Med Hyg 72: 605–609

Takemori T, Rajewsky K 1984 Mechanism of neonatally induced idiotype suppression and its relevance for the acquisition of self-tolerance. Immunol Rev 79: 103–117

von Lichtenberg F 1987 Consequences of infections with schistosomes. In: Rollinson D, Simpson A J G (eds) The biology of schistosomes from genes to latrines. Academic Press, London, pp 185–232

Warren K S 1982 The secret of the immunopathogenesis of schistosomiasis: in vivo models. Immunol Rev 61: 189–213

Weil G J, Hussain R, Kumaraswami V, Tripathy S P, Phillips K S, Ottesen E A 1983 Prenatal allergic sensitization to helminth antigens in offspring of parasite-infected mothers. J Clin Invest 71: 1124–1129

Discussion of paper presented by D. G. Colley

Discussed by J. R. David
Reported by M. Capron

Idiotypic–anti-idiotypic interactions in a chronic disease, such as schistosomiasis in endemic areas, might have regulatory functions on immunopathological processes, morbidity and resistance to infection.

The influence of a perinatal exposure to maternal schistosome-related idiotypes, on the response to infection of the neonates was discussed in relation to previous experiments of low-dose tolerance induced in newborn mice by schistosome antigens. This discussion illustrated the complexities of interactions, involving placental transfer of circulating antigens with multiple specificities, as well as antibodies bearing idiotypes. There are a number of studies in the past showing that antigens can influence the fetus or the young animal's responses, in schistosomiasis but also in nematode infections. Soluble antigens can go through the placenta or possibly through the milk. These maternal influences might account for the differences observed in the development of schistosomiasis in children from endemic countries, by comparison with schistosomiasis acquired by a 'tourist' (child). Very little is known regarding this problem, apart from observing more frequently the acute toxaemic form of schistosomiasis in children born and raised outside endemic areas.

The nature of the idiotypes was envisaged. Whereas a precise identification has not been achieved, most idiotype preparations, except for those isolated from acute patients are IgG, but the actual profile of IgG subclasses is not known. In idiotypes isolated from acute patients, there was a ratio of 50:50 IgM and IgG and the presence of IgM might be related to the absence of a stimulatory activity. Experiments using F(ab')2 and Sepharose-coupled Fab fragments suggested that the Fc portion was not essential for the stimulation. Idiotypes are not antigens, but the presence of contaminating antigens in purified preparations was not totally ruled out.

The specificity of the idiotypes was evaluated in terms of anti-lymphocyte reactivity. Only cells from schistosomiasis patients and not from uninfected individuals were stimulated by anti-SEA antibodies. Moreover, no cross-reactivity was found between anti-epimastigote versus anti-SEA antibodies, both on lymphocytes from patients with schistosomiasis or with Chagas' disease. As far as human monoclonal antibodies as idiotypes are concerned, their antigen specificity for carbohydrate peptide epitopes is not yet known. It was pointed out that most of IgG2 responses against egg antigens have carbohydrate specificities.

The functions of idiotypes were then discussed. First, idiotypes in parasitology have been used as a possible basis for producing vaccines: rather than giving antigens, anti-idiotypes were used for immunization. A significant protection by using such an anti-idiotype vaccine was reported in rat schistosomiasis. In a different study mice immunized by anti-egg monoclonal antibodies were shown to produce both AB2 and AB3 antibodies, suggesting the possible initiation of an idiotype network by monoclonal antibodies. One very important point which was discussed, concerned the suppression of granuloma formation in vitro by these idiotypes. It was recalled that schistosomiasis is caused largely by granulomatous inflammation and fibrous tissue formation in organs like the liver and the urinary tract, and such a mechanism of suppression might be crucial to the prevention or the regulation of the disease. An area of the discussion was to know the cellular response of patients with hepatosplenomegaly to idiotypes. In fact, the cells from hepatosplenic patients did not respond to idiotypes coming from patients with the intestinal form of the disease. Their interaction with these antibodies, even though it led to proliferation, did not lead to the regulatory response but this requires more careful examination. Another question was to know whether T cells within granulomas in the animal models were idiotype specific. T cells in the spleens have been shown to be idiotype specific but T cells in the lesions have not yet been studied.

Besides the effects of idiotypes on T-cell responses, they might also influence antibody-dependent mechanisms. In this respect, it was recalled that antigen–antibody complexes were shown to inhibit complement-dependent cytotoxic antibodies. Since levels of such 'lethal' antibodies differed in the groups of Brazilian patients with various clinical forms of schistosomiasis, one can suspect a regulatory role of idiotypes, in addition to blocking immune complexes or antibodies. Another aspect of the effects of idiotypes on effector mechanisms could be related to eosinophils and activating eosinophil factors. It has been shown previously that mononuclear cells from normal subjects were able to produce such an eosinophil-enhancing factor. However, most of the people who had mild schistosomiasis no longer made this eosinophil activating factor. The role of idiotypes in the suppression of the production of such a factor has to be envisaged.

Finally, a number of questions have still be to answered concerning especially the nature of antigens responsible for the production of such idiotypes. However, the bypassing of the usual mechanism of processing, the activation of T cells, together with the immunosuppressive effects, certainly represent interesting features of the idiotypic network.

11. Immunity and morbidity in human schistosomiasis

A. E. Butterworth   E. L. Corbett   D. W. Dunne
A. J. C. Fulford   G. Kimani   R. K. Gachuhi
R. Klumpp   G. Mbugua   J. H. Ouma
T. K. arap Siongok and R. F. Sturrock

INTRODUCTION

The possible existence of immunity to schistosome infection in man has two practical implications. First, the development of an age-dependent acquired resistance to infection, and its heterogeneous expression in different individuals, will influence the age-specific distribution of intensities of infection and of re-infection after treatment among communities living in endemic areas, and may therefore affect the design of chemotherapy-based control programmes (Anderson & May 1982, 1985, Anderson 1987). Second, the recent application of techniques in molecular biology has allowed the large-scale production of several schistosome antigens that might be candidates for inclusion in a vaccine (Lanar et al 1986, Balloul et al 1987). However, such a vaccine is unlikely to be completely effective in preventing infection, and its successful use in preventing schistosome-associated disease will depend critically on understanding both the relationship between infection and morbidity in schistosomiasis and the nature of the immune responses that are associated with the expression of resistance in man. In this paper, we describe some aspects of schistosomiasis in man, in particular: the relationship between infection and morbidity; the evidence that acquired immunity may limit schistosome infection in older individuals; and an analysis of some immune responses that may help to explain why immunity develops only slowly in older individuals.

BIOLOGY OF SCHISTOSOMIASIS: INFECTION AND MORBIDITY

As is the case with other helminth parasites in their definitive hosts, the adult schistosome does not replicate in its human host. The number of eggs that are produced therefore depends on the actual number of adult worms that mature within the host, and on the lifespan of these worms. Examination of the distribution of intensities of infection in a community reveals a high degree of aggregation or over-dispersion: a small proportion of individuals harbour most of the worms (Anderson 1987). Such over-dispersion is associated with a demonstrable predisposition of heavily infected individuals to become heavily re-infected following chemotherapy (Bensted-Smith et al 1987, Tingley et al 1988), and may be attributed to inherited differences in primary susceptibility or in the development of immunity to superinfection; to environmentally determined differences in primary susceptibility or in the development of immunity (for example, the simultaneous presence of immunosuppressive infections, or of infections that elicit a cross-reactive immunity); or to other environmental factors, in particular the level of exposure to infection.

Most of the morbidity associated with schistosome infection is due to the deposition of eggs in tissues, the ensuing granulomatous reaction leading to fibrosis (Warren 1987, Chen & Mott 1988). In schistosomiasis mansoni, fibrosis in the liver leads to portal hypertension, hepatosplenomegaly and the development of oesophageal varices, without gross loss of liver function: in schistosomiasis haematobia, fibrosis in the urinary tract leads to hydronephrosis or similar obstructive renal abnormalities. In addition, the granulomas that develop during late infection are smaller and lead to less fibrosis than those that develop during the initial stages. Such granulomas are described as 'modulated' (Warren 1987), a process that may be attributable to the development of T-suppressor cells or other immunoregulatory mechanisms (Colley 1987, Warren 1987).

The major factors that determine the extent of schistosome-associated morbidity are therefore the intensity of infection (Lehman et al 1976, Chen & Mott 1988) and its duration: in endemic communities, this in turn depends on age (Table 11.1). Severe disease therefore develops only in the small proportion of children who acquire heavy infections: and, even in such children, the extent of morbidity (provided that it has not reached the stage of irreversible portal hypertension) diminishes with age, as the adult worms of early infections die, the child becomes immune to re-infection (see later), and the amount of tissue damage elicited by eggs resulting from new infections becomes less marked.

However, the intensity and duration of infection may not be the only factors that determine the development of morbidity. We have recently identified a focus of unusually severe schistosome-associated morbidity in Kambu, Machakos District, Kenya (Mbugua et al in preparation). In general, *Schistosoma mansoni* infections in rural Kenya are relatively mild, causing hepatomegaly in 7–17% of infected schoolchildren, but hepatosplenomegaly in only 0.2–0.5% (Butterworth et al unpublished observations). In Kambu, in contrast, we have found that while 17% of children have simple hepatomegaly, an additional 16% have hepatosplenomegaly: in many patients the condition is gross, and associated with the development of demonstrable oesophageal varices.

Table 11.1 Factors that may influence the development of schistosome-associated morbidity

Intensity of infection
Duration of infection, usually reflected by age
Host genetic differences (e.g. HLA-DR or DQ)
Parasite strain differences
Age at first infection
Concomitant infections (e.g. malaria, hepatitis)
Host nutritional status
Maternal infection status, leading to variations in the
  induction of immunoregulatory mechanisms

The reasons for the difference in prevalence of severe hepatosplenomegaly between Kambu and a more typical area (Kangundo, Machakos Location) are not yet clear. Prevalence and intensities of infection among schoolchildren in the two areas are comparable and, in both areas, there is a similar relationship between the prevalence of hepatomegaly and intensity of infection (Fig. 11.1). In contrast, an associated splenomegaly is almost undetectable in Kangundo, but is strongly associated with intensity of infection in Kambu (Fig. 11.2). This indicates: first, that the splenomegaly in Kambu is attributable to schistosome infection; and second, that the lack of splenomegaly in Kangundo is not simply due to the lower intensities of infection.

The difference between the two areas is potentially of practical importance. Kangundo is typical of the long-settled rural areas of Kenya, being fertile, well-watered and relatively prosperous. In contrast, Kambu is characteristic of those areas in Kenya that have been more recently settled, being harsh, arid and poor. Such areas are assuming increasing importance, as population pressure drives families out of the more fertile valleys: if schistosomiasis is generally more severe in this type of environment, then it is important to understand the reason, and we are considering and have begun to test several optional, but not mutually exclusive, explanations (Table 11.1).

1. Since the people of both areas are of the relatively homogeneous Akamba tribe, host genetic differences (for example in HLA-DR or DQ haplotypes, leading to differences in immune responses to egg antigens (Kojima et al 1984)) are unlikely to account for the major differences between the two areas, although they might contribute to differences between individuals within the high morbidity area.

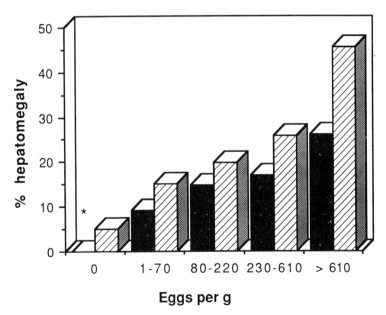

Figure 11.1 Distribution of hepatomegaly by stratified intensity of infection among children from Kakayuni, a low morbidity area in Kangundo, and Kambu, a high morbidity area (Mbugua et al in preparation). *: not examined. ■ Kakayuni liver; ▨ Kambu liver

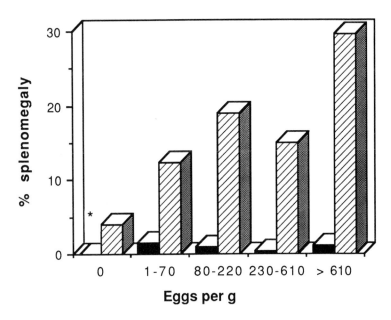

Figure 11.2 Distribution of splenomegaly by stratified intensity of infection among children from Kakayuni, a low morbidity area in Kangundo, and Kambu, a high morbidity area (Mbugua et al in preparation). *: not examined. ■ Kakayuni spleen; ▨ Kambu spleen

2. A difference in pathogenicity of local parasite strains, although not recorded in the literature, cannot at this stage be excluded.

3. Preliminary water contact observations suggest that children in Kambu are exposed to infected water at an earlier age than those in Kangundo (the mothers being reluctant to leave young children alone at home, from fear of baboons). Early exposure of the small liver of a young child to eggs may lead to more severe damage than later exposure of an older child.

4. Concomitant infections may interact with schistosomiasis in compounding the damage to the liver or spleen. For example, malaria is more prevalent in Kambu than in Kangundo. There is no direct correlation between malaria and schistosomiasis, allowing a distinction between splenomegaly attributable to malaria and hepatosplenomegaly attributable to schistosomiasis, but previous malarial infection might interact with schistosomiasis in enhancing splenic changes.

5. Liver damage may be enhanced by poor nutritional status. Children in the Kambu schools are less well nourished than those in Kangundo, and in all schools the presence of hepatomegaly is correlated with a low triceps skin-fold thickness (Fig. 11.3) as a measure of short-term nutritional status and with low height for age (Fig. 11.4) as a measure of long-term nutritional status (Corbett et al in preparation). It is assumed that the changes in short-term nutritional status are a consequence rather than a cause of hepatomegaly. It remains to be determined whether the long-term changes in nutrition precede or follow the onset of hepatomegaly, although examination of the age distribution of changes in height for age in patients with or without hepatomegaly suggests the latter (Fig. 11.5).

6. A child's T-cell-mediated granulomatous response to an initial egg burden may

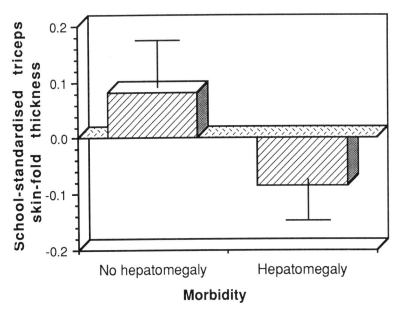

Figure 11.3 Skin-fold thicknesses, standardized for age and school, among children from Kangundo and Kambu with or without hepatomegaly (Corbett et al in preparation). Mean±95% confidence interval

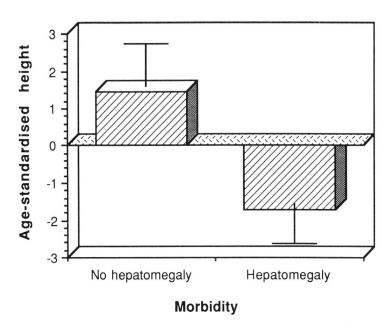

Figure 11.4 Height, standardized for age, among children from Kangundo and Kambu with or without hepatomegaly (Corbett et al in preparation). Mean ±95% confidence interval

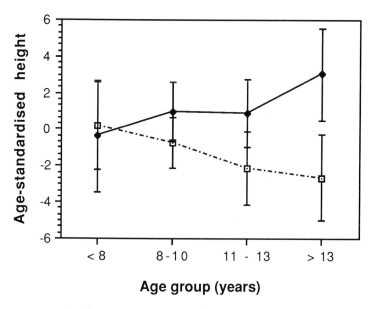

Age group (years)

Figure 11.5 Age distribution of age-standardized height among children from Kangundo and Kambu with or without hepatomegaly (Corbett et al in preparation). Mean ±95% confidence interval. □ hepatomegaly; ◆ no hepatomegaly

be modified by maternal infection status. Because of recent immigration into the area, a greater proportion of children from Kambu than from Kangundo schools are born of mothers who have had less than 5 years of potential exposure to schistosome infection at the time that the child was born (Corbett et al in preparation). Gazzinelli, Colley and colleagues have shown the existence of T cells with an anti-idiotypic specificity for anti-egg antibodies, in particular in patients without hepatosplenic disease (Lima et al 1986, Colley 1987, Gazzinelli et al 1988, Parra et al 1988), and have demonstrated the presence of such cells in the cord

Table 11.2 Lymphocyte proliferative responses to egg antigens (SEA) and to affinity-purified anti-SEA antibodies

Patient	Antigen	Concentration (μg/ml)			
		10	i	0.1	0
8	SEA	7 368	406	532	472
	Id-P2	7 683	1 575	874	–
	Id-P3	11 303	1 132	543	–
42	SEA	66 132	9 420	406	213
	Id-P2	3 219	1 453	432	–
	Id-P3	1 814	1 030	797	–
45	SEA	10 727	1 541	883	857
	Id-P2	3 532	1 982	3 846	–
	Id-P3	5 683	1 846	1 438	

Incorporation (counts/min) of [³H]-thymidine after 5 days of culture of lymphocytes from individual schistosome-infected patients in the presence of SEA or of one of two pools of anti-SEA antibodies affinity-purified from human infection sera (Id-P₂ and Id-P₃)

198

blood of neonates born of infected mothers. It is possible that previous maternal infection status, by stimulating the development of long-lived anti-idiotypic T cells in the infant through placentally transferred antibodies, might modify the child's subsequent response to any initial schistosome infection. We have confirmed the existence of such cells in some patients without hepatosplenomegaly (Table 11.2), and are currently testing their distribution in age-, sex- and intensity-matched patients with or without severe morbidity.

There is as yet no clear evidence that favours any one of the above hypotheses: they are not mutually exclusive, and the severity of disease may be determined by more than one factor other than the known criteria of intensity and duration of infection. The importance of the topic lies in the fact that, although it is necessary for control programmes (based either on chemotherapy or eventually on vaccination) to be directed towards reducing the prevalence of high-intensity infections, this by itself may not be a sufficient criterion for reducing morbidity.

EVIDENCE FOR IMMUNITY IN MAN

In spite of the possible influence of other factors, described above, in determining the extent of morbidity in infected individuals, the currently accepted criteria are intensity and duration of infection. It is also generally accepted that eradication of transmission is an impractical task, even at the local level, and the aim of any control programme is to reduce transmission to levels below which intensities of infection are insufficient to allow the development of morbidity.

Such control is currently achieved by chemotherapy, with or without snail control, health education, and improvements in water supplies and sanitation. The new drugs available for the treatment of schistosomiasis, in particular praziquantel, are both safe and highly effective, and the application of mass chemotherapy has successfully reduced both transmission and morbidity, in particular in areas of low endemicity (Jordan 1985, World Health Organization 1985). However, chemotherapy has several inherent problems. Re-infection occurs rapidly, especially among the younger children who are at risk of developing severe morbidity. Surveillance and retreatment must therefore be carried out at frequent intervals; and, since the newly available drugs are expensive, this may lead to unacceptably high costs for national control programmes. In addition, there is the risk that drug-resistant strains of parasite may eventually emerge, a problem that has already been described, under both laboratory and field conditions, for oxamniquine (Diaz et al 1982).

In this context, studies on immunity to schistosomes in man have two practical goals. First, the demonstration of an acquired immunity to re-infection after treatment may mean that chemotherapy programmes, in particular during the surveillance phase, need only be directed at young children. This would lead to a useful reduction in drug costs, as well as in the skilled labour required for diagnosis and delivery of treatment. Second, immunization programmes have generally proved to command long-term support by national health authorities: and the development of a schistosome vaccine, which could be incorporated into existing immunization programmes, would be a useful adjunct to control.

However, the development of such a vaccine will require not only the production of sufficient quantities of an appropriate vaccine antigen, but also its administration in an appropriate fashion – that is, in a manner that elicits immune responses which are known to be protective in man. Studies in experimental animal models of schistosome infection have yielded much useful information about possible mechanisms of immunity: but each model differs markedly from the next, and none can be accepted as an absolute indicator of events that may be important in man. The definition of those responses that must be elicited by an effective vaccine will therefore depend on the identification of individuals who are immune or susceptible to re-infection, and an analysis of their immune responses.

The commonly observed distribution of prevalence and intensity of schistosome infection, with a characteristic rise during the first two decades of life followed by a decline, suggests the development in older individuals of an immunity to superinfection, and various early studies supported this interpretation (Clarke 1966, Kloetzel & da Silva 1967, Bradley & McCullough 1973). However, these studies did not clearly distinguish between the possibilities that the lower levels of re-infection observed in older individuals might be due either to immunity or to an age-dependent reduction in exposure (Warren 1973, Dalton & Pole 1978). An approach to this problem was provided by the detailed studies of Wilkins et al (1984) on S. haematobium infections in the Gambia. They compared the change in intensities of infection over a 3-year period in two villages: in the first, transmission had been interrupted by the application of molluscicides, whereas in the second no intervention was undertaken. The changes with time in intensities of infection in the first village allowed the calculation of an approximate mean lifespan of the adult worm of 3.4 years. Application of this figure to egg counts for the second village allowed the authors to estimate the extent of new infections that were occurring among different age groups over the 3 year follow-up period. New infections in adults were 1000-fold less than in young children and, although direct observations of water contact were not made, this difference was considered to be far greater than could be attributed to differences in exposure between the age groups, and was more likely to be attributable to the development with age of an acquired immunity.

An alternative approach, which has been adopted in studies on S. haematobium in the Gambia (Hagan et al 1987, Wilkins et al 1987), and on studies on S. mansoni in Kenya (Sturrock et al 1983, 1987, Butterworth et al 1984, 1985, 1988a), Egypt (Colley et al 1986) and Brazil (Dessein et al 1988), has been to follow intensities of re-infection after chemotherapy in individuals whose levels of contact with water known to contain infected snails is simultaneously observed. The consensus that has emerged is that, although there is a slow reduction with age in levels of exposure, this is insufficient to account for the very marked reduction with age in intensities of re-infection after chemotherapy, which is instead largely attributable to the development of an age-dependent acquired resistance.

Treatment and re-infection studies of this type have generally taken two forms. In the first, observations have been made of a narrow age-band of children and young teenagers, who show little change with age in patterns of water contact, but very marked changes in levels of re-infection. An example is shown in Figures 11.6 and 11.7, which show the results for a cohort of children who were treated and followed for re-infection over a 1 year period during which intense transmission continued in the study area. Among younger children, aged 3–9, intensities of infection, expressed either as the geometric mean (Fig. 11.6) or as the percentage of individual pretreatment levels (Fig. 11.7), returned in 1 year to more than

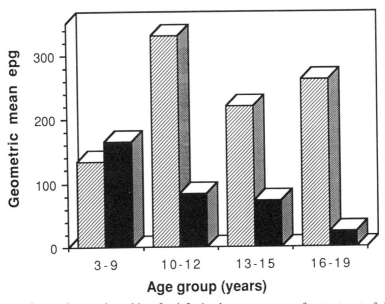

Figure 11.6 Geometric mean intensities of re-infection by age, one year after treatment of children in a high-transmission area (Mbugua et al in preparation). ▨ pretreatment; ■ 1 year post-treatment

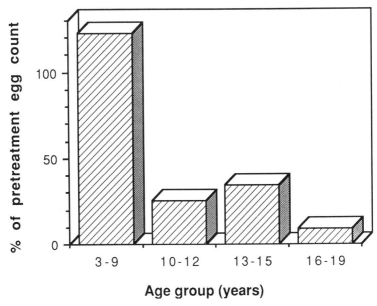

Figure 11.7 Intensities of re-infection following treatment of children in a high-transmission area, expressed as percentage of pretreatment intensity of infection (Mbugua et al in preparation)

pretreatment levels. Older children, in contrast, showed geometric mean intensities of re-infection of only 8–28% of pretreatment levels, a difference that cannot be accounted for by differences in water contact, and that implies a surprisingly clearcut development of a resistance to re-infection around the age of puberty. Immune responses in such children can then be studied either by comparing extreme subgroups of resistant or susceptible individuals (Butterworth et al 1985, Dessein et al 1988), or by analysis of correlations, for the study group as a whole, of intensities of re-infection with various immune responses (Hagan et al 1985, 1987, Butterworth et al 1987, 1988a, 1988b, Dunne et al 1988). Conclusions from such analyses of correlations are given below.

A second approach has been to follow intensities of re-infection after treatment among individuals of all ages, and to attempt to distinguish between a lack of re-infection attributable to reduced exposure in older individuals and a lack of re-infection attributable to an acquired resistance. In studies on *S. haematobium* infection in the Gambia, Wilkins et al (1987) were able to identify a group of older women who showed low intensities of infection in spite of high levels of observed exposure, and were therefore putatively immune. Similarly, we have followed intensities of re-infection 1 year after treatment in a community in which continued transmission was occurring (Butterworth et al 1988a). Mean intensities of re-infection reached a peak in children aged 8–12 years, declining in older individuals to very low levels. In contrast, levels of water contact, as reflected by mean duration of contact, reached a peak in individuals aged 20–24 years. It was considered possible that the difference in age distribution between intensity of re-infection and total duration of water contact might be attributable to the fact that adults have a less infective type of water contact than children. When the water contact data were weighted to take into account those activities (such as washing clothes) that are carried out mainly by adults and that might be less likely to lead to infection, then the distribution of estimated exposure by age corresponded more closely to the distribution of intensities of re-infection. However, the reduction with age in exposure was still insufficient to account for the reduction in re-infection. Young adults aged 20–24 years, for example, showed over half the level of estimated exposure that was observed in the 8–12 year olds, but only 1% of the level of re-infection.

A problem about this approach is that the weighting factors used, although based on biologically sensible criteria, are arbitrary. More recently, therefore, we have attempted to develop a model in which the water contact data themselves are used to generate weightings that give the maximum likelihood of predicting intensities of re-infection (Butterworth et al 1988a, Fulford et al in preparation): the effects of age can then be tested as an additional variable. Because of problems with the distribution of data for post-treatment egg counts, with large numbers of zeros, this model has so far proved sufficiently stable only for analysis of pretreatment data. The model is self-justifying, in that it yields weightings that predict the most infectious water contact sites, the times of day when cercariae are most abundant, and the nature and extent of activities (such as whole body immersion during swimming or bathing) that are most likely to lead to infection. In this model the effect of age is still very marked, implying again that there are age-dependent changes in susceptibility that are not dependent on the extent and nature of exposure.

Apart from the problem of imprecision in water contact observations, an inherent, although unlikely, difficulty is that there may be undetectable and age-dependent inaccuracies in observations of exposure. A possible approach to this difficulty is to compare intensities of infection, or of re-infection after treatment, between areas in which there are different observed age distributions in water contact, but otherwise similar patterns of transmission. The recently identified focus of high morbidity in Kambu (described earlier) offers an opportunity for this type of study, since preliminary observations indicate that, in comparison with Kangundo, adults maintain very high levels of exposure: this is associated with a need to travel long distances to collect large volumes of water for themselves and for their cattle, a task that is beyond the capacity of children. Such comparative studies are now in progress. In the meantime, the data available from our own studies and from those of others are not compatible with the hypothesis that the low levels of re-infection seen in older children and adults are solely attributable to reduced exposure: instead, they support the hypothesis that an acquired resistance plays a major role in limiting re-infection in older individuals.

STUDIES ON THE MECHANISMS OF ACQUIRED RESISTANCE TO RE-INFECTION

A notable feature of the epidemiological studies described above is the length of time required for the development of immunity after natural infection in man. In a typical community, children may acquire their first detectable infections around the age of 4 years, yet a resistance to re-infection cannot be demonstrated until about the age of 12 years. During the intervening period, children are most susceptible and most exposed, and they progressively accumulate a substantial worm burden, which slowly declines during later life. This slow development of immunity is in contrast to that seen in most rodent models of infection or immunization, but is comparable to that seen in chronically infected baboons (Sturrock et al 1978).

Two possible reasons for this slow development of immunity may be envisaged. The first is that under conditions of natural exposure in the field, in which children are infrequently infected with small numbers of cercariae, the antigenic stimulus is small and the appropriate protective responses take a long time to develop. In this context, it may be noted that most experimental situations, in which animals are challenged with large numbers of cercariae at limited skin sites, are highly unnatural. Cercarial densities in naturally infected bodies of water are commonly of the order of 0.1–1 per litre and it must be assumed that, even under conditions of heavy exposure, children will be challenged only with occasional cercariae penetrating the skin in widely separated sites. If protective responses are directed against antigens present only in the cercaria or young schistosomulum stages, then it is entirely conceivable that repeated exposure over many years would be required for the induction of the appropriate responses.

However, the evidence available so far does not support this hypothesis: a range of potentially protective responses can be demonstrated in young children who remain susceptible to infection. Studies in experimental animals have provided evidence for two main effector mechanisms of immunity. The first, which is important in the rat model of schistosomiasis, is an antibody-dependent cell-mediated cytotoxic reaction (ADCC) involving either IgE or IgG2a antibodies (Capron et al 1981, Grzych et al 1982) and either macrophages, eosinophils or platelets (Capron A et al 1975, Capron M et al 1979, 1981), the effect being directed primarily against young schistosomula expressing parasite antigens at their surface. The second, which is of importance in the mouse model, involves an antibody-independent effect of activated macrophages (James 1986a & 1986b): the antigens that elicit such activation need not be expressed on the parasite surface, and the reaction can be directed against older organisms. Studies in vitro with human materials have provided strong evidence for ADCC reactions of the type observed in the rat (Butterworth 1984): these involve primarily the eosinophil (Butterworth et al 1975, 1977) and either IgG (Vadas et al 1979) or IgE (Capron et al 1984) antibodies. In contrast, an effect of activated macrophages in man is controversial (Olds et al 1981, Remold et al 1988, Cottrell et al 1989). Therefore, although a role for other effector mechanisms cannot at this stage be excluded, eosinophil-mediated ADCC reactions are of potential importance in mediating immunity in man. This possibility is supported by the demonstration by Hagan et al (1985) of an association in children between resistance to re-infection with *S. haematobium* and increased circulating eosinophil levels.

The magnitude of the ADCC reaction mediated by eosinophils against schistosomula depends not only on the presence of appropriate antibodies, but also on the functional state of the cells. Eosinophils from eosinophilic individuals are activated and show, among a variety of functional changes, an enhanced capacity to kill schistosomula in the presence of suboptimal concentrations of anti-schistosomulum IgG (David et al 1980) or IgE antibodies (Capron et al 1984). This effect may be attributable to the production, in individuals with eosinophilia, of a variety of eosinophil activating moieties, including eosinophil activating factor (EAF) (Veith & Butterworth 1983, Thorne et al 1985, 1986), IL-5 (Clutterbuck & Sanderson 1988) and GM-CSF (Silberstein et al 1986).

It might therefore be expected that young children who remain susceptible to re-infection after treatment have either insufficient levels of anti-schistosomulum antibodies, or insufficiently active eosinophils, or both. However, this would appear not to be the case. In a study of 129 children, aged 9–15 years, who were treated for *S. mansoni* infections and followed for intensities of re-infection over a 21-month period (Butterworth et al 1984, 1985, 1987), we have found no correlation between the extent of resistance to re-infection and either the levels of circulating eosinophils (as an indirect estimate of eosinophil functional activity) or the levels of antibodies mediating killing of schistosomula by activated eosinophils. Young children show not only increased circulating eosinophil levels and antibodies mediating eosinophil-dependent killing of schistosomula, but also a wide range of both humoral and cell-mediated responses (lymphocyte proliferation and gamma-interferon production) against a variety of schistosome antigens: they may be described as being immunologically hyperactive.

The lack of potentially protective responses therefore does not seem to be the explanation for the continued susceptibility of young children to re-infection after treatment. Instead, an alternative explanation is that there may be, in such children, an inappropriate balance betwe·n protective and 'blocking' responses. Early experiments by Grzych et al (1982, 1984) in the rat model of schistosome infection showed that the capacity of an IgG2a monoclonal antibody to mediate eosinophil-dependent killing of schistosomula in vitro and to confer protection in vivo after passive transfer could be blocked by an IgG2c monoclonal antibody with specificity for the same schistosomulum surface antigen. In addition, a transient phase of susceptibility to re-infection in the rat, 7 weeks after a primary infection, was associated with high levels of IgG2c antibodies. In extending these observations to man, we have analysed the relationship (in rank correlation tests) between intensities of re-infection following treatment of the 129 children described above and various humoral responses (Khalife et al 1986, Butterworth et al 1987, 1988a, 1988b, Dunne et al 1988). We demonstrated initially a positive correlation between intensities of re-infection 9 months after treatment and (1) total anti-egg antibodies and (2) the levels of antibodies inhibiting the binding to antigens of the rat IgG2c monoclonal antibody described above (Butterworth et al 1987). This antibody recognizes a carbohydrate epitope that is expressed both in eggs and on the schistosomulum surfa · (Grzych et al 1984).

These find· igs suggested the following hypothesis. During prim·.·y infections in man, the main immunogenic stimuli are antigens released from the abundant eggs, rather than from the migrating larvae or adult worms. These egg antigens, which include a major polysaccharide component (Dunne et al 1987), bear carbohydrate epitopes that are also expressed on glycoproteins on the schistosomulum surface. Antibodies of an inappropriate isotype, elicited in response to egg polysaccharide antigens, may cross-react with the schistosomula of a challenge infection, and prevent the binding of anti-schistosomulum antibodies, of an appropriate 'effector' isotype, with specificity for the same or closely adjacent epitopes. These blocking antibodies may then decline with age, permitting the expression of the effector antibodies and hence of immunity.

Support for this hypothesis came from a series of additional observations:

1. IgM antibodies from human infection sera blocked the eosinophil-dependent killing of schistosomula mediated by IgG antibodies from the same sera (Khalife et al 1986).
2. Of the total anti-egg antibodies, IgG4 antibodies recognized primarily stage-specific glycoprotein or protein antigens, and correlated only with pretreatment intensity of infection (Butterworth et al 1988b, Dunne et al 1988).
3. In contrast, IgM and IgG2 antibodies recognized primarily polysaccharide antigens, including the major egg polysaccharide K3 (Dunne et al 1987), that bore epitopes also expressed on schistosomulum surface glycoproteins. IgM and IgG2 antibodies correlated with intensities of re-infection after treatment but not with pretreatment intensities. They were therefore predictive of *susceptibility* to re-infection and represented putative blocking antibodies.
4. IgM and IgG2 anti-egg antibodies also correlated with the levels of total antibodies against periodate-sensitive epitopes on schistosomulum surface antigens, and against the antigens (largely polysaccharide in nature) that are released from the schistosomulum during culture in vitro.
5. IgM anti-schistosomulum antibodies correlated with susceptibility to re-

infection. Total IgG anti-schistosomulum antibodies correlated with resistance to re-infection, this correlation becoming stronger when sera from individuals with high IgG2 anti-egg antibodies were eliminated from the analysis.

Although not providing direct proof, these results are consistent with the hypothesis that IgG antibodies (of an unidentified isotype) with specificity for schistosomulum surface antigens can mediate immunity, the effect being blocked by IgM and IgG2 antibodies of a similar specificity. Further analysis has suggested that the functional state of the eosinophil may also be of key importance. Khalife et al (1989) have found that activated eosinophils from moderately eosinophilic donors kill schistosomula in the presence of purified IgG1, IgG2 or IgG3, the effect being blocked by IgG4. In contrast, eosinophils from normal donors fail to kill schistosomula in the presence of any purified isotype. However, if such cells are partially activated, either by EAF or by the simultaneous presence of serum from an eosinophilic individual, then they are able to mediate killing in the presence of IgG1 and IgG3: in this case, the effect is blocked by both IgG4 and IgG2. These results suggest a complex interaction in which the capacity of different IgG isotypes to mediate or to block killing by eosinophils depends on the state of activation of the cells.

CONCLUSIONS: IMPLICATIONS FOR VACCINE DEVELOPMENT

The results summarized in this review have two implications for the eventual use in man of the recombinant vaccines currently being developed by several groups (Lanar et al 1986, Balloul et al 1987). First, the finding that older children and adults do develop an immunity to re-infection suggests that it should be possible, by appropriate immunization during early life, to overcome the prolonged phase of susceptibility that is observed in younger children and that is associated with the expression of severe morbidity. Second, however, it will be of key importance that such vaccines are administered in a manner which will elicit protective, rather than blocking, immune responses. Considerably more work is required on the nature of such responses, on their induction by active immunization in appropriate primate models, and on their regulation in man. It will be of particular importance to determine the effects of treatment on an established protective immunity, and the consequences, in terms of the subsequent development of blocking antibodies, of

Table 11.3 A rational approach to vaccine development

---

1. Identification of immune responses associated with protection in man
2. Identification of invariant antigens against which such responses may be directed
3. Large-scale preparation of antigens:
   – cloning and expression in *E. coli* or other hosts
   – synthetic peptides
4. Selective elicitation of appropriate immune responses:
   – adjuvants
   – fusion peptides with adjuvant properties
   – live vaccine cloning hosts (vaccinia, attenuated *Salmonella*)

---

the acquisition of low intensities of infection following incompletely effective immunization. Such information can only be gained by detailed and long-term investigations of naturally exposed communities. Table 11.3 summarizes the methodology of the development of a vaccine.

SUMMARY

Morbidity in human schistosomiasis is related primarily to intensity and duration of infection: severe disease develops mainly among heavily infected young children. In addition, however, further factors may be important in determining the prevalence of disease in particular geographical foci. These may include host and parasite genetic factors, concomitant infections and nutritional status of the host, and aspects of exposure that may affect immunoregulatory mechanisms, including age at first exposure and maternal infection status.

Children living in endemic areas slowly acquire an immunity to re-infection which, in addition to changes in exposure, is of major importance in limiting intensities of infection among older individuals. The slow acquisition of immunity with age appears to be attributable, not to the slow development of appropriate protective responses, but rather to the early rise and subsequent slow decline of inappropriate (blocking) antibodies that prevent the expression of the protective responses. These blocking antibodies may be elicited by egg polysaccharides released during early infections, may cross-react with schistosomulum surface antigens containing carbohydrate epitopes, and may include both IgM and IgG2 antibodies.

These findings are discussed in the context of the eventual use of recombinant vaccines in man.

ACKNOWLEDGEMENTS

Work by the authors and their colleagues reviewed in this paper was supported by grants from the Edna McConnell Clark Foundation, the Medical Research Council, the European Commission and the Rockefeller Foundation/WHO Joint Funding Venture. This paper is published with the kind permission of the Director of Medical Services of the Government of Kenya.

REFERENCES

Anderson R M 1987 Determinants of infection in human schistosomiasis. In: Mahmoud A A F (ed) Schistosomiasis: Bailliere's clinical tropical medicine and communicable diseases, Bailliere, London, pp 297–300

Anderson R M, May R M 1982 Population dynamics of human helminth infections: control by chemotherapy. Nature (Lond) 297: 557–563

Anderson R M, May R M 1985 Herd immunity to helminth infection and implications for parasite control. Nature (Lond) 315: 493–496

Balloul J M, Sondermeyer P, Dreyer D et al 1987 Molecular cloning of a protective antigen of schistosomes. Nature (Lond) 326: 149–153

Bensted-Smith R, Anderson R M, Butterworth A E et al 1987 Evidence for the predisposition of individual patients to reinfection with *Schistosoma mansoni* after treatment. Trans R Soc Trop Med Hyg 81: 651–654

Bradley D J, McCullough F S 1973 Egg output stability and the epidemiology of *Schistosoma haematobium*. Trans R Soc Trop Med Hyg 67: 491–500

Butterworth A E 1984 Cell-mediated damage to helminths. Adv Parasitol 23: 143–235

Butterworth A E, Sturrock R F, Houba V, Mahmoud A A F, Sher A, Rees P H 1975 Eosinophils as mediators of antibody-dependent damage to schistosomula. Nature (Lond) 256: 727–729

Butterworth A E, David J R, Franks D, Mahmoud A A F, David P H, Sturrock R F, Houba V 1977 Antibody-dependent eosinophil-mediated damage to 51Cr-labeled schistosomula of *Schistosoma mansoni*: damage by purified eosinophils. J Exp Med 145: 136–150

Butterworth A E, Dalton P R, Dunne D W et al 1984 Immunity after treatment of human schistosomiasis mansoni. I. Study design, pretreatment observations and the results of treatment. Trans R Soc Trop Med Hyg 78: 108–123

Butterworth A E, Capron M, Cordingley J S et al 1985 Immunity after treatment of human schistosomiasis mansoni. II. Identification of resistant individuals, and analysis of their immune responses. Trans R Soc Trop Med Hyg 79: 393–408

Butterworth A E, Bensted-Smith R, Capron A et al 1987 Immunity in human schistosomiasis: prevention by blocking antibodies of the expression of immunity in young children. Parasitology 94: 281–300

Butterworth A E, Fulford A J C, Dunne D W, Ouma J H, Sturrock R F 1988a Longitudinal studies on human schistosomiasis. Phil Trans R Soc Lond B 321: 495–511

Butterworth A E, Dunne D W, Fulford A et al 1988b Immunity in human schistosomiasis mansoni: cross-reactive IgM and IgG2 antibodies block the expression of immunity. Biochimie 70: 1053–1063

Capron A, Dessaint J P, Capron M, Bazin H 1975 Specific IgE antibodies in immune adherence of normal macrophages to *Schistosoma mansoni* schistosomules. Nature (Lond) 253: 474–475

Capron M, Torpier G, Capron A 1979 In vitro killing of *Schistosoma mansoni* schistosomula by eosinophils from infected rats: role of cytophilic antibodies. J Immunol 126: 2087–2092

Capron M, Bazin H, Joseph M, Capron A 1981 Evidence for IgE-dependent cytotoxicity by rat eosinophils. J Immunol 126: 1764–1768

Capron M, Spiegelberg H L, Prin L et al 1984 Role of IgE receptors in effector function of human eosinophils. J Immunol 132: 462–468

Chen M G, Mott K E 1988 Progress in assessment of morbidity due to *Schistosoma mansoni* infection. Trop Dis Bull 85: R1–R56

Clarke V de V 1966 Evidence of the development in man of acquired resistance to infection of *Schistosoma* spp. Cent Afr J Med 12 (suppl 1): 1–30

Clutterbuck E J, Sanderson C J 1988 Human eosinophil hematopoiesis studied in vitro by means of murine eosinophil differentiation factor (IL5): Production of functionally active eosinophils from normal human bone marrow. Blood 71: 646–651

Colley D G 1987 Dynamics of the human immune response to schistosomes. In: Mahmoud A A F (ed) Schistosomiasis: Bailliere's clinical tropical medicine and communicable diseases. Bailliere, London, pp 315–332

Colley D G, Barsoum I S, Dahawi H S S, Gamil F, Habib M, El Alamy M A 1986 Immune responses and immunoregulation in relation to schistosomiasis in Egypt. III. Immunity and longitudinal studies of in vitro responsiveness after treatment. Trans R Soc Trop Med Hyg 80: 952–957

Cottrell B, Pye C, Butterworth A 1989 Cytotoxic effects in vitro of human monocytes and macrophages on schistosomula of *Schistosoma mansoni*. Parasite Immunol 11: 91–104

Dalton P R, Pole D 1978 Water contact patterns in relation to *Schistosoma haematobium* infection. Bull WHO 56: 417–426

David J R, Vadas M A, Butterworth A E et al 1980 Enhanced helminthotoxic capacity of eosinophils from patients with eosinophilia. N Engl J Med 303: 1147–1152

Dessein A J, Begley M, Demeure C et al 1988 Human resistance to *Schistosoma mansoni* is associated with IgG reactivity to a 37-kDa larval surface antigen. J Immunol 140: 2727–2736

Diaz L C de S, Pedro R de J, Deberaldini E R 1982 Use of praziquantel in patients with schistosomiasis mansoni previously treated with oxamniquine and/or hycanthone: resistance of *Schistosoma mansoni* to schistosomicidal agents. Trans R Soc Trop Med Hyg 76: 652–658

Dunne D W, Bickle Q D, Butterworth A E, Richardson B A 1987 The blocking of human antibody-dependent, eosinophil-mediated killing of *Schistosoma mansoni* schistosomula by monoclonal antibodies which cross-react with a polysaccharide-containing egg antigen. Parasitology 94: 260–280

Dunne D W, Grabowska A M, Fulford A J C, Butterworth A E, Sturrock R F, Koech D, Ouma J H 1988 Human antibody responses to *Schistosoma mansoni*: the influence of epitopes shared between different life-cycle stages on the response to the schistosomulum. Eur J Immunol 18: 123–131

Gazzinelli R T, Parra J F C, Correa-Oliveira R, Cancado J R, Rocha R S, Gazzinelli G, Colley D G 1988 Idiotypic/anti-idiotypic interactions in schistosomiasis and Chagas' disease. Am J Trop Med Hyg 39: 288–294

Grzych J M, Capron M, Bazin H, Capron A 1982 In vitro and in vivo effector function of rat IgG2a monoclonal anti-*Schistosoma mansoni* monoclonal antibodies. J Immunol 129: 2739–2743

Grzych J M, Capron M, Dissous C, Capron A 1984 Blocking activity of rat monoclonal antibodies in experimental schistosomiasis. J Immunol 133: 998–1003

Hagan P, Wilkins H A, Blumenthal U J, Hayes R J and Greenwood B M 1985 Eosinophilia and resistance to *Schistosoma haematobium* in man. Parasite Immunol 7: 625–632

Hagan P, Blumenthal U J, Chaudri M et al 1987 Resistance to reinfection with *Schistosoma haematobium* in Gambian children: analysis of their immune responses. Trans R Soc Trop Med Hyg 81: 939–946

James S L 1986a Induction of protective immunity against *Schistosoma mansoni* by a nonliving vaccine. III. Correlation of resistance with induction of activated larvacidal macrophages. J Immunol 136: 3872–3877

James S L 1986b Activated macrophages as effector cells of protective immunity in schistosomiasis. Immunol Res 5: 139–147

Jordan P 1985 Schistosomiasis – the St Lucia project. Cambridge University Press, Cambridge

Khalife J, Capron M, Capron A, Grzych J M, Butterworth A E, Dunne D W, Ouma J H 1986 Immunity in human schistosomiasis mansoni: regulation of protective immune mechanisms by IgM blocking antibodies. J Exp Med 164: 1626–1640

Khalife J, Dunne D W, Richardson B A et al 1989 Functional role of human IgG subclasses in eosinophil-mediated killing of schistosomula of *S. mansoni*. J Immunol 1: 4422–4427

Kloetzel K, da Silva J R 1967 Schistosomiasis mansoni acquired in adulthood: behaviour of egg counts and the intradermal test. Am J Trop Med Hyg 16: 167–169

Kojima S, Yano A, Sasazuki T, Ohta N 1984 Association between H L A and immune responses in individuals with chronic schistosomiasis japonica. Trans R Soc Trop Med Hyg 78: 325–329

Lanar D E, Pearce E J, James S L, Sher A 1986 Identification of paramyosin as schistosome antigen recognized by intradermally vaccinated mice. Science 234: 593–596

Lehman J S, Mott K E, Morrow R H, Muniz T M, Boyer M H 1976 The intensity and effects of infection with *Schistosoma mansoni* in a rural community in northeastern Brazil. Am J Trop Med Hyg 25: 285–294

Lima M S, Gazzinelli G, Nascimento E, Carvalho Parra J, Montesano M A, Colley D G 1986 Immune responses during human schistosomiasis mansoni. Evidence for antiidiotypic T lymphocyte responsiveness. J Clin Invest 78: 983–988

Olds G R, Ellner J J, el-Kholy A, Mahmoud A A F 1981 Monocyte-mediated killing of schistosomula of *Schistosoma mansoni*: alterations in human schistosomiasis mansoni and tuberculosis. J Immunol 127: 1538–1542

Parra J C, Lima M S, Gazzinelli G, Colley D G 1988 Immune responses during human Schistosomiasis mansoni. XV. Anti-idiotypic T cells can recognize and respond to anti-SEA idiotypes directly. J Immunol 140: 2401–2405

Remold H G, Mednis A, Hein A, Caulfield J P 1988 Human monocyte-derived macrophages are lysed by schistosomula of *Schistosoma mansoni* and fail to kill the parasite after activation with interferon gamma. Am J Pathol 131: 146–158

Silberstein D S, Owen W F, Gasson J C et al 1986 Enhancement of human eosinophil cytotoxicity and leukotriene synthesis by biosynthetic (recombinant) granulocyte-macrophage colony stimulating factor. J Immunol 137: 3290–3294

Sturrock R F, Butterworth A E, Houba V, Karamsadkar S D, Kimani R 1978 *Schistosoma mansoni* in the Kenyan baboon (*Papio anubis*): the development and predictability of resistance to homologous challenge. Trans R Soc Trop Med Hyg 72: 251–261

Sturrock R F, Kimani R, Cottrell B J et al 1983 Observations on possible immunity to reinfection among Kenyan schoolchildren after treatment for *Schistosoma mansoni*. Trans R Soc Trop Med Hyg 77: 363–371

Sturrock R F, Bensted-Smith R, Butterworth A E et al 1987 Immunity after treatment of human schistosomiasis mansoni. III. Long-term effects of treatment and retreatment. Trans R Soc Trop Med Hyg 81: 303–314

Thorne K J I, Richardson B A, Veith M C, Tai P C, Spry C J F, Butterworth A E 1985 Partial purification and biological properties of an eosinophil activating factor (EAF). Eur J Immunol 15: 1083–1091

H

Thorne K J I, Richardson B A, Taverne J, Williamson D J, Vadas M A, Butterworth A E 1986 A comparison of eosinophil-activating factor (EAF) with other monokines and lymphokines. Eur J Immunol 16: 1143–1149

Tingley G A, Butterworth A E, Anderson R M et al 1988 Predisposition of humans to infection with *Schistosoma mansoni*: evidence from the reinfection of individuals following chemotherapy. Trans R Soc Trop Med Hyg 82: 448–452

Vadas M A, David J R, Butterworth A E, Pisani N T, Siongok T A 1979 A new method for the purification of human eosinophils and a comparison of the ability of these cells to damage schistosomula of *Schistosoma mansoni*. J Immunol 122: 1228–1236

Veith M C, Butterworth A E 1983 Enhancement of human eosinophil-mediated killing of *Schistosoma mansoni* larvae by mononuclear cell products in vitro. J Exp Med 157: 1828–1843

Warren K S 1973 Regulation of the prevalence and intensity of schistosomiasis in man: immunology or ecology? J Infect Dis 127: 595–609

Warren K S 1987 Determinants of disease in human schistosomiasis. In: Mahmoud A A F (ed) Schistosomiasis: Bailliere's clinical tropical medicine and communicable diseases. Bailliere, London, pp 301–313

Wilkins H A, Goll P H, Marshall T F de C, Moore P J 1984 Dynamics of *Schistosoma haematobium* infection in a Gambian community. III. Acquisition and loss of infection. Trans R Soc Trop Med Hyg 78: 227–232

Wilkins H A, Blumenthal U J, Hagan P, Hayes R J, Tulloch S 1987 Resistance to reinfection after treatment of urinary schistosomiasis. Trans R Soc Trop Med Hyg 81: 29–35

World Health Organization 1985 The control of schistosomiasis. WHO Tech Rep Ser 728. WHO, Geneva

Discussion of paper presented by A. E. Butterworth

Discussed by A. Capron
Reported by M. Capron

The convincing demonstration of an age-dependent immunity to re-infection in children living in endemic areas of schistosomiasis raised several important questions. Prior to debate about the effector mechanisms in human and experimental schistosomiasis, the influence of a heavy infection on the hormonal status of the children was discussed. A delay in puberty as well as hypogonadism have been reported previously in several endemic areas all over the world (Brazil, Egypt, the Philippines and China). Besides the consequences of a very severe hepatosplenic disease on the nutritional status and therefore on the development of the children, a different explanation was proposed. Following the demonstration that schistosomes can produce ecdysteroid hormones, it was shown recently (Duvaux et al in press) that schistosomes possess a gene encoding for proopiomelanocortin (POMC), the precursor of beta-endorphin and ACTH, and that there is a significant production of both beta-endorphin and ACTH by schistosomes. Since POMC-derived peptides are implicated in gonad endocrine regulation or gonadotropin release, this observation might be related to hypogonadism reported in human and experimental schistosomiasis.

Acquired immunity to re-infection against schistosomiasis seems to be attributable not only to the development of a protective response but to a decline in blocking antibodies preventing the expression of the protective response. Therefore indicators of susceptibility might be as important as potential markers of immunity in the understanding of protective immunity in the human population. Among the various antigens proposed as potential vaccines against schistosomiasis, two of them induced a strong proliferative response of lymphocytes from infected patients, TPI (triosephosphate isomerase) and P28. TPI, which has been cloned, was detected by monoclonal antibodies to the surface of the worm but also on transversal sections throughout the schistosome, in all cells except in the lumen of the intestine. On the other hand, P28, a protective antigen of schistosomes has been cloned and identified as a glutathione S-transferase (GST). Unlike a cloned GST of *S. japonicum* (SJ26), P28 has a rather modest homology with the rat glutathione transferase, the conserved region being mainly located in the N- and C-terminal domains of the molecule. Synthetic peptides modelled from the P28 molecule variable regions have been constructed and used to identify the major T- and B-cell epitopes and to explore the antibody response and cellular response to P28 in human populations.

Following the previous description of IgM- and IgG2-blocking antibodies, the function of IgG4 antibodies was discussed. IgG4 antibodies, purified by affinity chromatography were able to inhibit eosinophil-dependent cytotoxicity mediated by the three other isotypes. However, the precise mechanism is still obscure. In particular, it is not known whether the blocking effect is due to competition for Fc receptors on eosinophils rather than for target antigens. Further experiments are needed to compare Fc and F(ab')2 fragments of IgG4, as well as to evaluate their effects on non IgG-dependent effector mechanisms such as IgE-mediated cytotoxicity by hypodense eosinophils. It was also pointed out that, in spite of the fact that IgG4 usually represents a quantitatively minor subclass of IgG, the IgG4 responses towards schistosome adult and egg antigens were highly predominant, particularly in response to peptide epitopes. IgM and IgG2 tend to be directed against carbohydrate epitopes. A different approach allowed the evaluation, using an appropriate radio-immunoassay, of the antibody response to the recombinant P28 protein and to the various synthetic peptides in Kenyan children, according to the criteria of immunity or susceptibility. Whereas a strong IgE response (about 96% of the children) was demonstrated against P28, a large proportion of the children (around 70%), showed a specific IgG4-antibody response to the P28.

Among the various synthetic peptides, it has been possible to identify a particular construction which corresponds to the 115–131 amino-acid sequence as the major B-cell epitope recognized by IgE antibody not only in rats, but also in human infections. Interestingly, whereas no significant differences were seen between immune and susceptible individuals in the specific IgE levels to this peptide, a very significant increase of IgG4 antibody was observed in the susceptible group of children compared with the immune population, 5 weeks after treatment (sample B). (Fig. 11.8.) It has to be recalled that IgG4 is reputed as a blocking antibody in IgE-dependent reactions, such as allergy for instance. The association of an IgG4 response to the IgE response seems to be related to the susceptibility of the children to re-infection. Similarly, the existence of a significant antibody response of the IgA isotype was detected towards the P28 antigen, and this response increased 5 weeks after treatment by comparison with the low levels before treatment. In this study, it was also detected that a particular construction corresponding to the peptide 140–153 was able to discriminate the specific IgA response between immune and non-immune populations with increased levels in immune children (Fig. 11.9). Very little is known at the moment regarding the biological role of IgA antibodies, and especially their possible effector or regulatory function in schistosomiasis, and more generally in all parasitic diseases. The possible participation of these antibodies into protection mechanisms was recently supported by two sets of observations. In the perspective of optimization of the vaccine strategy which could be applied to the human population, a model of single-shot immunization of rats was recently developed (Grezel et al in preparation). A single injection of 25 µg of the recombinant P28 molecule in the presence of aluminium hydroxide could induce a mean level of protection up to 60% in immunized rats. When the antibody response of these immunized rats either with aluminium hydroxide or more recently with BCG as adjuvant was

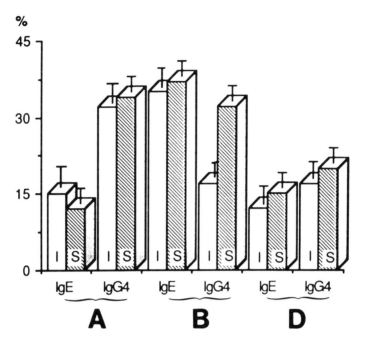

Figure 11.8 Human humoral response in infected patients from Kenya. IgE and IgG4 antibodies to synthetic peptide 115–131 derived from the amino-acid sequence of the P28 molecule. I, immune children; S, susceptible children. Samples A, before treatment; B, 5 weeks after treatment with oxamniquine; D, 1 year after treatment. The assay is a radioimmunoassay using beads coated with the peptide and ^{125}I-labelled specific antihuman IgE or IgG4 antibodies

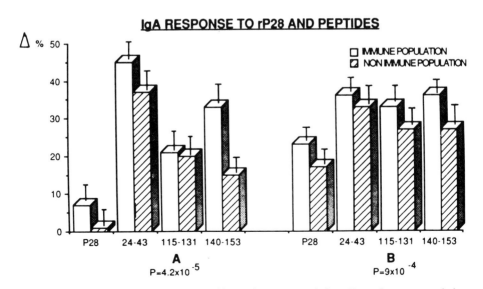

Figure 11.9 IgA response to rP28 and peptides. □ immune population; ▨ non-immune population

examined, a strong IgE-antibody response was observed. However, at the same time, an unexpected IgA-antibody response was obtained in these immunized animals. Not only were these two antibody isotypes, IgA and IgE, present in the serum of these protected animals, but they were also required in effector mechanisms depending upon the presence of eosinophils. These observations have to be related to the recent description of a receptor for IgA on the eosinophil membrane. Taken together, these findings raised the question of a possible role of IgA antibodies as effector or regulatory molecules in immune defence against parasites.

Studies in experimental animals provided evidence for at least two main effector mechanisms of immunity. The first, which is important in rats, is based on antibody-dependent cell-mediated cytotoxicity involving IgE or IgG subclasses and pro-inflammatory cells (macrophages, eosinophils and platelets). The second, which is important in the mouse model, involved antibody-independent effects of activated macrophages. The relevance of such experimental models to human immunity was actively discussed. It was agreed that each model differed markedly from the other and that none of them can be accepted as an absolute indicator of events that may be important in man. It might appear in some studies that eosinophils and antibodies are involved in pathology, whereas activated macrophages are involved in immunity. This is limited to one particular model system, which is schistosomiasis in the mouse. This does not seem to be the case in the rat or in the baboon, in which eosinophil-mediated reactions in the skin are of major importance for a protective response. Not only might the host species be of importance but also some differences can be related to the strain of *Schistosoma mansoni* itself. The experimental approach to demonstrate the participation of a given effector mechanism in protection was also debated. Several studies were reported concerning the use of specific reagents to eliminate eosinophils such as the use of antibodies to IL5 or to remove IgE with neutralizing antibodies to IL4 for instance. Again, the conclusions of such studies are only valuable for a given host-parasite interaction and for instance it is difficult to extrapolate from experiments performed in mice infected by *Nippostrongylus* to rat schistosomiasis. As well as depletion experiments, positive experiments can be performed by/on for instance adoptive transfer of immune cells or passive transfer of monoclonal antibodies which were shown to induce protection in experimental animals. It was also mentioned that even when one effector mechanism has been depleted, there are often alternative mechanisms, for instance subclasses of IgG which can share some effects with IgE. The discussion ended with agreement that such complicated infections are probably not related to only a single effector mechanism.

Plenary Lecture III

Chairman: P. K. Peterson

12. Selective primary health care and parasitic diseases

K. S. Warren

INTRODUCTION

The control of parasitic diseases in the developing world has been inhibited by a remarkable variety of environmental, social, economic and scientific factors. These include:

1. The tropical location of most of the developing world, with its warmth and humidity, which fosters transmission of infectious diseases, particularly those that are water and insect borne.
2. Poverty, which results in malnutrition, crowding, lack of water and sanitation, exposure to insects and close association with animal reservoirs.
3. The success of the developed world in controlling most infectious diseases through socio-economic development which has led to attempts to emulate this approach in the developing world with relative neglect of direct medical and public health interventions.
4. A series of global attempts to eradicate specific major tropical diseases such as hookworm and malaria, the failure of which has led to disillusionment with specific medical and public health measures.
5. The World Health Organization's Alma Ata declaration of 'health for all by the year 2000' which provided a general, relatively undifferentiated approach.
6. The narrow focus on parasitology by tropical medicine has led to the relative exclusion of other, in many cases, more important infectious diseases. This has been exacerbated by undue competition between biomedical research and public health.
7. A gross lack of support for research on all aspects of parasitology, from immunology to anthropology, and from laboratory to field investigation, which has improved only in the last decade.
8. The failure to set realistic priorities for the control of all diseases, infectious diseases and, within the latter category, the parasitic diseases themselves.

The tropical climates which are the norm for the most of the developing world are warm and usually have a high degree of humidity outside of the arid desert regions. These environmental conditions support the growth of bacteria and fungi and the transmission of protozoa and helminths. They also support the proliferation of a wide number of insect and snail vectors of disease. In many parts of the tropics transmission continues virtually unabated, on a year-round basis. Man-made environmental factors such as irrigation and urbanization facilitate the transmission of many parasite species. Finally, a crucial condition endemic to the tropics fostering the transmission of parasitic infections is poverty, resulting in lack of water for drinking and washing, lack of food storage facilities and indeed food itself, poor sanitation, and exposure to insects due to open housing and lack of screening. All of this is compounded by crowding, both in rural and urban environments. An additional devastating factor is internal conflict and war.

McKeown (1976), observed that the rise of population in Europe in the nineteenth and early twentieth centuries was the result of a remarkable decline in infectious diseases, due largely to socio-economic progress and not to specific medical interventions. 'There need be no disappointment with the conclusion that medical measures of immunization and treatment were relatively ineffective; they were also unnecessary.' He claimed that this was related principally to the availability of food and a drastic decrease in malnutrition. Other factors were water supplies/sanitation and decent housing. These results were extrapolated to the developing world of today, suggesting socio-economic development as the only strategy. This attitude was also reflected in major studies of Third World development over the last 20 years such as the Pierson Report of 1969 (Mission on International Development 1969) and the Brandt Report of 1980 (Independent Commission for International Development Issues 1980) both of which virtually ignored health as a factor and focused almost wholly on socio-economic development.

The most highly visible efforts to improve health in the developing world have been the great global attempts to eradicate specific diseases. This strategic approach began with the Rockefeller Foundation's campaign in 1913 to eradicate hookworm. It was then followed by General Gorgas' attempt, after his great success in controlling yellow fever in Cuba and the Panama Canal, to eradicate this devastating disease from its strongholds in Africa and South America. By far the largest such venture was the eradication of malaria which began in 1955 and ended in 1970 when the World Health Organization (WHO) decided to 'throw in the towel'. Disillusionment was so great that it led to a backlash against centrally planned programmes and medical technology.

In 1978 the WHO held a conference in Alma Ata to proclaim a comprehensive programme in primary health care in order to enable 'the attainment by all people of the world by the year 2000 of a level of health that would permit them to lead a socially and economically productive life. Primary health care includes at least: education concerning prevailing health problems and the methods of preventing and controlling them; promotion of food supply and proper nutrition; an adequate supply of safe water and basic sanitation; maternal and child health care, including family planning; immunization against the major infectious diseases; prevention and control of locally endemic diseases; appropriate treatment of common diseases and injuries; and provision of essential drugs' (World Health Organization 1978). This diffusion of responsibility for health in a vast pro-gramme which was not economically feasible led to a decade of relative inaction.

The field of tropical medicine, which began around the turn of the century, was a response largely to the exploration and colonization of the developing world. It became identified with parasitic diseases (protozoan and helminth), almost to the exclusion of other infectious diseases. This led to the isolation of parasitology from the bacterial and virological diseases that contributed so much to the revolution in the field of infectious diseases through the development of immunology and molecular biology and of antibiotics and vaccines. Negative effects were many, resulting in a relatively low quantity and quality of research on all aspects of these important problems (Warren in press (a)).

One related difficulty has been a gross lack of funding for research in parasitology until the last decade when the WHO and several foundations began to provide significant, though still relatively low levels of support in this area. The Tropical Disease Research Programme of WHO which was limited to six diseases – malaria, leishmaniasis, trypanosomiasis, schistosomiasis, filariasis and leprosy – involved researchers from the developing world with a particular focus on institution strengthening. It ranged from basic laboratory investigation to clinical and field research, including the social sciences. The Clark Foundation developed a unique long-term research plan for schistosomiasis, later switching to the blinding diseases, onchocerciasis and trachoma. The Rockefeller Foundation's (RF) Great Neglected Diseases of Mankind programme brought in outstanding laboratories and scientists, largely from the developed world, to work in any of the important diseases of the tropics, bacterial and viral as well as parasitic. The MacArthur Foundation's Biology of Parasitic Diseases programme provided long-term support for basic research in major laboratories throughout the world. Recently, WHO and RF began a joint collaborative programme between major research groups from the developed and developing world.

SETTING PRIORITIES

A major problem with the diseases of the developing world has been the failure to set realistic priorities, with respect to both research and control. This, of course, should be put in the context not only of the parasitic diseases but infectious diseases in general and, indeed, all of the diseases of the developing world.

The relative importance of a problem requiring control must be balanced with the availability of cost-effective means of control. While acute diarrhoea can be alleviated by oral rehydration therapy, a problem of equal importance, viral respiratory infections, suffers from a dearth of adequate methods of diagnosis, treatment and control. Other diseases of relatively different levels of priority for control (as described below) also lack cost-effective control measures; these include tuberculosis, leprosy, Chagas' disease, African trypanosomiasis and amoebiasis, among others. Major campaigns to control these diseases are both costly and relatively ineffective.

In 1979 Walsh & Warren published a paper called 'Selective primary health care: an interim strategy for disease control in developing countries.' They observed that 'faced with the vast number of health problems of mankind, one immediately becomes aware that all of them cannot be attacked simultaneously.' Four factors, they suggested, should be assessed for each disease: prevalence, morbidity, mortality and feasibility of control (including efficacy and cost). Data were gathered not only from the official figures supplied to the WHO but from numerous studies of specific problems which were extrapolated to a broader level. This resulted in Table 12.1 based on 1977 data in which the diseases were ranked by relative importance based on prevalence, mortality and morbidity. In general, these rankings were well accepted by the international health community. Table 12.2 presents the 10 principal causes of death for individuals of all ages in the developing world in 1986 (Walsh 1988), and also the 10 major causes of death due to parasitic infections. This clearly demonstrates that the latter form only a fraction of the major causes of mortality in the developing world today.

The study published in 1979 (Walsh & Warren) grouped the diseases on the basis of high, medium and low priorities based not only on prevalence, mortality, and morbidity but on feasibility of control (Table 12.3). These groupings led to the development of a selective strategy to control many of the major diseases of

Table 12.1 Prevalence, mortality and morbidity of the major infectious diseases of Africa, Asia and Latin America, 1977–78[a]

Infection	Infections (10^3/year)	Deaths (10^3/year)	Disease (10^3/year)	Average no. of days of life lost (per case)	Relative personal disability[b]
Diarrhoeas	3–5000 000	5–10 000	3–5000 000	3–5	2
Respiratory infections		4–5000		5–7	2–3
Malaria	800 000	1200	150 000	3–5	2
Measles	85 000	900	80 000	10–14	2
Schistosomiasis	200 000	500–1000	20 000	600–1000	3–4
Whooping cough	70 000	250–450	20 000	21–28	2
Tuberculosis	1000 000	400	7000	200–400	3
Neonatal tetanus	120–180	100–150	120–180	7–10	1
Diphtheria	40 000	50–60	700–900	7–10	3
Hookworm	7–900 000	50–60	1500	100	4
South American trypanosomiasis	12 000	60	1200	600	2
Onchocerciasis					
skin disease		Low	2–5000	3000	3
river blindness	30 000	20–50	200–500	3000	1–2
Meningitis	150	30	150	7–10	1
Amoebiasis	400 000	30	1500	7–10	3
Ascariasis	800 000–1 000 000	20	1000	7–10	3
Poliomyelitis	80 000	10–20	2000	3000+	2
Typhoid	1000	25	500	14–28	2
Leishmaniasis	12 000	5	12 000	100–200	3
African trypanosomiasis	1000	5	10	150	1
Leprosy		Very low	12 000	500–3000	2–3
Trichuriasis	500 000	low	100	7–10	3
Filariasis	250 000	low	2–3000	1000	3
Giardiasis	200 000	Very low	500	5–7	3
Dengue	3–4000	0.1	1–2000	5–7	2
Malnutrition	500–800 000	2000			

[a]Based on estimates from the WHO and its Special Programme for Research and Training in Tropical Diseases, confirmed or modified by extrapolations from published epidemiological studies performed in well defined populations (see references). Figures do not always match those officially reported, because under-reporting is great.
[b]Denotes: 1 bedridden, 2 able to function on own to some extent, 3 ambulatory and 4 minor.

Table 12.2 The 10 principal causes of all deaths and parasitic disease deaths for individuals of all ages in the developing world in 1986

Deaths (all causes—10^3/yr)		Deaths (parasitic diseases—10^3/yr)	
Respiratory diseases	10 000	Malaria	1500
Circulatory system	8 000	Schistosomiasis	500
Diarrhoea	4 300	Amoebiasis	70
Measles	2 000	Chagas' diseases	60
Neoplasms	2 000	Hookworm	50
Injuries	2 000	Ascariasis	10
Malaria	1 500	Giardiasis	10
Tetanus	1 200	Leishmaniasis	1
Tuberculosis	900	Trichuriasis	1
Hepatitis B	800	Filariasis	1
Total	32 700		2203

Table 12.3 Priorities for disease control in the developing world, based on prevalence, mortality, morbidity and feasibility of control

Priority group	Reasons for assignment to this category
High	High prevalence, high mortality or high morbidity, effective control
Diarrhoeal diseases	
Measles	
Malaria	
Whooping cough	
Schistosomiasis	
Neonatal tetanus	
Medium	
Respiratory infections	High prevalence, high mortality, no effective control
Poliomyelitis	High prevalence, low mortality, effective control
Tuberculosis	High prevalence, high mortality, control difficult
Onchocerciasis	Medium prevalence, high morbidity, low mortality, control difficult
Meningitis	Medium prevalence, high mortality, control difficult
Typhoid	Medium prevalence, high mortality, control difficult
Hookworm	High prevalence, low mortality, control difficult
Malnutrition	High prevalence, high morbidity, control complex
Low	
South American trypanosomiasis (Chagas' disease)	Control difficult
African trypanosomiasis	Low prevalence, control difficult
Leprosy	Control difficult
Ascariasis	Low mortality, low morbidity, control difficult
Diphtheria	Low mortality, low morbidity
Amoebiasis	Control difficult
Leishmaniasis	Control difficult
Giardiasis	Control difficult
Filariasis	Control difficult
Dengue	Control difficult

childhood at a reasonable cost: immunization for tetanus, diphtheria, pertussis, polio, measles and tuberculosis; oral rehydration for all acute diarrhoeal diseases; breast feeding; and antimalarial drugs for episodes of fever in children under 3 years of age in areas where malaria is prevalent.

In 1982 the United Nation Children's Fund (UNICEF) declared a 'children's revolution' offering 'four vital new opportunities for improving the nutrition and health of the world's children' (Grant 1983). For all of these actions, 'the cost of the supplies and technology would be no more than a few dollars per child. Yet they could mean that literally hundreds and millions of young lives would be healthier. And within a decade, they would be saving the lives of 20 000 children each day. It is not the possibility of this kind of progress that is now in question. It is its priority.' UNICEF recommended universal child immunization, oral rehydration therapy, the promotion of breast feeding and the use of growth charts to follow the nutritional status of children. Some of the data that led to these decisions are shown in Figures 12.1 and 12.2 (Grant 1984).

Later that year a group of international agencies, UNICEF, WHO, the World Bank, United Nations Development Programme (UNDP) and RF decided to work together to focus on immunizing all of the world's children. At a meeting in Bellagio, Italy in March of 1984 a Task Force for Child Survival was developed to co-ordinate these activities (Rockefeller Foundation 1984). Subsequent meetings were held in Cartagena, Colombia in October 1985 and in Talloires, France in 1988 to assess progress. When the Task Force began to co-ordinate the efforts of the five sponsoring agencies late in 1984 only 20% of the world's children were immunized. By May 1987, only 2½ years later, WHO affirmed that immunization had exceeded 50%. It is now expected that early in the 1990s at least 80% of the world's children will be immunized (Warren 1988a). In the decade, research may add new vaccines for diarrhoeal and respiratory diseases, as well as the major parasitic infections, malaria and schistosomiasis.

As early as the meeting in Cartagena, plans were being made to foster other key strategies for improving health in the developing world. These included oral rehydration therapy and family planning (Rockefeller Foundation 1986). By the time of the meeting in Talloires there had been remarkable progress on oral rehydration with use of ORS packets reaching 23% (Warren 1988a). WHO has

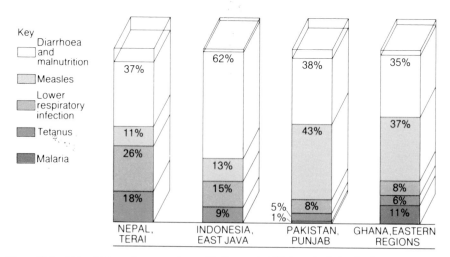

Figure 12.1 Why children die: percentages of infant and child (ages 0–4) deaths due to preventable diseases in selected countries (Reproduced with permission from UNICEF)

222

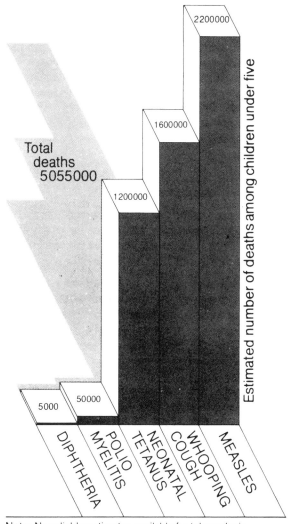

Total
deaths
5055000

2200000

1600000

1200000

50000

5000

DIPHTHERIA

POLIO MYELITIS

NEONATAL TETANUS

WHOOPING COUGH

MEASLES

Estimated number of deaths among children under five

Note: No reliable estimates available for tuberculosis

Figure 12.2 Total child deaths from immunizable diseases, 1980 (Based on WHO estimates)

recently announced a new programme entitled 'Safe Motherhood' which totally changes perceptions from the control of population as macro-socio-economic priorities to that of maintenance of the health and wellbeing of the individual mother and child. Finally, it is worthy of note that chronic disease and injuries are now well entrenched in the top 10 causes of mortality in the developing world (Table 12.2).

While the parasitic diseases are not major causes of mortality, with the exception of malaria, and perhaps schistosomiasis (Table 12.2), they remain major causes of morbidity in the developing world. Most of them are chronic infections which are debilitating, contribute to malnutrition, may cause blindness and are grossly disfiguring. It is within the realm of possibility that with proper planning many of the parasitic diseases can be controlled at relatively low cost. At present, however, because of the lack of vaccines, insecticide resistance, drug resistance, difficult and expensive diagnostic tests and/or relatively ineffective and toxic drugs, significant control of protozoan diseases does not appear to be possible. In contrast, it now appears that we can control most of the major helminth diseases with a simple annual regimen involving two or three broad-spectrum and anthelmintic drugs.

LEVELS OF CONTROL

We have seen at the beginning of this paper how the vast global campaigns to eradicate hookworm and malaria, while clearly of value (the former fostering sanitation and the latter insect control), led to disillusionment and a backlash against 'technological means' of controlling these diseases when they failed to reach their lofty objectives. As is well known, many of these infections have complex life cycles in which control measures can be instituted at several different stages. If the strategy of eradication is adopted this means that most diseases must be attacked at several vulnerable points (Walsh & Warren 1986). In the case of hookworm this involved sanitation, the wearing of shoes and treatment with anthelmintic drugs. For the control of malaria the principal means used were control of mosquitos through larvicides, insecticides and water management systems, and the use of antimalarial drugs. The more methods used, the higher the cost, particularly when they are capital intensive, such as sewerage and water systems. In the 1950s the Chinese government instituted a massive attempt to eradicate schistosomiasis. This was particularly complex, involving sanitation, water supplies not only for drinking but for bathing and washing, the use of molluscicides for killing the intermediate vector snails and antischistosome drugs not only for humans but for reservoir animals. Following these efforts the prevalence of this infection in China was reduced to approximately two-thirds of its original level (Warren in press (b)).

Another approach to these problems is control of infection (transmission), which while falling short of the complexity of eradication programmes still involves major effort. In the case of schistosomiasis WHO had recommended until very recently the use of all the methods used in eradication attempts. 'Current integrated control methods employ all the available forms of chemo-therapy, the latest mollusciciding techniques, methods to meet basic health needs such as the supply of potable water at village level and the provision of sanitation, as well as continuing health education and socio-economic improvement' (World Health Organization 1980). A major attempt to control schistosomiasis using this approach was instituted in Brazil several years ago at a cost of $300 million and was, at best, only moderately successful.

The most cost-effective strategy is to focus, wherever possible, on the control of disease rather than infection. While this may not seem self-evident it has been a major approach to the control of helminth infections since RF's global hookworm campaign which began in 1913. In Fosdick's *The Story of the Rockefeller Foundation* (1952), he observed 'in the earlier days, Rose and his colleagues spoke of the eradication of hookworm; the original Rockefeller sanitary commission used that word in its title. It is a goal that has never been reached. Social patterns and habits cannot be changed overnight and discouraging reinfection can occur where adequate sanitary arrangements are not maintained. Moreover, as the years went by, it began to be clear that there was a distinction between hookworm disease and a comparatively harmless hookworm infection. Laboratory investigation proved that people with a limited number of hookworms are not necessarily ill.'

The reason for this distinction in the case of helminths is well described by the population ecologists Anderson & May (1979) who termed these organisms macroparasites 'which tend to have much longer generation times than the microparasites (protozoa, bacteria and viruses), and direct multiplication within the host is either absent or occurs at a low rate. The immune response elicited by these metazoans generally depends upon the number of parasites present in a given host, and tends to be of relatively short duration. Macroparasitic infections, therefore, tend to be of a persistent nature, with hosts being continually re-infected.' Almost 20 years ago, Crofton (1971) noted that the parasite populations within the host are greatly overdispersed in that the majority of helminth infections are light and that only a small minority bear heavy worm burdens; it is in this small population that the infection is associated with disease. In an editorial in *The New England Journal of Medicine* entitled 'The guerrilla worm' (Warren 1970) it was pointed out that 'many patients invaded by schistosomes, trichinellae, ascarides, filariae and hookworms never had and never will have overt signs or symptoms of disease. The respective manifestations caused by these worms – liver fibrosis, myositis, intestinal obstruction, elephantiasis and anaemia – occur only when there is an unusually heavy attacking force or when large numbers of parasites have accumulated.'

Early in the hookworm campaigns it was realized that disease was related to intensity of infection which could be measured by egg counts. Since even the most virulent hookworms suck only about 250 μl of blood per day it requires large numbers of such worms to produce anaemia, particularly when there is adequate iron in the diet. As Smillie noted in 1924 'hookworm infection is slowly acquired and slowly lost. Thus a severe degree of infection is rare in a child under 5 years of age, and even in a heavily infected zone the number of hookworms harbored by a child does not increase and decrease with each season, but increases gradually in number year by year. As a rule, therefore, the older the child, the heavier the infection... Massive infection from a single or occasional exposure to hookworm infected soil is rare.' He then observed that 'hookworm disease, that is, an infection which is severe enough and widespread enough to be an important economic factor in the lives of the people, should be found almost exclusively in the rural children of school age (6–16 years) because their barefeet are almost continually exposed to hookworm infected soil throughout the warm season of the year.' Smillie added that 'It is true that sanitation alone will control hookworm disease. But this method is extremely slow. To be effective, at least 80% of the rural homes and all the rural schools must have sanitary toilets, and these must be used. This necessitates a changing of habits and customs of a lifetime and can scarcely be accomplished in a decade.' He concluded, 'hookworm disease can best be controlled by mass treatment of the heavily infected group of individuals. One single treatment of the rural school children will reduce the actual number of worms harbored by more than 90%. New infection is slowly acquired. The children are relieved immediately of the great burden they have been carrying and sanitary measures can be undertaken to prevent reinfection.' Thus, 'we may establish the axiom that hookworm treatment should be used to control hookworm disease; the infection rate is controlled by sanitation.'

After the RF campaigns ended, this remarkable strategy was essentially forgotten. It is particularly sad, because it is relevant to virtually all of the helminth infections. In the case of schistosomiasis, which many consider to be the most important of these, this approach had to be completely rediscovered. Several factors led to this realization. A long-term study of the ecology and control of schistosomiasis on the island of St Lucia, which continued for a period of 16 years, provided vast amounts of integrated data (Jordan 1985). Ecologically, schistosomiasis was shown to have slow infection rates that were seasonally

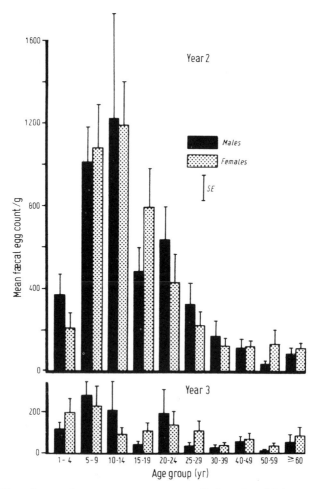

Figure 12.3 Effect of targeted mass treatment on age-specific intensity of *Schistosoma mansoni* infection

related. The worms were found to have a relatively short lifespan of about 5 years. Both on St Lucia and in many other endemic areas, disease was clearly shown to be related to intensity of infection. With the use of the Kato technique for schistosomiasis mansoni and japonica and the Peters technique for schistosomiasis haematobia, determination of the intensity of infection was simple and rapid. During this period, excellent single dose oral drugs became available.

In 1976 an approach called 'targeted mass treatment' was described and its use in Kenya delineated (Warren & Mahmoud 1976). The effectiveness of this approach was demonstrated in a village in Kenya in which the infection rates were exceedingly heavy and there was a relatively high proportion of disease. As can be seen in Figure 12.3, the intensity of infection was highest in school-age children. Following treatment of all those with moderate and heavy infections in a Kenyan village, egg counts remained at about 10% of their pretreatment level (Fig. 12.3), and those with hepatosplenic disease showed a marked reduction in liver size over a period of 1 to 2 years (Mahmoud et al 1983). Studies in an area of extremely heavy infection in north-east Brazil have demonstrated that following a single course of treatment, there is a marked reduction in liver disease in spite of continuing re-infection (Bina & Prata 1984). A method of controlling schistosomiasis in Kenya has been recommended based on these principles (Warren 1982). Since the groups most heavily infected are schoolchildren (ages 5–19) and they are the easiest to reach for treatment, they were designated as the target population. In areas of heavy infection all schoolchildren might be treated with the new single-dose, non-toxic drugs, but in areas of lighter infection, rapid quantitative diagnostic techniques such as the quick Kato or the Peters technique might be used to decide treatment.

HOOKWORM REVISITED

The year 1988 was the 75th anniversary of the beginning of the RF's global campaign to eradicate hookworm. At the suggestion of Dr Gerhard A Schad, of the University of Pennsylvania School of Veterinary Medicine, a conference on the present status and future of hookworm control was held. Given that there are still 900 million people in the world with this infection, this meeting concluded with a discussion of the control of hookworm today. While the public health measures of sanitation and health education have changed relatively little, we now have better drugs which are single-dose and non-toxic, and, of particular interest, are broad-spectrum, being effective against both *Ascaris* and *Trichuris*. Controlled studies with the use of these drugs in Kenya have revealed a positive effect on the nutritional status of treated children (Crompton & Stephenson in press). As was noted in a report of this conference, it became evident that all of the geohelminths could be controlled simultaneously using a strategy similar to that of the hookworm campaigns of the 1920s 'when it was realized that treatment targeted towards those most heavily infected – rural school children' was the most cost-effective approach. It was then noted that 'a similar approach to the control of schistosomiasis by use of a single dose, broad spectrum, antitrematode drug' might be used in conjunction with the antigeohelminth drugs (Warren 1988b).

227

Roy Anderson, the population ecologist, and colleagues (Anderson & May 1982, Anderson & Medley 1985) have done a series of studies of the population dynamics of the control of helminth infections by chemotherapy using a combination of mathematical simulation and data from field investigations. He has made a distinction between targeted and selective mass treatment, the former being directed toward specific age groups at high risk, the latter to 'wormy' individuals identified by laboratory tests. Anderson (Anderson & Medley 1985) did note that 'targeting is more likely to be cost-effective when aimed at specific age groups within the community who are at major risk of infection and suffer the associated morbidity.' He then stated that age-targeted treatment 'is unlikely to be very effective in the overall control of transmission,' but, as noted above, the purpose of this programme is to control morbidity.

Anderson later wrote, 'our understanding of the transmission dynamics of the major helminth infections of man is probably sufficient at present to provide qualitative guidelines for the design of community-based chemotherapy programmes (despite the inadequacy of current epidemiological knowledge concerning the issues of predisposition and the generation of parasite aggregation). The question of how frequently to mass treat, for example, can be answered in broad terms. In the case of short-lived parasites such as *Ascaris* and *Trichuris*, the interval between mass treatments should be around 4–6 months. For hookworms with an intermediate reproductive lifespan, the interval should be around 1 year or so, while for the comparatively long-lived schistosome species the interval can be extended to 2–3 years... The effective application of these principles, however, will depend on the resources available for community-based chemotherapy programmes. This in turn will depend on the priority given by public health authorities in developing countries to helminth control. In terms of visible morbidity, and immediate mortality following infection, diseases such as measles and pertussis clearly demand high priority. The toll exacted by the life-time presence of helminths is difficult to quantify at present but common sense argues that it must be of great significance to overall community health.'

TREATMENT STRATEGY

A specific plan which I would like to propose at this point would prevent the morbidity caused by virtually all of the major helminths of man, as shown in Table 12.4, by an integrated programme of treatment at appropriate intervals, with only three drugs. Treatment at 6-month intervals with albendazole in a single dose would drastically reduce the intensity of infection with the three geohelminths plus *Enterobius*. Studies suggest that the single-dose antitrematode drug praziquantel will maintain infection at low levels not only of all species of the human schistosomes, but also of most other trematodes as well, including the liver flukes, *Clonorchis* and *Opisthorchis*, the intestinal fluke *Fasciolopsis* and the lung fluke *Paragonimus*. It will also control the three major human intestinal tapeworm infections. Although the time intervals have not been worked out adequately yet, use of the new drug ivermectin would control many of the tissue nematode infections, including *Onchocerca*, *Brugia* and *Wuchereria*, when given at intervals of approximately one year.

Table 12.4 Major helminth infections of man

Organism	Common name	Means of infection	Major disease manifestation[a]
Nematodes			
Ancylostoma duodenale	Hookworm	Skin	Anaemia
Ascaris lumbricoides	Giant roundworm	Oral	Intestinal obstruction
Enterobius vermicularis	Pinworm	Oral	Anal pruritus
Onchocerca volvulus	River blindness	Insect	Blindness
Strongyloides stercoralis	Strongyloidiasis	Skin	Auto-infection
Trichinella spiralis	Trichinosis	Oral	Myositis
Trichuris trichiura	Whipworm	Oral	Rectal prolapse
Wuchereria bancrofti	Filariasis	Insect	Elephantiasis
Trematodes			
Clonorchis sinensis	Liver fluke	Oral	Biliary obstruction
Fasciola hepatica	Liver fluke	Oral	Hepatomegaly
Fasciolopsis buski	Intestinal fluke	Oral	Diarrhoea
Paragonimus westermani	Lung fluke	Oral	Cough
Schistosoma haematobium	Blood fluke	Skin	Hydronephrosis
Schistosoma japonicum	Blood fluke	Skin	Hepatosplenomegaly
Schistosoma mansoni	Blood fluke	Skin	Hepatosplenomegaly
Cestodes			
Diphyllobothrium latum	Fish tapeworm	Oral	Anaemia
Taenia saginata	Beef tapeworm	Oral	None
Taenia solium	Pork tapeworm	Oral	Cysticercosis
Echinococcus granulosis	Hydatid cyst	Oral	Cyst

[a]These manifestations are relatively infrequent and tend to be related to the intensity of infection; exceptions are *Strongyloidiasis* and *Echinococcosis*.

The programme will be tailored to the needs of individual countries. The dosages and time intervals will be selected, the proper targets will be aimed at and campaign material will be prepared to educate the public. Such an approach to the control of virtually all of the major helminth infections of the children of this world and, in some cases the adults, will coincide with the cost-effective approach to selective primary health care and might be one of the next major targets of this strategic approach to achieving health throughout the world.

ERADICATION REDUX

To achieve eradication, a proper target at a proper time needs to be chosen. Obviously, eradication of hookworm in the 1920s and yellow fever as well, and malaria in the 1950s and 1960s was not feasible given the tools available. Neither is it feasible today. But in the 1970s and early 1980s, the world did eradicate its first disease, smallpox. This was rendered possible by a vaccine which, though available for more than 200 years, had been recently improved. It was also rendered possible by the fact that every single case of smallpox develops a recognizable rash. And it was rendered possible by the absolute dedication of field workers throughout the world and a myriad of small improvements in the system gained from experience in the field. At the meeting in Talloire, in March 1988, a new goal of eradication was announced (Warren 1988a). 'By 1985 polio immunization had progressed to the point that the director of the Pan American Health Organization proposed eradication of the indigenous transmission of wild polio virus from the Americas by 1990.' This advanced at Talloires to a consensus that the global eradication of polio was attainable. In addition, there is an attempt now being made to eradicate the helminth infection, dracunculiasis (Hopkins 1988). The infection is localized to a relatively small number of countries in Asia and Africa. It is vulnerable because 'it has no animal reservoir; its prevalence is highly seasonal in most areas; it is only contracted by drinking water which must have been contaminated by human beings in the first place; its distribution is limited and focal; and there are at least three known ways to prevent it completely: health education, water supply and vector control.' For Asia, eradication goals have been set for the year 1990 in both India and Pakistan; for Africa, for 1993 in Cameroon and Ghana, for 1994 in Burkina Faso and for 1995 in the Ivory Coast and Nigeria.

CONCLUSION

In spite of environmental problems, poverty and past failures, parasitic diseases can be controlled in the developing world. Of course, the ultimate means of doing so is by socio-economic development. Unfortunately, this is not possible in the near future. One of the necessary factors to enable this is setting priorities not only in terms of the importance of these diseases as determined by their prevalence, morbidity and mortality, but also whether cost-effective means of controlling them are available. Modern biomedical research is giving us more new and powerful means of dealing with these problems all the time. Immunology and molecular biology are moving towards the development of vaccines against most major infectious diseases, including many of the helminth and protozoan parasites. Using biochemistry and molecular and structural biology, we should soon move into an era of rational design of drugs. Even public health measures, in some cases, have been made more effective.

A major development on the global scene is the political will to make health a high priority by the governments of the developing world. This began with the great Alma Ata declaration of 'health for all by the year 2000' which was disseminated throughout the world by the determined ambassadors of the World Health Organization led by its great Director General, Dr Halfdan Mahler. In recent years Dr Mahler's fervor has been complemented by the energy and drive of Dr James Grant, Executive Director of UNICEF which has demonstrated that by focusing on certain highly effective, low-cost measures, it can drastically reduce childhood morbidity and mortality throughout the developing world. Working together WHO, UNICEF, UNDP and the World Bank, assisted by bilateral agencies and foundations, have involved the leaders of many of the countries of the Third World in their efforts to improve health, not only of children, but also of all of the peoples of the developing world. As new and better vaccines, drugs and public health measures become available and reach a level of effectiveness that is affordable for the developing world, control of more and more diseases can be achieved.

In this paper, it is suggested that by using targeted mass chemotherapy it will be possible to control most of the major helminth infections of the developing world at a reasonable cost. In spite of past failures in the eradication campaigns for hookworm and malaria we have been heartened by the successful eradication of smallpox, and there is now hope that we may be able to eradicate polio and the parasitic infection dracunculiasis, often called 'the fiery serpent.'

REFERENCES

Anderson R M, May R M 1979 Population biology of infectious diseases: Part I. Nature 280: 361–367
Anderson R M, May R M 1982 Population dynamics of human helminth infections: control by chemotherapy. Nature 297: 557–563
Anderson R M, Medley G F 1985 Community control of helminth infections of man by mass and selective chemotherapy. Parasitology 9: 629–660
Bina J C, Prata A R 1984 Evolucao natural da esquistossomose huma area endemica In: Aspectos Peculiares da Infeccao por Schistosoma mansoni Centro Editorial a Didatico da UFBA, Salvador, pp 13–33
Crofton H D 1971 The quantitative approach to parasitism. Parasitology 62: 179–193
Crompton D W T, Stephenson L S 1989 Hookworm infection, nutritional status and productivity In: Schad G A, Warren K S (eds) Hookworm disease: present status and new directions. Taylor & Francis, London (in press)
Fosdick R B 1952 The Story of the Rockefeller Foundation. Harper & Brothers, New York
Grant J P 1983 The State of the World's Children 1982–83. Oxford University Press, Oxford
Grant J P 1984 The State of the World's Children 1984. Oxford University Press, Oxford
Grosse R N 1980 Interrelation between health and population: observations derived from field experiences. Soc Sci Med 14: 103
Hopkins D R 1988 Dracunculiasis eradication: the tide has turned. Lancet ii: 148–150
Independent Commission on International Development Issues 1980 North-South: A program for Survival. Chairman Brandt W, MIT Press, Cambridge, MA
Jordan P 1985 Schistosomiasis: The St Lucia Project. Cambridge University Press, Cambridge
McKeown T 1976 The modern rise of population. Academic Press, New York
Mahmoud A A F, Siongok T A, Ouma J, Houser H B, Warren K S 1983 Effect of targetted mass treatment on intensity of infection and morbidity in schistosomiasis mansoni: three year follow up of a community in Machakos, Kenya. Lancet i: 849–851
Mission on International Development 1969 Partners in development: Report. Chairman Pierson L B. Praeger, New York
Rockefeller Foundation 1984 Protecting the world's children: vaccines and immunization within primary health care. The Rockefeller Foundation, New York
Rockefeller Foundation 1986 Protecting the world's children 'Bellagio II' at Cartagena, Colombia, October 1985. The Rockefeller Foundation, New York
Smillie W G 1924 Control of hookworm disease in south Alabama. South Med J 17: 494–499
Walsh J A 1988 Establishing health priorities in the developing world. United Nations Development Programme, New York
Walsh J A, Warren K S 1979 Selective primary healthcare: an interim strategy for disease control in developing countries. N Engl J Med 301: 967–974
Walsh J A, Warren K S 1986 Strategies for primary health care: technologies appropriate for the control of disease in the developing world, University of Chicago Press, Chicago
Warren K S 1970 The guerrilla worm. N Engl J Med, 282: 810–811
Warren K S 1982 The present impossibility of eradicating the omnipresent worm. Rev Infect Dis 4: 955–959
Warren K S 1988a Protecting the world's children. An agenda for the 1990s. Lancet i: 659
Warren K S 1988b Hookworm control. Lancet ii: 897–898
Warren K S 1989a Tropical medicine and tropical health. The Heath Clark Lectures 1988. Rev Infect Dis (in press).
Warren K S 1989b Farewell to the plague spirit: chairman Mao's crusade against schistosomiasis. In: Bowers J Z (ed) Research and Education in 20th Century China. Center for Chinese studies, University of Michigan Press (in press)
Warren K S, Mahmoud A A F 1976 Targetted mass treatment: a new approach to the control of schistosomiasis. Trans Ass Am Phys 89: 195–204
World Health Organization 1978 Declaration of Alma Ata (Report on the International Conference on Primary Health Care, Alma Ata, USSR), September 6–12, 1978 World Health Organization, Geneva
World Health Organization 1980 Epidemiology and control of schistosomiasis, Report of a WHO Expert Committee. WHO Tech Rep Ser 643, World Health Organization, Geneva

Discussion of paper presented by K. S. Warren

Discussed by G. T. Keusch

Warren has consistently promoted a rational approach to tropical medicine, based on the twin pillars of (i) support of basic research to improve understanding of parasitic diseases in order to develop effective new drugs or preventive agents such as vaccines, and (ii) the setting of priorities for both laboratory and clinical endeavours. Together with Walsh, Warren has selected four criteria for determining priorities for disease control in developing countries, namely disease prevalence, morbidity, mortality and the feasibility of control. With this analysis as the basis, Walsh and Warren developed a strategy for selective primary health care in the developing world. The measures which emerged from this analysis included immunization, oral rehydration therapy (ORT) for watery diarrhoeas, promotion of breast feeding and anti-malarial treatment for fevers in young children. International and bilateral assistance agencies later took up this strategy, for example UNICEF's GOBI programme (which included growth monitoring as a guide to action to prevent malnutrition, oral rehydration therapy, promotion of breast feeding for its nutritional and immunological benefits and immunization) and the CCCD effort in Africa (a programme to control childhood communicable diseases) undertaken by the US Agency for International Development and the Centers for Disease Control (which promote development of the infrastructure to improve the delivery of immunizations, oral rehydration therapy (ORT) and malaria treatment). These programmes have attempted to meld science with politics and sociology, in particular the motivation of populations to change health-related behaviour.

Science operates on principles of rational thought, although this process may falter occasionally. However, it regularly falters in politics, and within the realm of social interactions, for example the popular perceptions of health and disease, cause and effect, diagnosis and therapy, the rational process is often based on erroneous data and can lead to the wrong conclusions or inappropriate actions. There is an inherent rationality in the GOBI and CCCD programmes. However, it is still difficult to find evidence of a major effect on either childhood morbidity or mortality at the present time. The immunization programme cannot yet be declared a success even though it has, without any doubt, significantly increased immunization coverage in the past decade. It is difficult to believe in reports of 50% coverage being reached globally by 1987 or of the possibility of reaching the goal of 80% coverage by the early 1990s. In many places the number of children receiving any immunization has certainly increased, but the number receiving more than the initial dose of the EPI (expanded programme of immunization) vaccines is disappointingly low, and the efficacy of the labile and heat-sensitive vaccines remains uncertain. One Asian country has made spectacular progress in its health infrastructure, with both an impressive record in delivering vaccines and in assuring the cold chain of the vaccines it uses, but these vaccines are all shipped in via the airports of nearby countries, where goods of all sorts (including EPI vaccines) regularly bake or age on the tarmac because of bureaucratic failures. Moreover, even though the technology exists, Keusch claimed that he never saw a single dose of a vaccine that had a temperature marker to indicate whether or not the cold chain of the vaccine can be preserved.

There is room to discuss whether or not the application of the Walsh/Warren test criteria of morbidity and mortality to parasitology will justify the selective programme of helminth control suggested by Warren. This is especially true if the target of primary health care is deemed to be the young child under 5 years of age, the most vulnerable renewable global resource that there is! Morbidity and mortality in developing countries are not spread evenly across the age spectrum; rather, the short life expectancy at birth which characterizes so many developing countries is primarily determined by the excess of early childhood deaths. If you make it to 5 years of age, you probably will live to at least 60. Helminths, even Warren's favourite schistosomes, are not the striking problem in this target age group. Thus, adding age to the criteria for setting priorities for selective primary health care is an important factor in public health planning.

The Walsh/Warren approach as described has been applied only to certain specific diseases. There is still another, very often overlooked, perspective to consider. For example, in the first meeting of the tropical diseases biomedical research network developed by Warren for the Rockefeller Foundation, he quoted the Foundation's President, John Knowles, who said in 1976 that 'we need a resurgence of interest in public health and tropical medicine, for we share with the less-developed countries the fact that the next major advances in health will be based on the elements of nutrition, family planning, control of infectious diseases, and a massive change in individual and national life styles.' Changes in life style may influence all the other factors, for example: At a recent regional Asian meeting on the dysenteries, the Asian participants were asked to answer a questionnaire concerning the adequacy of teaching on the diarrhoeal diseases at their own medical schools, about literature resources available, and about 'pharmacist' advice, because so much drug therapy is actually dispensed by shopkeepers selling drugs, whether or not they are trained pharmacists. The participants were asked to visit five 'pharmacies' and present a brief case of a sick 18-month-old child with a febrile bloody diarrhoea and anorexia, and to request advice. The results of this 'not-so-random' study were that not one responder reported satisfaction with his own medical curriculum and its practical applications to diarrhoeal disease therapy and control. Few reported regular access to key journals, but worse yet, few even had regular access to reports, reviews, or manuals from international organizations, such as the World Health Organization or International Centre for Diarrhoeal Disease Research in Bangladesh. Concerning drug therapy for the test patient, 20% of the pharmacy owners surveyed recommended taking the baby directly to a physician. This high referral rate is probably due in large part to the non-randomness of the study and to the obviously higher socio-economic status and educational level of the 'client'. Of the remaining 80%, half recommended an anti-amoebic drug, usually with one or more other drugs including a variety of appropriate or inappropriate antibiotics for *Shigella* dysentry, as well as ORT, herbal therapy, multivitamins, and antipyretics. The other half used a similar array of medications but did not include metronidazole for the amoebas. The likelihood of recommending an appropriate antibiotic was greater when anti-amoebic therapy was not included (50% vs 20%). In many of the developing countries, most health care is frequently obtained at the level of non-physician 'practitioners', such as traditional, sprititual and herbal healers. Patients or caretakers generally have a rationale for seeking care but rarely does it coincide with perceptions of Western medicine and schemes for selective primary health care. This being the case, we need to know how to enter into this decision-making process, how to influence practitioners' behaviour and how to utilize already functioning and accepted systems of health care to improve the standards of care in the community. It is often the medical profession which resists any such rapprochment.

This symposium is a demonstration of how much progress we have made in the science of parasitology and in new strategies of treatment or control. These advances need to be supported vigorously and pursued. At the same time, it is essential that we also move to address the last and perhaps most important part of the challenge offered by Knowles, to effect a massive change in individual and national life styles. As a laboratory scientist working on basic science approaches to solving health problems, Keusch expressed the opinion that without behavioural changes scientific accomplishments fall short of their potential. Attention must be paid to the social issues, and this means finding a way to integrate biomedical and social science approaches, particularly at the field level. This is difficult to do, as biomedical and social scientists often do not or cannot even talk with one another. But this dialogue is necessary as a start. For example, prevalence and incidence data for diarrhoeal diseases may be flawed without a knowledge of descriptions of illness in the community. In Bangladesh, one folk term for a cholera-like dehydrating illness is 'diarrhoea'. If a health worker asks whether or not a household member has had diarrhoea within the past 3 days, the answer may well be no even if somebody has just died of dysentary. Similarly, when interventions are being planned, understanding the basis for client and provider behaviour will ensure the best chance to influence that behavior towards appropriate health care decisions. One place to begin is behaviour relating to drug selection and use in developing countries, a subject of relevance not only for the patient but also for the future health of the pharmaceutical industry. In the context of selective primary health care, this would mean not only selecting the drugs to be given but also paying attention to the educational needs to ensure that they are used as intended and for the proper indications.

Section V:
AIDS-associated parasitic diseases

Chairman: H. C. Neu

13. Anticoccidial agents in the treatment of toxoplasmic encephalitis

E. R. Pfefferkorn

INTRODUCTION: ALTERNATIVE DRUGS IN AIDS PATIENTS

Toxoplasma gondii is an obligate intracellular protozoan parasite. Human infection with *T. gondii* is usually asymptomatic and results in the formation of dormant encysted bradyzoites that remain in the brain and elsewhere for life. Only the developing fetus and the immunosuppressed patient are at substantial risk of severe disease. Even among the immunosuppressed, toxoplasmic encephalitis was once comparatively rare, seen predominantly in patients who had leukaemia or lymphoma. The current AIDS epidemic has brought to the fore a number of once rare opportunistic infections, among them toxoplasmic encephalitis. The high incidence of toxoplasmic encephalitis in AIDS patients, first noted by Luft et al (1983), has been widely reported. Luft & Remington (1988) project that by 1991 there will be 20 000–40 000 AIDS patients with toxoplasmic encephalitis in the USA alone.

Early diagnosis of toxoplasmic encephalitis in AIDS patients may be difficult even with the advantages offered by computed axial tomography and magnetic resonance imaging. Conventional serology may not be useful because nearly all cases in the USA appear to be recrudescent disease resulting from the inability to suppress the multiplication of tachyzoites which arise from spontaneously excysted bradyzoites in the brain. Thus, there is no IgM response and the patients have antitoxoplasma IgG before the first symptoms of toxoplasmic encephalitis. Suzuki et al (1988) have reported that a serological test based on the agglutination of fixed tachyzoites will distinguish the antibodies characteristic of recrudescent toxoplasmic encephalitis from those found in all chronically infected persons. Their test may become the method of choice for serological diagnosis. Isolation of infectious *T. gondii* from a biopsy will not distinguish between the encysted bradyzoites of chronically infected patients and the actively multiplying tachyzoites which cause toxoplasmic encephalitis. Since this distinction can often be made in Giemsa-stained specimens, histological examination of biopsies may be useful.

The prognosis of toxoplasmic encephalitis is poor. In one series of cases the median survival from the initiation of therapy was 4 months (Haverkos 1987). This poor outcome cannot be entirely ascribed to the lack of potent antitoxoplasmic drugs. The standard therapeutic regimen of pyrimethamine and sulphadiazine is highly effective against the tachyzoites of *T. gondii*. These drugs act synergistically since pyrimethamine inhibits dihydrofolate reductase while sulphadiazine reduces the synthesis of functional folic acid. The response of the first episode of toxoplasmic encephalitis to pyrimethamine–sulphadiazine is so often good that a therapeutic trial has been advocated as a diagnostic procedure in AIDS patients who have a CNS mass lesion of uncertain aetiology. Since most AIDS patients with toxoplasmic encephalitis have recurrent disease when the pyrimethamine–sulphadiazine treatment is withdrawn, treatment with these drugs must be continued. Unfortunately, the prolonged use of these drugs results in a remarkably high incidence of bone marrow suppression and severe skin cutaneous reactions (Haverkos 1987). The onset of these side-effects often precludes further use of pyrimethamine–sulphadiazine.

Thus, there is an urgent need for alternative treatments for toxoplasmic encephalitis in AIDS patients. Prophylactic immunization can be ruled out since most cases arise from encysted bradyzoites and the patients already have antibodies to *T. gondii*. Perhaps lymphokines or other modulators of the immune response could reverse some of the immunological defects which characterize AIDS and thus prevent toxoplasmic encephalitis, but this is beyond the scope of our discussion. Several new approaches to the treatment of toxoplasmic encephalitis are currently under investigation. Clindamycin, which is effective against *T. gondii* in mice, has shown substantial promise in uncontrolled trials (Dannemann et al 1988). Also under investigation is trimetrexate, a potent inhibitor of dihydrofolate reductase which may reach intracellular parasites more readily because of its hydrophobicity (Kovacs et al 1987).

RATIONALE FOR CONSIDERING ANTICOCCIDIAL AGENTS IN THE CHEMOTHERAPY OF TOXOPLASMOSIS

A possible source of antitoxoplasma drugs is the large catalogue of anticoccidial agents which has been accumulated by the veterinary pharmaceutical industry. Anticoccidial drugs are designed to prevent the morbidity caused in chickens by intracellular protozoan parasites of the genus *Eimeria*. *Eimeria* species have a relatively simple life cycle in the intestinal epithelial cells of a single host species. Chickens are infected by the ingestion of faecal oocysts excreted during the acute phase of disease. When chickens are raised on a large and crowded commercial scale, coccidial infections can spread rapidly. The resulting morbidity would be a serious economic problem were it not for the widespread use of anticoccidial agents to block the growth of *Eimeria*. However, when very large populations of chickens are all treated with the same anticoccidial agent, the conditions are optimal for the selection of drug-resistant mutant parasites. The emergence of such mutants has curtailed the usefulness of many anticoccidial agents introduced during the past several decades (reviewed by McDougald 1982). The strategy of the veterinary pharmaceutical industry to counter the rapid obsolescence of their anticoccidial agents has been a vigorous search for new drugs. This search has focused on two sources, both of which have proved to be profitable, new antimetabolites prepared by organic synthesis and new antimicrobials isolated from the culture medium of soil organisms. The result of this search has been the development of an extensive and diverse catalogue of anticoccidial agents. We suspected that this catalogue might contain useful antitoxoplasma drugs for two reasons. First, many anticoccidial agents would be expected to be active against *T. gondii* because this parasite is a close phylogenetic relative of *Eimeria*. Second, the anticoccidial agents have been extensively tested not only for therapeutic efficacy, but also for low toxicity in chickens. The fact that the use of many of these drugs has been abandoned because of the emergence of resistant parasite mutants may not be a major concern. The population of actively multiplying *T. gondii* within any one patient is probably low enough that the appearance of a resistant mutant is unlikely. Even if such a resistant mutant were to arise, it would be a problem only for a single patient because human infections are nearly always dead-ends in terms of transmission of the parasite.

We decided, therefore, to examine the antitoxoplasma activity of various anti-coccidial agents and present here our experience with one product of organic synthesis and one product of soil microbiology. We have studied these anticoccidial agents in mice and in human fibroblasts infected with *T. gondii* in order to determine their antitoxoplasma activity and mechanism of action. One of the easiest ways to explore the mechanism of a drug is to compare the biochemistry of the wild-type parasite with that of a drug-resistant mutant. Such mutants are readily obtained from suitably mutagenized populations of *T. gondii* because this parasite is haploid (Pfefferkorn & Pfefferkorn 1980).

Arprinocid

The drug arprinocid (9-(2-chloro-6-fluorophenyl)-9H-purine-6-amine) is one of a series of purine analogues synthesized at the Merck Institute. Arprinocid was patented by Lire et al (1976) because it showed substantial promise as an anticoccidial agent. It never achieved much commercial success because the emergence of resistant mutants curtailed its usefulness. In the course of their studies of the pharmacology of arprinocid in chickens, workers at the Merck Institute discovered a minor metabolite, arprinocid-*N*-oxide, which was probably produced by the cytochrome P_{450} system of the liver. The structures of both substances are shown in Fig. 13.1. Interestingly, both arprinocid and arprinocid-*N*-oxide showed activity against *Eimeria tenella*, the usual parasite for testing anticoccidial agents.

Luft (1986) observed that arprinocid was remarkably effective in treating mice infected with the hypervirulent RH strain of *T. gondii*. We confirmed these data and attempted to determine the biochemical basis for the antitoxoplasma activity of arprinocid. Our in vitro experiments depended upon measuring the growth of *T. gondii* in human fibroblast cultures by determining the incorporation of [³H]uracil into acid precipitable form. This incorporation was specific for *T. gondii* because the parasites, but not the host cells, are able to salvage uracil (Pfefferkorn & Pfefferkorn 1977a). Labelling with [³H]uracil has been shown to be directly proportional to the number of parasites present (Mellors et al 1989). When the antitoxoplasma effects of arprinocid and arprinocid-*N*-oxide were measured by the incorporation of [³H]uracil, both proved to be active, with the *N*-oxide notably more potent. Figure 13.2 shows that 50% inhibition of parasite growth measured

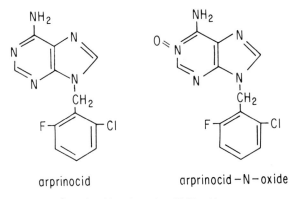

arprinocid   arprinocid −N−oxide

Figure 13.1   The structures of arprinocid and arprinocid-*N*-oxide

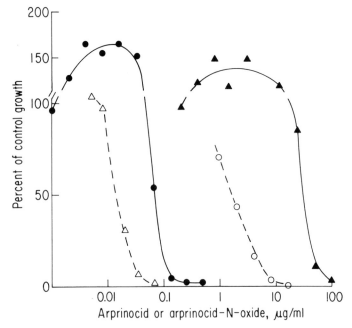

Figure 13.2   The effects of arprinocid and arprinocid-*N*-oxide on the growth of human fibroblasts and of wild-type RH *T. gondii*. Growth of the parasite was measured by the incorporation of [³H]uracil during a 4-h period 48 h after drug treatment. Growth of the human fibroblasts was measured by the incorporation of [³H]thymidine in a 6-h period 48 h after drug treatment of uninfected non-confluent cultures. Arprinocid vs human fibroblasts (▲); arprinocid-*N*-oxide vs human fibroblasts (●); arprinocid vs *T. gondii* (○); arprinocid-*N*-oxide vs *T. gondii* (△). (Reproduced with permission from Pfefferkorn et al (1988))

2 days after treatment was achieved by arprinocid at 2 µg/ml and by arprinocid-*N*-oxide at 20 ng/ml. For both substances the growth of the host cell, measured by the incorporation of [³H]thymidine, proved to be notably less sensitive than growth of the parasite, confirming the favourable therapeutic index seen in the treatment of murine toxoplasmosis. The relative insensitivity of the host cell to

arprinocid or arprinocid-*N*-oxide suggested that the drugs were affecting the parasite directly rather than acting indirectly through effects on the host cell.

In order better to understand the in vivo and in vitro antitoxoplasma activity of arprinocid and its *N*-oxide, we attempted to isolate single-step, drug-resistant mutants. Actively growing intracellular parasites were treated with the alkylating agent ethylnitrosourea and grown in human fibroblasts with normal medium for three daily subcultures. High concentrations of the resulting mutagenized parasites were allowed to make plaques in cultures incubated with medium that contained arprinocid, 10 µg/ml, or arprinocid-*N*-oxide, 100 ng/ml; concentrations which were twice the minimal amount required to block plaque formation by *T. gondii*. Several attempts with independently mutagenized preparations of *T. gondii* failed to yield any plaques in the cultures incubated with arprinocid. A total of approximately 3×10^8 parasites yielded no resistant mutants. The adequacy of the mutagenesis was confirmed in each case by the demonstration that mutants resistant to 5-fluorodeoxyuridine were induced at the expected frequency of $5-45/10^6$ mutagenized *T. gondii*. In contrast to our failure to isolate mutants resistant to arprinocid, we found a number of mutants that were resistant to arprinocid-*N*-oxide. Their frequency in mutagenized populations ranged from 1 to 8 per 10^6 *T. gondii*. The observation that mutants resistant to 5-fluorodeoxyuridine or arprinocid-*N*-oxide were induced by ethylnitrosourea at roughly the same frequencies suggests that arprinocid-*N*-oxide-resistant mutants might resemble 5-fluorodeoxyuridine-resistant mutants in having lost a non-essential function. This kind of mutant would be expected to be much more frequent than mutants with an altered but still functional enzyme. We chose a single clone of parasites resistant to arprinocid-*N*-oxide (R-Ano^R-1) for detailed in vitro and in vivo studies. As shown in Figure 13.3, R-Ano^R-1 was roughly 20-fold more resistant to arprinocid-*N*-oxide than was the wild-type parasite when growth was measured by the incorporation of [^{3}H]uracil 2 days after drug treatment. Surprisingly, R-Ano^R-1 retained the wild-type sensitivity to arprinocid (Fig. 13.3). Thus, despite their similar structures, arprinocid and arprinocid-*N*-oxide are likely to have some critical difference in their antitoxoplasma mechanisms. If the mechanisms of these two drugs were identical, R-Ano^R-1 should be cross-resistant to arprinocid. The lack of cross-resistance also rules out the possibility that arprinocid had antitoxoplasma activity only by virtue of the artefact that it was contaminated with a small amount of arprinocid-*N*-oxide. In this case, the mutant R-Ano^R-1 should also appear to be resistant to the impure arprinocid. Mutant R-Ano^R-1 is unlikely to differ from the wild type in being impermeable to arprinocid-*N*-oxide but not to arprinocid because the halogenated benzene ring makes both substances highly hydrophobic and because the *N*-oxide is more hydrophobic than arprinocid itself.

We realized that studying a mutant resistant only to arprinocid-*N*-oxide might allow us to determine the form of the drug that was active in experimental murine toxoplasmosis. We treated mice with chow pellets impregnated with a known amount of arprinocid. By daily weighing of the uneaten food we were able to calculate accurately the amount of arprinocid ingested. Treatment was begun immediately after infection of the mice by the intraperitoneal injection of about 2000 infectious *T. gondii*. In our hands this inoculum of the RH strain of *T. gondii* kills all mice within 8 days. The mouse LD$_{50}$ is a single viable parasite (Pfefferkorn

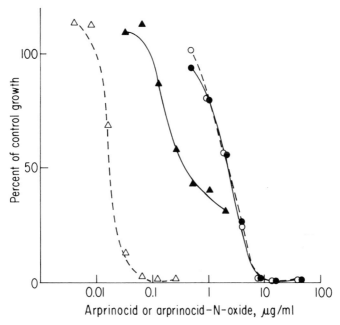

Figure 13.3 The effects of arprinocid and arprinocid-N-oxide on the growth of wild-type *T. gondii* and of a mutant parasite, R-Ano^R-1, selected for resistance to arprinocid-N-oxide. Growth of the parasites was measured by the incorporation of [^{3}H]uracil during a 4-h period 48 h after drug treatment. Arprinocid vs wild-type *T. gondii* (○); arprinocid vs R-Ano^R-1 *T. gondii* (●); arprinocid-N-oxide vs wild-type *T. gondii* (△); arprinocid-N-oxide vs R-Ano^R-1 *T. gondii* (▲). (Reproduced with permission from Pfefferkorn et al (1988))

& Pfefferkorn 1976). Mice that survived 3 weeks on a daily regimen of oral arprinocid were withdrawn from treatment and maintained for an additional 3 weeks. This interval would have been ample for a fatal infection caused by a single surviving parasite. None of the mice that survived the *T. gondii* challenge during the 3 weeks of treatment died during the subsequent 3 weeks without drug. However, without knowing the murine pharmacokinetics of arprinocid and arprinocid-N-oxide, we cannot be sure that all parasites were eradicated during the 3 week treatment. Parasite inhibitory concentrations of the drugs could have been retained during the 3 weeks in which treatment was withdrawn.

The data from several independent experiments confirmed Luft's (1986) observation that arprinocid was effective against the hypervirulent RH strain of *T. gondii* (Table 13.1). The critical experiment was to compare the therapeutic effect of arprinocid on wild-type *T. gondii* with the effect on R-Ano^R-1. If the form of the drug active in vivo was the ingested arprinocid, the mice should have been cured of their infection with R-Ano^R-1 because this mutant was fully sensitive to arprinocid (Fig. 13.3). The results of the two experiments presented in Table 13.1 show that arprinocid was totally ineffective in treating mice infected with R-Ano^R-1. Not only did all of the infected mice die but the time from infection to death was indistinguishable for the controls and the treated mice. The difference between the curative effects of arprinocid on the wild-type *T. gondii* and on mutant R-Ano^R-1 was significant ($p < 0.001$, pooling data from both experiments). Thus we conclude

Table 13.1 The effect of arprinocid on mice infected with wild-type *T. gondii* or with the arprinocid *N*-oxide-resistant mutant R-Ano[R]-1 derived from it

Arprinocid (μg/mouse per day)[b]	Deaths/infected mouse[a] (days to death)	
	Wild-type *T. gondii*[c]	R-Ano[R]-1 *T. gondii*[c]
	Experiment 1	
0	3/3 (8,8,8)	3/3 (7,8,8)
59 ± 11	1/3 (12,18)	3/3 (8,8,8)
135 ± 27	0/3	3/3 (8,8,8)
374 ± 57	0/3	3/3 (7,8,8)
	Experiment 2	
0	3/3 (6,8,8)	3/3 (7,7,8)
52 ± 11	2/3 (9,12)	3/3 (7,8,8)
137 ± 5	1/4 (15)	4/4 (7,8,8,9)
351 ± 47	0/4	4/4 (7,7,7,9)

[a] Difference between wild-type and R-Ano[R]-1 significant for each experiment ($p < 0.01$, χ^2 test with Yate's correction), pooling all arprinocid-treated mice
[b] Treatment with arprinocid incorporated into chow began at the time of infection and was continued for 3 weeks
[c] 2.0 to 2.6×10^3 infectious parasites per mouse, injected intraperitoneally
Reproduced with permission from Pfefferkorn et al (1988)

that in vivo the ingested arprinocid was converted to arprinocid-*N*-oxide, probably by the cytochrome P_{450} system of the liver, and that it was this N-oxide that cured the mice infected with *T. gondii*. Although arprinocid has a substantial antitoxoplasma effect in infected cultured cells we have no evidence for therapeutically important activity in vivo.

We know little of the biochemical basis of the action of arprinocid-*N*-oxide. Early work on the anticoccidial activity of arprinocid concentrated on disturbances of purine metabolism because the drug was originally synthesized as a purine analogue. The initial suggestion from these experiments was that arprinocid blocked the growth of *E. tenella* by inhibiting the transport of hypoxanthine and other purines (Wang et al 1979). This is a plausible mechanism because both *T. gondii* and *E. tenella* are incapable of de novo purine synthesis and thus dependent on their host cells for these essential metabolites. We therefore tested the effect of adding 25 μg/ml hypoxanthine to the medium of infected cultures treated with various concentrations of arprinocid or arprinocid-*N*-oxide. No reversal of parasite inhibition was seen even at drug concentrations that were minimally effective (Pfefferkorn et al 1988). We conclude that neither drug has any effect on purine metabolism that can be reversed by a high concentration of hypoxanthine, a purine that is readily used by intracellular *T. gondii* (Pfefferkorn & Pfefferkorn 1977b).

Although inhibition of hypoxanthine transport is unlikely to explain the antitoxoplasma effect of arprinocid-*N*-oxide, some other effect on purine metabolism at the base, nucleoside, or nucleotide level remains a reasonable hypothesis. If arprinocid-*N*-oxide had an effect on purine metabolism by *T. gondii* it should also probably have a prompt effect on nucleic acid synthesis by the parasite. Therefore we measured the effect of arprinocid-*N*-oxide on DNA and RNA synthesis by actively growing intracellular *T. gondii* using the parasite-specific

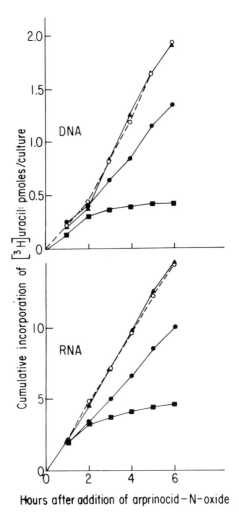

Figure 13.4 The effect of arprinocid-N-oxide on DNA and RNA synthesis by exponentially growing intracellular *T. gondii*. Heavily infected human fibroblast cultures with 8 parasites per infected cell were treated with various concentrations of arprinocid-N-oxide and the incorporation of [³H]uracil into DNA and RNA was measured at hourly intervals. Arprinocid-N-oxide 0 ng/ml (○), 15 ng/ml (▲), 30 ng/ml (●), 90 ng/ml (■). (Pfefferkorn unpublished)

precursor [³H]uracil. Figure 13.4 shows that both DNA and RNA synthesis were suppressed 30 min after treatment with arprinocid-N-oxide at 30 ng/ml. It should be noted that this inhibition of parasite nucleic acid synthesis could be secondary to some other effect of arprinocid-N-oxide. In addition to inhibiting parasite nucleic acid synthesis, arprinocid-N-oxide was parasiticidal for the entire 24-h period over which viable intracellular parasites were assayed by a plaque method (Pfefferkorn et al 1988). The observed rate of parasite death was more than enough to account for the prolonged survival of infected mice after treatment was halted.

Emimycin

Natural products with demonstrated anticoccidial activity may also hold promise for the treatment of toxoplasmic encephalitis. We have begun to study emimycin, an antimicrobial product of a *Streptomyces* species that was isolated by Terao et al (1960) and, independently, by DeZeeuw & Tynan (1969). Terao (1963) determined the structure of emimycin to be 2-hydroxypyrazine-4-oxide (Fig. 13.5). The first important clue as to the antimicrobial mechanism of emimycin came from the observation of DeZeeuw & Tynan (1969) that various pyrimidines could counter its activity. Emimycin was patented because of its anticoccidial activity (Patchett & Wang 1976). More recently, synthetic derivatives of emimycin, including emimycin riboside and carboxyemimycin have been shown to be useful anticoccidial agents (Kobayashi et al 1986; Mano et al 1980).

We observed that emimycin had potent antitoxoplasma activity in infected human fibroblasts (Pfefferkorn et al in press) without any marked effect on the host cell and set out to determine its mechanism of action. We could not use [^{3}H]uracil in the measurement of parasite growth in cultures treated with emimycin because pyrimidines were known to reverse its antimicrobial effect. Instead, we used the incorporation of [^{3}H]xanthine to measure the growth of *T. gondii*. This purine was incorporated, as guanine, into DNA and RNA by intracellular *T. gondii*, while the human fibroblast host cells were not labelled because only the parasite has a phosphoribosyltransferase that recognizes xanthine as a substrate. Human fibroblast cultures were infected with *T. gondii* and incubated for 18 h, at which time most infected cells contained 8 parasites. At this time emimycin was added and quadruplicate treated and control cultures were labelled with [^{3}H]xanthine for successive 60 min intervals to measure the rate of parasite nucleic acid synthesis. As shown in Figure 13.6, emimycin immediately inhibited both DNA and RNA synthesis by *T. gondii*.

We began our search for the mechanism of the antitoxoplasma activity of emimycin by selecting a parasite mutant resistant to the drug. Actively growing intracellular *T. gondii* were treated with ethylnitrosourea as described above. From this mutagenized population we isolated a number of mutants which were able to make plaques in human fibroblast cultures in the presence of 100 μmol/l emimycin, a concentration that completely suppressed plaque formation by the wild-type parasite. One such mutant, R-Emi^R-1, was recloned and further characterized biochemically. Figure 13.7 shows the effect of emimycin on the growth of the wild-type and mutant *T. gondii*, measured by the incorporation of

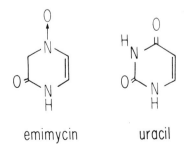

emimycin   uracil

Figure 13.5 The structures of emimycin and uracil

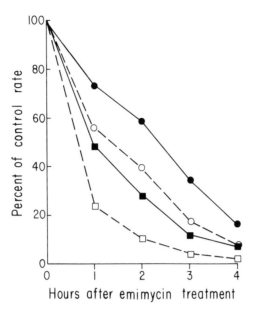

Figure 13.6 The effect of emimycin on the rates of DNA and RNA synthesis by exponentially growing intracellular *T. gondii*. Heavily infected human fibroblast cultures with 8 parasites per infected cell were treated with emimycin or served as untreated controls. The incorporation of [³H]xanthine into DNA and RNA during 60-min intervals was used to measure the rates of nucleic acid synthesis, which are presented as the percentage of untreated control values. Emimycin 30 µmol/l, DNA (■) and RNA (●). Emimycin 90 µmol/l, DNA (□) and RNA (○). (Reproduced in modified form with permission from Pfefferkorn et al (in press))

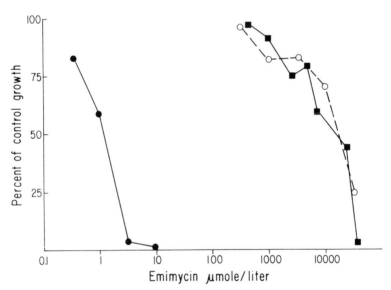

Figure 13.7 The effect of emimycin on the growth of wild-type *T. gondii* (●), R-Emi^R-1 *T. gondii* (○), and uninfected non-confluent human fibroblast cultures (■). Parasite growth was measured by the incorporation of [³H]uracil 48 h after treatment. Fibroblast growth was measured by the incorporation of [³H]thymidine 48 h after treatment. (Reproduced in modified form with permission from Pfefferkorn et al (in press))

[³H]xanthine, and on the growth of human fibroblasts, measured by the incorporation of [³H]thymidine. Emimycin had a substantial therapeutic index of about 1000 in this in vitro system. The mutation in R-Emi^R-1 made it as insensitive as the host cell to the inhibitory effect of the drug. We examined R-Emi^R-1 for cross-resistance to other antiparasitic drugs which we had studied and found that this mutant was highly resistant to 5-fluorodeoxyuridine. Since we had previously shown that resistance to 5-fluorodeoxyuridine in *T. gondii* was correlated with a defect in the salvage enzyme uracil phosphoribosyltransferase (Pfefferkorn 1978), we measured this enzyme in the wild-type and the mutant. As shown in Table 13.2, R-Emi^R-1 had no detectable uracil phosphoribosyltransferase activity. The wild-type *T. gondii* had more than 500 times the enzyme activity of the mutant parasite or of the host cells. The level of uracil phosphoribosyltransferase correlated well with the drug sensitivity.

One explanation for the correlation between emimycin resistance and the loss of uracil phosphoribosyltransferase activity was that emimycin was a substrate of this enzyme and that an emimycin nucleotide was the active form of the drug. In order to study its further metabolism, emimycin was labelled by catalytic tritium exchange and purified to radiochemical homogeneity by thin-layer chromatography. The resulting [G-³H]emimycin was as good a substrate for the uracil phosphoribosyltransferase as was uracil itself. Figure 13.8A shows that, when supplied at 10 μmol/l, emimycin and uracil were converted to the corresponding nucleoside 5'-phosphate at the same rate. The specific activity of our [³H]emimycin did not allow it to be used at concentrations low enough to measure the K_m of the parasite enzyme. Since the specific activity of our [³H]uracil was suitable for K_m determination, we used this substrate in an alternative approach which should detect significant differences in the K_m values for emimycin and uracil. In this approach, [³H]uracil was used to assay the enzyme by our usual radiometric procedure. In one set of reactions, the substrate concentration was raised by adding increasing amounts of non-radioactive uracil. The data from these reactions were used to measure the K_m of uracil. In a second set of reactions the non-radioactive supplement was emimycin instead of uracil but the reaction was still measured by the conversion of [³H]uracil to [³H]UMP. The data derived from the reactions supplemented with non-radioactive emimycin were used to calculate an approximate K_m for emimycin. Although the reaction was actually measured by the production of [³H]UMP, this procedure should yield a reasonably valid measurement of the K_m for emimycin because emimycin greatly predominated in

Table 13.2 Uracil phosphoribosyltransferase activity and emimycin sensitivity of human fibroblasts and of wild-type and emimycin-resistant *T. gondii*

Organism	Uracil phosphoribosyltransferase activity: pmol uridylic acid per mg protein[a]	Concentration of emimycin (mmol/l) required for 50% inhibition of growth[b]
Human fibroblast	< 5	13
Wild-type *T. gondii*	2800	0.012
R-Emi^R *T. gondii*	< 5	12

[a] Measured in sonic extracts
[b] Measured 48 h after addition of emimycin

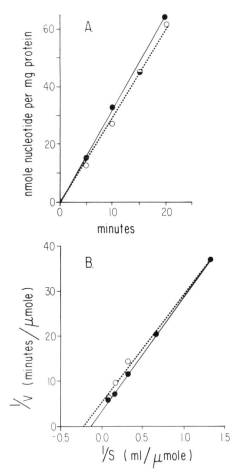

Figure 13.8 Comparison of the kinetic properties of the uracil phosphoribosyltransferase of *T. gondii* with uracil and emimycin as substrates. A. Reaction velocity with 10 μmol/l [³H]uracil (●) or [³H]emimycin (○). B. K_m determination for uracil (●) and emimycin (○). As explained in the text, the K_m measurement for emimycin depended upon the assay of the enzyme by the formation of [³H]UMP from [³H]uracil in the presence of progressively higher concentrations of unlabelled emimycin. (Reproduced with permission from Pfefferkorn et al (in press) and unpublished)

concentration. Figure 13.8B shows that the uracil phosphoribosyltransferase of *T. gondii* had similar K_m values (about 5 μmol/l) for uracil and for emimycin.

We next attempted to follow the fate of [³H]emimycin in actively growing intracellular parasites. Since emimycin was a good substrate for the parasite uracil phosphoribosyltransferase, emimycin should enter the nucleotide pool of *T. gondii* as emimycin riboside 5′-phosphate (EMP). The components of the nucleotide pool, particularly the nucleoside di- and triphosphates are labile and thus pool extracts must be made quickly. This lability posed a problem for the study of the nucleotide pool of an intracellular parasite. During the lengthy purification of *T. gondii* from its host cell, partial degradation of nucleotides in the soluble pool would be inevitable. We chose therefore to extract the total nucleotide pool of infected cultures rapidly. In such an extract, the contribution of the uninfected and infected host cells would far outweigh that of the intracellular parasites. Thus, we could not use spectrophotometric methods to measure parasite nucleotides. However, we took advantage of the observation that the human fibroblast host cells were devoid of uracil phosphoribosyltransferase. Since our host cells were thus incapable of inserting either [³H]uracil or [³H]emimycin into their nucleotide pools, we could be sure that any radioactive nucleotides found in the extract of an infected culture were indeed in the nucleotide pool of the intracellular *T. gondii*. We have previously shown that the pyrimidine nucleotide pool of *T. gondii* is not available to the host cell (Pfefferkorn 1978).

Cultures infected with *T. gondii* for 18 h were incubated with [³H]uracil or [³H]emimycin at a concentration of 30 μmol/l for 60 min. At this concentration emimycin partially inhibited nucleic acid synthesis by *T. gondii* (Fig. 13.6). The solution used for extraction of the pool contained unlabelled pyrimidine nucleotides to serve as optical density markers. The extract was analysed by high performance liquid chromatography on a partisil-SAX anion exchange column. A computer-driven gradient elution resolved all eight of the carrier nucleotides (Pfefferkorn et al in press). The effluent from the column was analysed sequentially by a flow-through spectrophotometer and a flow-through liquid scintillation counter. Both the optical density and radioactivity peaks were recorded and integrated. The resulting data could not be used to calculate the specific activity of parasite nucleotides but the radioactivity in each nucleotide peak was normalized to the number of parasites present in the culture to permit comparisons among experiments. [³H]Uracil was incorporated into all of the expected pyrimidine nucleotides of *T. gondii*. As shown in Table 13.3, the largest amount of label was found in UDP-hexose and UDP-*N*-acetylhexosamine.

Table 13.3 Incorporation of [³H]uracil or [³H]emimycin into pyrimidine nucleotides in the soluble pool of *T. gondii*

Nucleotide (or nucleotide analogue containing emimycin)	pmol [³H]nucleotide per 10^7 parasites in cultures incubated with [³H]uracil[a]	pmol [³H]nucleotide analogue per 10^7 parasites in cultures incubated with [³H]emimycin[a]	Ratio of [³H]emimycin-labelled nucleotide analogue: [³H]uracil-labelled nucleotide
UTP (or ETP)	57	173	3.0
UDP (or EDP)	36	104	2.9
UMP (or EMP)	60	53	0.9
UDP-hexose (or EDP-hexose)	125	64	0.5
UDP-*N*-acetyl-hexosamine (or EDP-*N*-acetyl-hexosamine)	108	6	0.06
CTP (or the emimycin analogue of CTP)	20	<2	<0.0
CDP (or the emimycin analogue of CDP)	13	<2	<0.2
CMP (or the emimycin analogue of CMP)	22	<2	<0.1

[a] Heavily infected human fibroblast cultures with 8 parasites per infected cell were incubated for 60 min with the radioactive precursor (30 μmol/l, 2.3 MBq/μmol) before extraction of the nucleotide pool

We did not have available emimycin-containing nucleotides to serve as optical density markers for the analysis of the extract of infected cultures labelled with [³H]emimycin. The nucleotides labelled with [³H]emimycin were identified by comparing their retention times with those of the absorbance peaks contributed by the uracil-containing nucleotides. We synthesized EMP and found that it eluted 1.2 min before UMP. All of the other [³H]emimycin-containing nucleotide peaks were found to elute 1.2 ± 0.1 min before the corresponding uracil-containing nucleotides. The extract of infected cultures labelled with [³H]emimycin showed a simpler pattern of radioactive peaks than that of the extract of [³H]uracil labelled cultures. No radioactive peaks corresponding to emimycin-based analogues of CMP, CDP or CTP were found (Table 13.3). Thus ETP cannot be converted to the emimycin analogue of CTP by the enzyme CTP synthase. We are currently investigating the possibility that ETP is an inhibitor of this enzyme and thus starves the parasite of cytidine nucleotides.

Intracellular *T. gondii* labelled with [³H]emimycin contained analogues of all of the uracil-containing nucleotides. However, we observed consistent qualitative differences between the pattern of labelling with [³H]uracil and [³H]emimycin (Table 13.3). The incorporation of [³H]emimycin into the analogues of the UDP-sugar cofactors essential for hexose interconversions was less than that observed for the incorporation of [³H]uracil. In particular, very little [³H]emimycin was found in the analogue of UDP-*N*-acetylhexosamine suggesting that emimycin might distort hexose interconversions in *T. gondii*. We refer to this peak as *N*-acetylhexosamine because our chromatographic procedure does not resolve the *N*-acetylgalactosamine and *N*-acetylglucosamine nucleotides. Once we learn how to separate these nucleotides, we may find that one of the *N*-acetylhexosamine nucleotides is completely unlabelled by [³H]emimycin. Such a result would further implicate emimycin as an inhibitor of hexose interconversions.

Two nucleotides were more heavily labelled by emimycin than they were by uracil. The intracellular parasites labelled with [³H]emimycin incorporated approximately three times as much label into EDP and ETP as the parasites labelled with [³H]uracil incorporated label into UDP and UTP (Table 13.3). Thus the UMP and UDP kinases of *T. gondii* appear to accept EMP and EDP readily as substrates. Since the parasites incubated with [³H]emimycin contained large quantities of [³H]ETP, we attempted to measure the incorporation of labelled emimycin into parasite nucleic acids. The conditions used to trace [³H]emimycin and [³H]uracil into the nucleotide pool (Table 13.3) were reproduced in our studies of nucleic acid synthesis to be sure that [³H]ETP would exceed [³H]UTP in the nucleotide pool of the parasite. Despite the preponderance of [³H]ETP in the parasites, repeated experiments showed much greater incorporation of [³H]uracil than of [³H]emimycin into both the DNA and the RNA of *T. gondii*. Since we have not yet been able reliably to measure the incorporation of [³H]emimycin into the deoxynucleotide pool of *T. gondii*, we concentrated our analyses upon RNA. The nucleotides which we can measure, UTP and ETP, are direct precursors of RNA. The incorporation of [³H]emimycin into parasite RNA was only about 0.5% of the incorporation of [³H]uracil even though the [³H]ETP content of the emimycin-labelled parasites was greater than the [³H]UTP content of the uracil-labelled parasites (Table 13.4). Before these rates of incorporation into parasite

Table 13.4 Incorporation of [³H]uracil and [³H]emimycin into the nucleoside triphosphate pool and the nucleic acids of *T. gondii*[a] and inhibition of parasite nucleic acid synthesis by 30 μmol/l [³H]emimycin measured by the incorporation of [³H]xanthine

Labelling conditions	[³H]UTP or [³H]ETP in the soluble pool, pmol/10⁷ parasites	pmol incorporated per hour per 10⁷ parasites	
		RNA	DNA
[³H]uracil (30 μmol/l)[b]	57	32	3.8
[³H]emimycin (30 μmol/l)[b]	173	0.17	0.032
[³H]xanthine (0.38 μmol/l)[c]		1.9	0.24
[³H]xanthine (0.38 μmol/l)[c] plus [³H]emimycin (30 μmol/l)[b]		0.75[d]	0.058[d]

[a] Heavily infected fibroblast cultures with 8 parasites per infected cell were incubated with radioactive medium for 1 h for labelling of the nucleotide pool or 2 h for incorporation into nucleic acids
[b] 2.34 MBq/μmol; 0.07 MBq/ml
[c] 185 MBq/μmol; 0.07 MBq/ml
[d] Calculated as [³H]xanthine incorporation because [³H]xanthine accounted for > 99.8% of the observed radioactivity
Reproduced in modified form with permission from Pfefferkorn et al (in press)

RNA could be compared, two correction factors had to be included and one potential artefact, excluded. The first correction was essential because [³H]uracil labelled both the uridine and cytidine nucleotide pools of *T. gondii* (Table 13.3) and thus was incorporated into RNA as both cytidylic and uridylic acid. However, no cytidine-nucleotide-like analogues of emimycin were formed. Thus, the proper comparison was between the incorporation of [³H]uracil into the uridylic acid residues of *T. gondii* RNA and the total incorporation of [³H]emimycin into *T. gondii* RNA. We measured the fraction of the total [³H]uracil incorporated into *T. gondii* RNA that was in uridylic acid residues and found it to be 58%. This factor was used to convert the total RNA incorporation of uracil into the incorporation that was specific for uridylic acid. A second correction factor was required because the [³H]emimycin was used at a concentration (30 μmol/l) that was partially inhibitory to RNA synthesis by *T. gondii* (Fig. 13.6). This inhibition would, of course, result in proportionately less incorporation of [³H]emimycin. We initially measured the inhibition of parasite RNA synthesis by unlabelled emimycin through the incorporation of [³H]xanthine. These studies confirmed that parasite RNA synthesis was about 50% of control values in infected cultures treated with 30 μmol/l emimycin.

Before these two corrections could be applied, we had to exclude one potential artefact. The possibility remained that our [³H]emimycin was contaminated by some substance produced during the tritium exchange labelling and that this substance was more inhibitory than was emimycin itself. The presence of such an inhibitory substance would markedly reduce the incorporation of [³H]emimycin into parasite nucleic acids. We excluded this artefact by directly measuring the inhibitory effect of our [³H]emimycin. Since so little labelling of parasite nucleic acids was observed in infected cultures incubated with [³H]emimycin, we were able to label these cultures simultaneously with enough [³H]xanthine so that virtually all of the incorporated radioactivity was derived from the [³H]xanthine. This specific precursor for parasite nucleic acids showed that 30 μmol/l [^{3}H]emimycin and 30 μmol/l unlabelled emimycin had the same inhibitory effect (Table 13.4 and Fig. 13.6).

The results of several experiments, presented in Table 13.4, show that very little [^{3}H]emimycin was incorporated into either the DNA or the RNA of *T. gondii* despite the presence of large amounts of ETP in the nucleotide pool of the parasite. After application of the two correction factors noted above, only about 2% of the level of incorporation predicted by the data from [^{3}H]uracil was actually observed. Thus the three parasite enzymes that make ETP from emimycin, uracil phosphoribosyltransferase, UMP kinase and UDP kinase all readily recognized emimycin analogues as substrates. Their combined activity served to produce the large amounts of [^{3}H]ETP seen in the nucleotide pool of cultures infected with *T. gondii* and incubated with [^{3}H]emimycin. However, the RNA polymerases of *T. gondii* had only a low capacity to use ETP. Although little emimycin was incorporated into the nucleic acids of *T. gondii*, the emimycin that made its way into nucleic acids may still have a profound effect on the parasite. We are currently considering the possibility that the insertion of an emimycin is a chain-terminating event.

SUMMARY AND PROSPECTS

Our initial in vivo and in vitro studies with arprinocid and emimycin are consistent with the suggestion that some anticoccidial agents may be clinically useful in toxoplasmic encephalitis. At a minimum their study should reveal new insights into parasite metabolism and the mechanism of antitoxoplasma drugs. For example, if arprinocid were to be considered for phase 1 testing, the pharmacokinetic data should include measurement of serum concentrations of both arprinocid and the active metabolite arprinocid-*N*-oxide.

Our in vivo test of potential antitoxoplasmic drugs used the intraperitoneal injection of the highly virulent RH strain. Promising drugs should also be tested in a recently described murine model that more closely approximates toxoplasmic encephalitis in AIDS patients (Vollmer et al 1987). In this model, chronically infected mice with bradyzoites encysted in their brains are treated repeatedly with a rat monoclonal antibody specific for murine helper T cells. As the helper T cells are depleted, the mice die of recrudescent toxoplasmic encephalitis. This model requires that the drug under investigation be able to cross the blood–brain barrier and effect a cure without the aid of an intact immune response. Both of these requirements mimic therapeutic problems posed by toxoplasmic encephalitis in AIDS patients.

This discussion has focused on the prospects for improving the chemotherapy of toxoplasmic encephalitis. Perhaps an alternative approach should be considered. Toxoplasmic encephalitis in AIDS patients is a recrudescent disease which has its origin in bradyzoites encysted within the brain. Instead of waiting for the cysts to open and release bradyzoites that will become invasive tachyzoites, a preventive strike designed to kill the encysted parasites would be preferable. At present no drug effective against bradyzoites is known. Indeed, it could be argued that this essentially dormant stage should not be sensitive to chemotherapy. This pessimistic assumption may well not be valid. Note that the hypnozoite of *Plasmodium vivax*, which is probably about as metabolically inert as the bradyzoite of *T. gondii*, is exquisitely sensitive to a single dose of primaquine. We plan to test various anticoccidial agents for their ability to kill bradyzoites.

ACKNOWLEDGEMENTS

This research was supported by grants AI-25817 and AI-14151 from the National Institutes of Health. We are indebted to the Merck Research Laboratories for support that allowed the purchase of a flow-through scintillation counter and for a gift of emimycin.

REFERENCES

Dannemann B R, Israelski D M, Remington J S 1988 Treatment of toxoplasmic encephalitis with intravenous clindamycin. Arch Int Med 148: 2477–2482
DeZeeuw J R, Tynan E J 1969 Pyrimidine reversal of emimycin inhibition of *Escherichia coli*. J Antibiot 22: 386–387
Haverkos H W 1987 Assessment of therapy for toxoplasma encephalitis. Am J Med 82: 907–914
Kobayashi N, Matsuno T, Hariguchi F, Yamazaki T, Imai K 1986 *Eimeria tenella, E. necatrix, E. acervulina, E. maxima*, and *E. brunetti*: potent anticoccidial activity of a uridine analogue, 1-β-D-ribofuranosyl)-2-(1*H*)-pyrazinone -4-oxide. Exp Parasitol 61: 42–47
Kovacs J A, Allegra C J, Chabner B A, Swan J C, Drake J, Lunde M, Parillo J E, Masur H 1987 Potent effect of trimetrexate, a lipid-soluble antifolate, on *Toxoplasma gondii*. J Infect Dis 155: 1027–1032
Lire E P, Barker W M, McCrae R C 1976 Use of 6-amino-9-(substituted benzyl) purines and their corresponding N'-oxides as coccidiostats. US Patents 3, 953, 597
Luft B J 1986 Potent in vivo activity of arprinocid, a purine analogue, against murine toxoplasmosis. J Infect Dis 154: 692–694
Luft B J, Remington J S 1988 Toxoplasmic encephalitis. J Infect Dis 157: 1–6
Luft B J, Conley F, Remington J S 1983 Outbreak of central-nervous-system toxoplasmosis in western Europe and North America. Lancet i: 781–783
McDougald L 1982 Chemotherapy of coccidiosis. In: Long PL (ed) The biology of the coccidia. University Park Press, Baltimore, pp 373–427
Mano M, Seo T, Hattori T, Kaneko T, Imai K 1980 Anticoccidials. V. Synthesis and anticoccidial activity of 2(1H)-pyrazinone 4-oxide derivatives. Chem Pharm Bull 28: 2734
Mellors J W, Debs R J, Ryan J L 1989 Incorporation of recombinant gamma interferon into liposomes enhances its ability to induce peritoneal macrophage antitoxoplasma activity. Infect Immun 57: 132–137
Patchett A A, Wang C C 1976 Methods for treating coccidiosis with emimycin and its derivatives. US Patent 3, 991, 185
Pfefferkorn E R 1978 *Toxoplasma gondii*: The enzymic defect of a mutant resistant to 5-fluorodeoxyuridine. Exp Parasitol 44: 26–35
Pfefferkorn E R, Pfefferkorn L C 1976 *Toxoplasma gondii*: Isolation and preliminary characterization of temperature-sensitive mutants. Exp Parasitol 39: 365–376
Pfefferkorn E R, Pfefferkorn L C 1977a Specific labeling of intracellular *Toxoplasma gondii* with uracil. J Protozool 24: 449–453
Pfefferkorn E R, Pfefferkorn L C 1977b *Toxoplasma gondii*: Specific labeling of nucleic acids of intracellular parasites in Lesch-Nyhan cells. Exp Parasitol 41: 95–104
Pfefferkorn E R, Pfefferkorn L C 1980 *Toxoplasma gondii*: Genetic recombination between drug resistant mutants. Exp Parasitol 50: 305–316
Pfefferkorn E R, Eckel M E, McAdams E 1988 *Toxoplasma gondii*: *in vivo* and *in vitro* studies of a mutant resistant to arprinocid-*N*-oxide. Exp Parasitol 65: 282–289

Pfefferkorn E R, Eckel M E, McAdams E 1989 *Toxoplasma gondii*: The biochemical basis of resistance to emimycin. Exp Parasitol 69: 129–139

Suzuki Y, Israelski D M, Dannemann B R, Stepic-Biek P, Thulliez P, Remington J S 1988 Diagnosis of toxoplasmic encephalitis in patients with acquired immunodeficiency syndrome by using a new serologic method. J Clin Microbiol 26: 2541–2543

Terao M 1963 On a new antibiotic, emimycin. II. Studies on the structure of emimycin. J Antibiot 16A: 182–186

Terao M, Karasawa K, Tanaka N, Yonehara H, Uzezawa H 1960 On a new antibiotic, emimycin. J Antibiot 13A: 401–405

Vollmer T L, Waldor M K, Steinman L, Conley F K 1987 Depletion of T-4[+] lymphocytes with monoclonal antibody reactivates toxoplasmosis in the central nervous system: a model of superinfection in AIDS. J Immunol 138: 3737–3741

Wang C C, Tolman R L, Simashkevich P M, Stotish R L 1979 Arprinocid, an inhibitor of hypoxanthine–guanine transport. Biochem Pharmacol 28: 2249–2260

Discussion of paper presented by E. R. Pfefferkorn

Discussed by R. Pierce
Reported by H. C. Neu

Following Pfefferkorn's presentation a number of questions were raised that bear on the future of compounds used to treat toxoplasmosis. Concern was expressed that resistance of *Toxoplasma* to drugs could develop in the same way as occurs with anticoccidial drugs. But Pfefferkorn felt that this was less of a problem since it was unlikely that a patient in early stages of encephalitis would have as many as 10^8 organisms. This number had been necessary to select mutants by the mutagenesis methods he used to select the arprinocid-resistant isolate. Others, however, felt that lesions in AIDS patients reflected large numbers of organisms. It was also mentioned that patients treated with trimetrexate, although they responded initially, inevitably had progressive CNS disease. There are no data to indicate whether *Toxoplasma gondii* with altered dihydrofolate synthetase enzymes exist in nature.

The potential role of other antitoxoplasma agents was discussed. There is no explanation of the effect of clindamycin, and whether a metabolic product of clindamycin is the active compound is unknown. *Toxoplasma* exists in a vacuole which is not acidified, so it is not reasonable to suspect that collapse of a pH gradient by the drug is the mechanism of activity. Studies with a series of 14- and 16-membered macrolides which included spiramycin, roxithromycin, azithromycin, and dithromycin have failed to show activity against toxoplasma either in cell culture or in mice. Indeed even though spiramycin is used in Europe to prevent placental transmission, it is the least active macrolide agent in the cell culture models.

To date none of the compounds tested has had activity on the bradyzoite stage of toxoplasma. Emimycin does not inhibit this stage. Overall much work needs to be done with the older coccidial agents, even those to which resistance rapidly developed, to determine if any agents will inhibit the zygozoite or bradyzoite stages of this important parasite.

Pierce addressed the problem of a *Toxoplasma* vaccine. This would not be of value in HIV infected patients, but could be useful in prophylaxis of women of childbearing age who have never had *Toxoplasma*. Congenital toxoplasmosis occurs in the fetus of mothers who develop acute toxoplasmosis during pregnancy. Primary infection leads to a state of solid immunity toward re-infection. It is not known, however, whether bradyzoites are necessary for continuing immunity.

Pfefferkorn has a mutant blocked in the formation of bradyzoites that produces only acute infection. This mutant may answer this question.

The approach Pierce and colleagues used was to examine the excretory–secretory antigens of the tachyzoite infectious stage. Similar to schistosomiasis, it appears that secretory antigens rather than surface antigens are important in the immune response to *Toxoplasma* tachyzoites, and that the immune response is maintained by release of antigens from the breakdown of the cyst structure of bradyzoite stage. The animal model chosen by Pierce and co-workers was the athymic rat which is susceptible to as few as 1000 tachyzoites. The athymic rat can be immunologically reconstituted with either non-specific T lymphocytes or with T lymphocytes from animals immunized with excretory–secretory antigens from the tachyzoite stage. Serum from immunized rats will also protect the athymic rat. A 24-kD excretory–secretory antigen was discovered which was a major tachyzoite product and which was recognized by human serum and antisera from the immunized animals. Furthermore, immunoprecipitation reactions with antisera could be blocked by bradyzoite material suggesting the 24-kD material was a common antigen for both stages of the parasite. Cloning studies revealed that this material was a calcium-binding protein which is synthesized de novo and is not a membrane-bound molecule since it lacks an anchor sequence or a transmembrane sequence. This material is excreted by tachyzoites into serum-containing medium.

To date it has not been possible to achieve good expression of this antigen in *E. coli*, but that work is ongoing. Other excretory–secretory antigens have also been cloned and may provide leads for a vaccine.

Important unknown factors about a vaccine such as this are the length of immunity or whether there is a cytotoxic T-cell response. Synthetic peptides from the primary sequence of the antigen stimulate T cells in immunized and infected mice and rats but the identity of the T-cell population is still unknown.

The ultimate goal is to use this material to immunize selected populations such as young women. Another possible use would be in sheep in which toxoplasmosis is a problem.

14. Cryptosporidiosis

W. L. Current

INTRODUCTION

Organisms of the genus *Cryptosporidium* are small (2–6 µm, depending on stage of life cycle) coccidian parasites which invade and then replicate within the microvillous region of epithelial cells lining the digestive and respiratory organs of vertebrates (Angus 1983, Current 1986, 1989, Fayer & Ungar 1986, Tzipori 1983). Recognized and named more than 80 years ago (Tyzzer 1907, 1910, 1912), these obligate intracellular protozoans remained until recently nothing more than a biomedical curiosity. Prior to 1980, infections with species of *Cryptosporidium* were considered rare in animals and in man they were thought to be the result of a little-known opportunistic pathogen of immune-deficient individuals outside its normal host range. In 1982, our concept of these protozoan parasites began to change into that of important, widespread causes of diarrhoeal illness in several animal species, including humans. At the time of writing, no effective therapy for cryptosporidiosis has been identified; thus, the finding of this parasite in the immunocompromised host, especially patients with AIDS, usually carries an ominous prognosis. Reports of infections of the respiratory tract (Forgacs et al 1983) and biliary tree (Pitlik et al 1983) demonstrate that the developmental stages of this protozoan are not confined to the gastrointestinal tract and suggest that *C. parvum* may be an under-reported cause of respiratory and biliary tract disease, especially in the immune-deficient host.

Recent recognition of the importance of *Cryptosporidium* spp. as pathogens of man and his domesticated animals can be confirmed easily by the number of relevant publications that have appeared in the biomedical literature. Fewer than 30 papers addressing these parasites were published prior to 1980; however, currently, more than 630 papers on *Cryptosporidium* spp. and cryptosporidiosis exist. Among the many recent papers are several reviews of the biology of *Cryptosporidium* spp. infecting man and his domesticated animals (Current 1986, Fayer & Ungar 1986, Crawford & Vermund 1988). In this brief communication those aspects of most importance to the clinical microbiologist and the immunologist will be addressed.

HISTORY AND TAXONOMY

Clarke (1895) may have been the first to observe a species of *Cryptosporidium* which he described as 'swarm spores lying upon the gastric epithelium of mice.' In retrospect, these small organisms were probably the motile merozoites of *C. muris*, the type species named and described approximately 12 years later by the well-known American parasitologist, E. E. Tyzzer (1907). This protozoan, infecting the gastric epithelium of laboratory mice used in Tyzzer's research programme, was placed in a new genus (*Cryptosporidium* = hidden sporocysts) because, unlike the previously known coccidia, the oocyst of this parasite did not have sporocysts surrounding the sporozoites. Three years later, Tyzzer (1910) described many of the life-cycle stages of *C. muris* and in 1912 he described much of the morphology and life cycle of a second species, *C. parvum*, found in the small intestine of laboratory mice (Tyzzer 1912). During the ensuing 70 years, approximately 19 additional species of *Cryptosporidium* were named from a variety of vertebrate hosts (Levine 1984, Current 1986, Fayer & Ungar 1986). Only a few of these named species, including the two originally described by Tyzzer, are now considered valid (Table 14.1).

Interest in *Cryptosporidium (C. parvum)* by the veterinary medical profession has increased significantly since 1971 when this protozoan was first reported to be associated with bovine diarrhoea (Panciera et al 1971). Numerous case reports from many different animals are now present in the literature and one species, *C. parvum*, is recognized as an important cause of neonatal diarrhoea in calves and lambs (Angus 1983, Current 1986, Tzipori 1983). Another species, *C. baileyi*, is now recognized as an important cause of respiratory disease in poultry (Current et al 1986, Blagburn et al 1987, Current & Snyder 1988).

The first cases of human cryptosporidiosis were reported in 1976 (Miesel et al 1976, Nime et al 1976), and subsequent reports were rare until it was recognized that *Cryptosporidium* (now believed to be *C. parvum*) may produce a short-term diarrhoeal illness in immunocompetent persons and a prolonged, life-threatening, cholera-like illness in immune-deficient patients, especially those with acquired immune deficiency syndrome (AIDS) (Current et al 1983, Current 1986, Fayer & Ungar 1986). Additional details of the historical events outlined above can be found in review papers published between 1983 and 1988 (Angus 1983, Tzipori 1983, Current 1986, Fayer & Ungar 1986, Crawford & Vermund 1988).

The taxonomic classification of small intracellular protozoans assigned to the genus *Cryptosporidium* is presented in Table 14.2. Species of *Plasmodium*, causing

Table 14.1 Species of *Cryptosporidium*

Species	Hosts	Oocyst size
C. muris	Mice, cattle	7.4 × 5.6
C. parvum	Mammals	5.0 × 4.5
C. baileyi	Poultry	6.2 × 4.6
C. meleagridis	Poultry	5.2 × 4.6
C. species	Quails	Approx. 5.0
C. species	Guinea pigs	Approx. 5.0

Table 14.2 The taxonomic classification of *Cryptosporidium*

Classification	Name	Biological characteristics
Phylum	Apicomplexa	Invasive forms have apical complex with polar rings, rhoptries, micronemes, conoid, and subpellicular microtubules
Class	Sporozoasida	Locomotion of invasive forms by body flexion gliding, or undulation
Subclass	Coccidiasina	Life cycle with merogony, gametogony, and sporogony
Order	Eucoccidiorida	Merogony present; in vertebrate hosts
Suborder	Eimeriorina	Male and female gametes develop independently
Family	Cryptosporidiidae	Homoxenous (one host life cycle), with developmental stages just under the membrane of the host cell; oocyst without sporocysts and with four sporozoites; microgametes without flagella

malaria in man, are in the same order (Euccodiorida) but in a different suborder (Haemospororina) than are species of *Cryptosporidium*. More closely related to *Cryptosporidium* spp. are the other true coccidia (suborder Eimeriorina), *Isospora belli, Sarcocystis* spp. and *Toxoplasma gondii*, which infect human beings and *Eimeria* spp. which infect other mammals and birds. Most species of *Cryptosporidium* named in the biomedical literature following Tyzzer's creation of the genus were classified with the assumption that these coccidia were as host specific as the closely related (taxonomically) species of *Eimeria* infecting mammals and birds. However, cross-transmission studies conducted in the early 1980s demonstrated little or no host specificity for 'species' of *Cryptosporidium* isolated from mammals. The lack of host specificity exhibited by mammalian isolates prompted Tzipori et al (1980) to consider *Cryptosporidium* as a single species genus. A more realistic approach was presented by Levine (1984) who consolidated the 20 named parasites into 4 species; one each for those infecting fishes (*C. nasorum*), reptiles (*C. crotali*), birds (*C. meleagridis*), and mammals (*C. muris*). Information currently available indicates that this consolidation is not entirely correct. *Cryptosporidium crotali* is now considered to be a species of *Sarcocystis*, a genus of coccidian parasites found commonly in snakes. There are at least two valid species, *C. baileyi* and *C. meleagridis*, infecting birds (Current et al 1986). There are also at least two valid species infecting mammals (*C. muris* infecting the small intestine and *C. parvum* infecting the stomach) and on the basis of oocyst morphology it is *C. parvum*, not *C. muris*, that is associated with all of the well-documented cases of cryptosporidiosis in mammals (Upton & Current 1985). Thus, the species with oocysts measuring 4–5 μm which produces clinical illness in man and other mammals should be referred to as *C. parvum*, or *Cryptosporidium* sp. if there are not enough morphological, life-cycle, and/or host specificity data to relate it to Tyzzer's original description. I have adopted this conservative approach realizing that careful studies of proposed differences in host specificity, sites of infection and pathogenicity among mammalian isolates (Tzipori 1983, Current 1986, Fayer &

Ungar 1986) may result in the validation of additional species. In the light of present uncertainties in the taxonomy of *Cryptosporidium* spp., the designation of a particular parasite obtained from a mammalian host as an isolate rather than a strain is preferable.

LIFE CYCLE

Studies of different isolates (human and calf) of *C. parvum* in the suckling mouse model (Current & Reese 1986), in chicken embryos (Current & Long 1983) and in cell cultures (Current & Haynes 1984) revealed that the life cycle of this parasite (Fig. 14.1) is similar to that of other true coccidia (eg. *Eimeria* and *Isospora* spp.) infecting mammals in that it can be divided into six major developmental events: excystation (release of infective sporozoites), merogony (asexual multiplication within host cells), gametogony (formation of micro- and macrogametes), fertilization, oocysts wall formation and sporogony (sporozoite formation). The life cycle of human and calf isolates of *C. parvum* differs somewhat from that of other

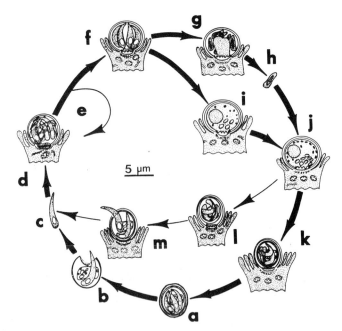

Figure 14.1 Proposed life cycle of *Cryptosporidium parvum* as it occurs in experimentally infected mice. (a) Sporulated, thick-walled oocyst in faeces. (b) Excystation within the small intestine. (c) Free sporozoite in the small intestine prior to penetration of an enterocyte. (d) Mature type I meront with 6 or 8 merozoites. (e) Recycling of a type I merozoite to produce additional type I meronts. (f) Type II meront with 4 merozoites that do not recycle, they develop into the sexual stages. (g) Microgamont with approximately 16 microgametes. (h) Free microgamete that fertilizes macrogamete (i) to form a zygote (j). Most of the zygotes (~80%) form thick-walled oocysts that sporulate within the parasitophorous vacuole of the host cell (k) before being passed in the faeces as the environmentally resistant form that transmits the infection to another host. Some (~20%) of the zygotes do not form an oocyst wall; their sporozoites are surrounded only by a unit membrane. These thin-walled, auto-infective oocysts (l) rupture and release sporozoites (m) that re-initiate the endogenous cycle (at c)

260

monoxenous (one host in life cycle) coccidia (*Eimeria* and *Isospora* spp.). Each intracellular stage of *C. parvum* resides within a parasitophorous vacuole confined to the microvillous region of the host cell, whereas comparable stages of *Eimeria* or *Isospora* spp. occupy parasitophorous vacuoles usually deep (perinuclear) within the host cells. Oocysts of *C. parvum* undergo sporogony while they are within the host cells and are infective when released in the faeces, whereas oocysts of *Eimeria* or *Isospora* spp. do not sporulate until they are passed from the host and exposed to oxygen and temperatures below 37° C. Studies, using experimentally infected mice, have also shown that approximately 20% of the oocysts of *C. parvum* within host enterocytes do not form a thick, two-layered, environmentally resistant oocyst wall; the four sporozoites of this auto-infective stage are surrounded only by a single unit membrane. Soon after being released from the host cell, the membrane surrounding the four sporozoites ruptures and these invasive forms penetrate into the microvillous region of other enterocytes and re-initiate the life cycle (Current & Reese 1986). The majority (approximately 80%) of the oocysts of *C. parvum* found in enterocytes of suckling mice were similar to those of *Eimeria* and *Isospora* spp. in that they develop thick, environmentally

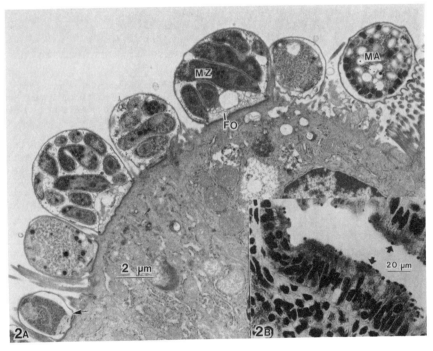

Figure 14.2 Developmental stages of *Cryptosporidium parvum* in the microvillous region of ileal enterocytes. (A) Transmission electron micrograph of infected enterocytes of experimentally infected mouse. Three of the meronts contain merozoites (MZ) and a feeder organelle (FO) at the base of the parasitophorous vacuole; one macrogamete (MA) contains the characteristic amylopectin granules near the centre and wall-forming bodies near the periphery; and the arrow points to a newly formed uninucleate meront. (B) Light micrograph of a histological section of the ileum of a small bowel biopsy of an immunocompromised patient with prolonged cryptosporidiosis. Arrows point to two of the many developmental stages of the parasite in the brush border of the enterocytes

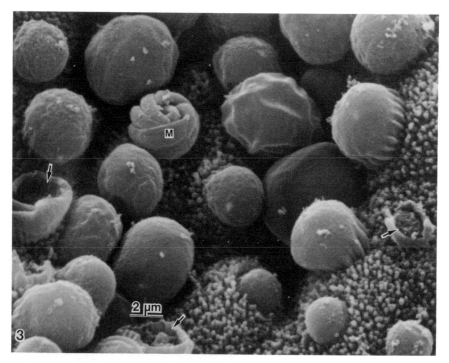

Figure 14.3 Scanning electron micrograph of intestinal mucosa containing many developmental stages of *Cryptosporidium*. The host cell and parasitophorous vacuole membrane of one of the meronts (M) was removed during processing allowing visualization of the merozoites. Arrows point to craters left in the microvillous border after parasites are released from the host cells

resistant oocyst walls and are passed in the faeces. Thick-walled oocysts are the life-cycle forms that transmit the infection from one host to another. The presence of auto-infective, thin-walled oocysts and type I meronts that can recycle are believed to be the life-cycle features of *C. parvum* responsible for the development of severe infections in hosts exposed to only a small number of thick-walled oocysts, and for persistent, life-threatening disease in immune-deficient persons who are not exposed repeatedly to these environmentally resistant forms. Ultra-structural features of some of the developmental stages of *Cryptosporidium* in enterocytes of the experimentally infected host are shown in Figures 14.2 and 14.3.

Subsequent studies (Current et al 1986) of *C. baileyi* in experimentally infected chickens revealed that this species has a life cycle similar to that described above for *C. parvum* in the suckling mouse model. The major difference in the life cycle of these two species is that *C. baileyi* has three distinct types of meronts rather than the two types found in *C. parvum*.

EPIDEMIOLOGY OF HUMAN CRYPTOSPORIDIOSIS

Transmission

Studies of experimental infections in farm and laboratory animals clearly demonstrate that *C. parvum* is transmitted by environmentally resistant oocysts that are fully sporulated and infective at the time they are passed from the host (Current et al 1983, Current 1986). As long as the thick, two-layered wall remains intact, *Cryptosporidium* spp. oocysts are remarkably resistant to most common disinfectants and they can survive for months if kept cold and moist. One study (Sundermann et al 1987) designed to evaluate the efficacy of commercial disinfectants demonstrated that ammonia (50% or higher) and formalin (10% or higher) for 30 min can kill *Cryptosporidium* spp. oocysts. When these disinfectants and others used commonly in hospitals and laboratories were evaluated at the lower concentrations recommended by the manufacturers, none was effective against *Cryptosporidium* spp. oocysts. Freeze-drying and exposure (30 min) to temperatures above $+60°$ C and below $-20°$ C have also been reported to kill *Cryptosporidium* spp. oocysts (Tzipori 1983, Anderson 1985). Most *C. parvum* oocysts stored at $4°$ C in 2.5% (weight/volume) aqueous potassium dichromate remain viable for 3–4 months, and some may remain infective for cell cultures and suckling mice for more than one year (Current 1986). A procedure used routinely in several laboratories to sterilize *Cryptosporidium* spp. oocysts prior to obtaining viable sporozoites by in vitro excystation involves incubation in 10–25% commercial bleach (5.25% sodium hypochlorite) for 10–15 min in an ice bath. Since oocysts of *Cryptosporidium* spp. are resistant to this sterilization procedure, routine chlorination of drinking water should have little or no effect on their viability.

Data published from several laboratories during the early 1980s demonstrated that calves are a source of human infection (Anderson et al 1982, Reese et al 1982, Current et al 1983). Companion animals such as rodents, puppies and kittens may also serve as reservoir hosts (Current et al 1983). These findings in conjunction with reports of more than 40 mammals that harbour the parasite (Current 1989) and the realization that *C. parvum* readily crosses host species barriers, led to the concept that most human infections are a result of zoonotic transmission. This view is probably correct for persons living and working in environments where exposure to faecal contamination from potential reservoir hosts is likely. However, zoonotic transmission does not explain the large number of infections reported from persons living and working in urban areas where exposure to animal faeces is minimal. Evidence currently available indicates that person-to-person transmission of cryptosporidiosis is common. In 1983, an accidental laboratory infection demonstrated that a human isolate of *C. parvum* could be transmitted from one person to another (Blagburn & Current 1983). Since that time, outbreaks of cryptosporidiosis have been reported among children in day-care centres (Alpert et al 1984, Anonymous 1984, Driscoll et al 1988), hospital-acquired infections have been investigated (Koch et al 1985), at least two large waterborne outbreaks have been well documented (D'Antonio et al 1985, D. Juranik personal communication CDC, Atlanta), and this protozoan is now recognized as a cause of travellers' diarrhoea (Jokipii et al 1983, Soave & Ma 1985).

After the first large waterborne outbreak (D'Antonio et al 1985) was investigated, we (Current & Schaefer unpublished data) demonstrated that oocysts of *C. parvum* can be recovered from water samples by high volume filters that were designed to trap cysts of the enteric protozoan, *Giardia lamblia*. Application of similar filtration techniques in conjunction with immunofluorescent detection methods has since been used to demonstrate *Cryptosporidium* spp. oocysts in surface and drinking waters, and sewage effluent samples obtained from different geographical regions of the United States and from several other countries (Stibbs & Ongereth 1985, Madore et al 1987).

The epidemiological features of cryptosporidiosis emphasized above – transmission by environmentally resistant cysts (oocysts), existence of numerous potential reservoir hosts for zoonotic transmission, documentation of person-to-person transmission in settings such as day-care centres, and documentation of water-borne transmission – are similar to those of human giardiasis that were revealed during the past decade. *Cryptosporidium parvum* is now gaining the recognition it deserves as an important, widespread cause of diarrhoeal illness in man.

Prevalence

Prevalence data contained in published surveys relying on standard stool examination techniques to detect *C. parvum* oocysts are quite variable from one geographical location to another. Direct comparison of these data is often difficult because study populations may not be comparable and because different stool sampling and oocyst detection procedures were used. In spite of these difficulties, a data base is being compiled from which a limited understanding of the geographical distribution and prevalence of human cryptosporidiosis is beginning to emerge.

A review (Fayer & Ungar 1986) of 36 large-scale surveys of selected populations, such as children and adults seeking medical attention for diarrhoea and other gastrointestinal symptoms, demonstrates that *Cryptosporidium* spp. are associated with diarrhoeal illness in most areas of the world and that the prevalence of cryptosporidiosis is highest in poorly developed regions. For example, prevalence rates reported in surveys from Europe (1–2%) and North America (0.6–4.3%) are lower than those reported in surveys from Asia, Australia, Africa, and Central and South America (3–20%). In most of the surveys reviewed by Fayer & Ungar (1986), *Cryptosporidium* was the most common parasite found and, in several, this protozoan was considered to be the most significant of all known enteropathogens causing diarrhoeal illness. Other findings common to many of the surveys were that children usually had a significantly higher prevalence than did adults and that infections were often seasonal, with a higher prevalence during warmer, wetter months. Another interesting finding from the standpoint of infection control was that a small number of oocysts may be present in faeces for up to 2 weeks following resolution of diarrhoea.

Several, more recent reviews (Crawford & Vermund 1988, Garcia & Current in press) of the published reports of cryptosporidiosis in persons residing in industrialized and developing countries support the overall conclusions presented above, and may also provide a more global view of the prevalence of human infection. Crawford & Vermund (1988) compared the worldwide occurrence of *Cryptosporidium* infection compiled by Navin (1985) from studies prior to 1985 with that obtained from studies published after 1985. Data compiled from the pre- and post-1985 studies were similar. Navin reported that studies prior to 1985 suggested that the overall occurrence of *Cryptosporidium* infection in individuals with diarrhoea was 2.5% (19 of 7779) for persons living in industrialized countries and 7.2% (82 of 1135) for persons residing in developing countries. The more recent studies summarized by Crawford & Vermund suggested an infection rate for individuals with diarrhoeal illness was 2.2% (285 of 11 716) for individuals in industrialized countries and 8.5% (532 of 6295) for individuals in developing countries. Estimates provided by Walsh & Warren (1979) suggest that in Asia, Africa, and Latin America alone there are as many as 5 billion episodes of diarrhoea and 5–10 million diarrhoea-associated deaths annually. If the estimates of Walsh & Warren are accurate and if the *Cryptosporidium* prevalence data summarized by Navin (1985) and Crawford & Vermund (1988) are correct, then one may predict 360 million to 425 million *Cryptosporidium* infections annually in persons living in Asia, Africa, and Latin America.

Limited serological surveys also support the concept that *Cryptosporidium* infection is common, especially in developing countries. For example, approximately 64% of 389 children and adults in Lima, Peru and 84 children in Maracaibo and Caracas, Venezuela had serological evidence of previous infection, i.e. their sera contained antibodies (IgG and/or IgM) specific for *Cryptosporidium* (Ungar et al 1988).

In the light of the epidemiological information just reviewed, it is essential that health care professionals emphasize the importance of *Cryptosporidium* in training programmes so that cryptosporidiosis is considered in the differential diagnosis of diarrhoeal illness. This educational role should be approached aggressively because of the common occurrence of the disease, because of the large number of potential reservoir hosts, and because persons with impaired immune function may develop life-threatening cryptosporidiosis.

CLINICAL FEATURES

The most common clinical feature of cryptosporidiosis in immunocompetent and immunocompromised persons is diarrhoea; it is this symptom that most often leads to diagnosis. Characteristically, the diarrhoea is profuse and watery, it may contain mucus but rarely blood and leucocytes, and it is often associated with weight loss. Other less common clinical features include abdominal pain, nausea and vomiting, and low-grade fever ($< 39°$ C). Occasionally, non-specific symptoms such as myalgia, weakness, malaise, headache and anorexia occur. Severity of these symptoms may wax and wane in individuals and usually parallels the intensity of oocyst shedding. Both the duration of symptoms and the outcome typically vary according to the immune status of the host. AIDS patients usually experience a prolonged, life-threatening illness, whereas most immunocompetent persons experience a short-term illness with complete, spontaneous recovery. However, the clinical presentation of gastrointestinal cryptosporidiosis does not always fit within one of these two divergent categories. Persons with the clinical and laboratory features of AIDS have been reported to clear infections after several months of diarrhoea, and individuals reported to be immunocompetent have had infections lasting more than one month (Current 1986). Mild and asymptomatic infections have been reported in immunocompetent persons and in several patients with AIDS (Current 1986).

Immunocompetent persons

Most of the 18 cases of cryptosporidiosis in immunocompetent humans reported prior to 1983 and the numerous cases reported since then (see Current in press, Fayer & Ungar 1986, Crawford & Vermund 1988, Garcia & Current in press for a list of case reports) describe a self-limited, cholera-like or flu-like gastrointestinal illness. The most common symptoms reported are profuse, watery diarrhoea (cholera-like), and abdominal cramping, nausea and vomiting, low-grade fever, and headache (flu-like). In their review of the symptoms reported for 586 persons in 36 large-scale surveys, Fayer & Ungar (1986) reported that diarrhoea was the most commonly listed clinical feature (92%), followed by nausea and vomiting (51%), abdominal pain (45%), and low-grade fever (63%).

In most well-nourished persons, diarrhoeal illness due to *C. parvum* infections lasts from 3 to 12 days. Occasionally, these patients may require fluid replacement therapy, and occasionally the diarrhoeal illness may last for more than 2 weeks. In poorly nourished children with cryptosporidiosis, oral and parenteral rehydration therapy are often required because of excessive fluid loss that may last more than 3 weeks. One study (Sallon et al 1988) from a hospital in Jerusalem revealed that children with diarrhoea and *Cryptosporidium*-positive stools were significantly more malnourished than children with diarrhoea and no *Cryptosporidium* spp. oocysts in their stools. Also, children with severe malnutrition and with *Cryptosporidium* spp. oocysts in their stools had a significantly longer duration of diarrhoea than similarly malnourished children without cryptosporidiosis. Diarrhoeal illness is a major cause of morbidity and mortality, especially in young children living in developing countries. Based on the limited prevalence data from stool and serological surveys (reviewed above), it is likely that *Cryptosporidium* plays an important role in the overall health status of these children.

Immunodeficient persons

In the most severely immunocompromised host, such as a patient with AIDS, diarrhoeal illness due to *Cryptosporidium* infection of the gastrointestinal tract becomes progressively worse with time and may be a major factor leading to death. It is believed that the infection usually begins with organisms colonizing the ileum or jejunum and develops into a life-threatening condition when a large portion of the gastrointestinal mucosa is covered with what has been described as a monolayer of parasites. Fluid loss in patients with AIDS and cryptosporidiosis is often excessive; 3–6 litres of diarrhoeic stool per day is common, and as much as 17 litres of watery stool per day has been reported.

In the immune-deficient patient, *Cryptosporidium* spp. infections are not always confined to the gastrointestinal tract. Acute and gangrenous cholecystitis in AIDS patients has been attributed to *Cryptosporidium* spp. infections of biliary tree and gall bladder epithelium (Pitlik et al 1983). Respiratory tract infections with this parasite have been associated with chronic coughing, dyspnoea, bronchitis, and pneumonitis in persons with AIDS and in an infant with severe combined immune deficiency (Forgacs et al 1983, Lewis et al 1985). In children, symptomatic intestinal and respiratory infections with *Cryptosporidium* spp. have also been associated with the acute phase of measles, a cause of transient immuno-suppression (Bogaerts et al 1984). The role of *C. parvum* as a cause of respiratory

266

illness in persons whose immune function is compromised because of congenital or acquired immune deficiencies or because of malnutrition and/or other infectious diseases remains to be determined.

PATHOGENICITY

At present, the pathophysiological mechanisms of *Cryptosporidium*-induced diarrhoea are poorly defined. Studies in germ-free calves mono-infected with *C. parvum* suggest that malabsorption and impaired digestion in the small bowel coupled with malabsorption in the large intestine are major factors responsible for diarrhoea in calves with cryptosporidiosis (Heine et al 1984). This malabsorption and impaired digestion may result in an overgrowth of intestinal microflora, a change in osmotic pressure across the gut wall, and an influx of fluid into the lumen of the intestine. Malabsorption and impaired digestion have also been reported in humans infected with *C. parvum*. However, the secretory (often described as cholera-like) diarrhoea common to most immune-deficient patients with cryptosporidiosis suggests a toxin-mediated hypersecretion into the gut. Definitive, systematic studies are needed to determine the mechanisms by which *C. parvum* and its metabolites or toxins may alter normal intestinal function of a susceptible animal model.

DIAGNOSIS

Prior to 1980, diagnosis of human cryptosporidiosis required identification of the small spherical life-cycle stages of *C. parvum* in the microvillous region of the intestinal mucosa obtained by biopsy and subsequently processed for examination by light or electron microscopy. Such invasive and time-consuming procedures are no longer required since a variety of techniques have been developed for identifying *C. parvum* oocysts in faecal specimens.

For the diagnosis of cryptosporidiosis, stool specimens should be submitted as fresh material or in 10% formalin or sodium acetate–acetic acid–formalin (SAF) preservatives. Most recommended stains for *Cryptosporidium* spp. oocysts cannot be performed on stools preserved in polyvinyl alcohol (PVA) fixative. The routine stains (trichrome, iron haematoxylin) used for stool diagnosis of other parasites are not acceptable for the identification of *Cryptosporidium* spp. oocysts. Several widely used techniques (Fig. 14.4) for demonstrating *Cryptosporidium* spp. oocysts in faecal specimens from humans and animals are modified acid-fast staining (Garcia et al 1983, Ma & Soave 1983), negative staining (Current 1983), and Sheather's sugar flotation (Reese et al 1982, Current et al 1983). Although the last two procedures are useful in the research laboratory, acid-fast staining is usually the method of choice for the clinical microbiology laboratory. Considerable experience is often required with the concentration and staining methods to obtain an accurate diagnosis. For this reason, immunofluorescent antibody (IFA) procedures employing *Cryptosporidium*-specific polyclonal or monoclonal antibodies have been developed to aid in the identification of oocysts in stool specimens (Stibbs & Ongereth 1985, Garcia et al 1987).

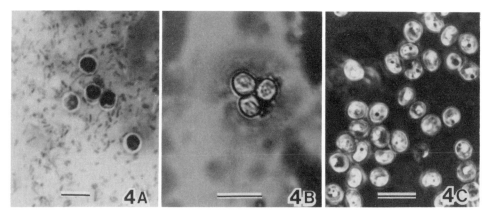

Figure 14.4 Light micrographs of oocysts of *Cryptosporidium parvum* demonstrated by three common stool diagnostic techniques. (A) Acid-fast staining (Garcia et al 1983) results in oocysts appearing bright red against the counter-stained background. Yeast stain darkly with the background stain. (B) Carbol fushsin negative staining (Current 1983) resulting in bright and refractile oocysts which do not take up the stain. Yeast stain darkly. (C) Sheather's sugar flotation and phase-contrast microscopy (Current et al 1983) result in bright and refractile oocysts containing dark granules. Yeast are not bright and refractile

The use of serodiagnostic techniques for monitoring exposure to *Cryptosporidium* has thus far been limited to a few laboratories. Antibodies specific to *Cryptosporidium* have been detected, using an IFA procedure, in sera obtained from persons who recovered from confirmed infections (Campbell & Current 1983, Casemore 1987) and an IFA assay has been used for the presumptive diagnosis of cryptosporidiosis in two clusters of cases (D'Antonio et al 1985, Koch et al 1985). Specific anti-*Cryptosporidium* IgG and/or IgM were also detected, by an enzyme-linked immunosorbent assay (ELISA), in the sera of 95% of patients with cryptosporidiosis at the time of medical presentation and in 100% within 2 weeks of presentation (Ungar et al 1986). Several serological surveys have reported that more than 50% of persons with no known infection may have anti-*Cryptosporidium* IgG, suggesting recent exposure to the parasite (Tzipori & Campbell 1981, Koch et al 1985, Ungar et al 1988). Additional evaluations are needed to confirm the utility of these serological procedures for diagnosing and monitoring infections, for determining the prevalence of prior exposure in selected study populations, and to determine if there is any correlation between the presence of *Cryptosporidium*-specific serum antibodies and resistance to re-infection.

TREATMENT

Chemotherapy
The lack of an effective treatment for cryptosporidiosis in previously healthy, immunocompetent persons has not resulted in a great deal of concern within the biomedical community since, in such patients, the duration of diarrhoea is almost

always less than 20 days and since clinical symptoms and oocyst shedding generally resolve spontaneously. However, reports (Bogaerts et al 1984, Sallon et al 1988) demonstrating an association between cryptosporidiosis and severe malnutrition in children may warrant a change of perception. Regardless of one's present perception, if a safe and effective therapy was available, most clinicians would probably treat the severe diarrhoeal illness that often develops in immuno-competent persons following oral exposure to oocysts.

Because immunocompromised persons often develop a prolonged life-threatening infection following exposure to the parasite, an effective therapy is desperately needed for the treatment of cryptosporidiosis in this patient population. To date, treatment of cryptosporidiosis in immune-deficient persons has been frustrating and unsuccessful in most cases. No controlled studies have been published and all therapeutic information is based on isolated reports. The list of unsuccessful attempts to treat cryptosporidiosis in immunocompromised persons is growing rapidly and these attempts include the use of more than 80 different drugs (Hart & Baxby 1985, Soave 1985, Current 1986, Fayer & Ungar 1986, Current 1989). Of the antimicrobial agents used to treat AIDS patients with cryptosporidiosis, spiramycin has been the only one suspected of having efficacy; it was reported to control diarrhoea in some individuals but not in others. This macrolide antibiotic may help control the diarrhoea in some patients treated for cryptosporidiosis while in an early stage of AIDS but does not appear to have any effect on the course of clinical cryptosporidiosis in patients who have progressed into the later stages of AIDS (Soave 1985).

In the absence of an effective treatment for cryptosporidiosis, supportive therapy appears to be the only intervention available to most clinicians. Oral and parenteral rehydration therapy is often required by both immunodeficient and immunocompetent persons, especially young children, with severe cryptosporidial diarrhoea. Parenteral nutrition may also help sustain the nutritional status of some patients with persistent cryptosporidiosis.

Immunological intervention
Since immune status of the host appears to be the major factor determining the severity and duration of infection following oral exposure to *C. parvum* oocysts (Current & Bick in press) and since an effective therapy is not available (Current 1989), immunological intervention may be a reasonable approach to the control of cryptosporidiosis. Discontinuation of immunosuppressive chemotherapy, allowing restoration of immune function, has resulted in complete resolution of intestinal cryptosporidiosis in several patients (Miller et al 1983). One other approach directed toward restoration of immune function has also been reported to be of some value in treating cryptosporidiosis in AIDS patients. In one small study, 5 of 8 patients with AIDS and prolonged cryptosporidiosis exhibited a marked decrease in the number of daily bowel movements and developed formed stools following oral administration of an uncharacterized dialysable extract prepared from lymph node cells obtained from calves immune to *C. parvum* infection (Louie et al 1987). Oocyst shedding was eradicated from the stools of 4 patients; 2 of the 4 remained parasite-free following therapy and the other 2 had subsequent relapses after the termination of therapy. Additional studies are

needed to confirm the findings reported for a small number of AIDS patients and to determine the feasibility and utility of transfer factor therapy in the treatment of immunocompromised hosts with persistent cryptosporidiosis.

Although there appear to be *Cryptosporidium*-specific IgA, IgM and IgG responses detectable in the sera by ELISA and IFA procedures (Campbell & Current 1983, Casemore 1987, Ungar et al 1986, 1988), it is likely that these antibodies play only a minor role in protective immunity. Because the parasite appears to be confined to the mucosal surface and because numerous studies have failed to demonstrate a protective role for serum antibodies against closely related species of coccidia (Rose 1987), it is more probable that secretory antibodies coupled with cell-mediated immune mechanisms are responsible for the clearance of parasites from the infected mucosa and for rendering the immunocompetent host resistant to re-infection. I am not aware of studies addressing the presence or function of secretory antibodies in hosts during or following infection. Mata et al (1984) reported that breast-fed infants in Costa Rica had a significantly lower incidence of cryptosporidiosis than did age-matched babies in the same study populations that were fed artificial diets, and they proposed that lactogenic immunity may play an important role in controlling *C. parvum* infections. This concept was subsequently tested in several studies to determine if antibodies in milk or colostrum can prevent or abrogate intestinal infections with *C. parvum.*

Colostrum or milk from dairy cows that are exposed naturally to the parasite does not appear to protect calves or humans from *C. parvum* infection; however, colostrum from hyperimmunized cows may provide some protection. We routinely administer oocysts of *C. parvum* to one-day-old calves along with the first of 3 litres of colostrum. The subsequent course of infection is not affected by the presence of high titres of *Cryptosporidium*-specific antibody in the colostrum; the parasites excyst, invade, and then replicate within the intestinal mucosa when high levels of colostrum antibody are present in the gut lumen. The fact that most calves will experience cryptosporidiosis while they are nursing from cows, most of which have colostrum antibodies to *C. parvum*, also supports the concept that natural exposure to the parasite does not result in significant lactogenic immunity. Oral administration of colostrum from a non-immunized, naturally exposed dairy cow that contained antibodies to *C. parvum* did not alter the course of infection in an AIDS patient with cryptosporidiosis (Saxon & Weinstein 1987). A similar lack of lactogenic immunity was also reported in infant mice whose dams were immunized by oral inoculation of *C. parvum* oocysts (Moon et al 1988).

In contrast to the above reports, several studies indicate that colostrum obtained from cows hyperimmunized with oocyst/sporozoite antigens of *C. parvum* may protect humans and mice from cryptosporidiosis. Tzipori et al (1986) reported that three immune-deficient patients recovered from cryptosporidiosis within 3–5 days after initiation of oral administration of hyperimmune cow colostrum produced by immunizing pregnant cows with concentrated *C. parvum* oocyst/sporozoite antigens. Two of the patients had subclinical infections following treatment and the other remained free of infection for several months after the treatment was stopped. Fayer et al (1989) demonstrated that hyperimmune bovine colostrum, obtained from cows immunized with purified *C. parvum* oocysts, neutralized sporozoites and protected mice from oocyst challenge. Significantly fewer stages of *C. parvum* were found in suckling mice that were given whey from hyperimmune colostrum (undiluted or diluted 1:20 or 1:50) before and after oocyst inoculation than in mice given whey from control colostrum. Significantly fewer stages were also found in mice following intrarectal inoculation of sporozoites incubated in hyperimmune whey (diluted 1:20 or 1:50) than in mice receiving sporozoites incubated in similar dilutions of control whey. Fayer et al (in press) also reported that this hyperimmune colostrum provided prophylaxis against cryptosporidiosis in calves. Calves given hyperimmune colostrum 2 days after oral inoculation of *C. parvum* oocysts had less diarrhoea and shed oocysts for a shorter period of time than did calves given non-hyperimmune colostrum 2 days after oocyst inoculation. Although these studies indicate that some component of hyperimmune bovine colostrum may exhibit anti-*Cryptosporidium* activity, additional studies are needed to further define the role of lactogenic immunity in preventing and treating cryptosporidiosis and to isolate and characterize the components of hyperimmune colostrum or milk that are responsible for the reported protective effects.

CONCLUSIONS

It is exciting to be involved in some of the basic research that is responsible in part for changing our concept of *Cryptosporidium* from that of a mere biomedical curiosity to that of an important, widespread enteropathogen of man and his domesticated animals. Now that a number of laboratories throughout the world are devoting significant resources into cryptosporidiosis research, our understanding of this protozoan should increase dramatically during the next decade. Some of the most important areas of cryptosporidiosis research that should be addressed include: the taxonomy, natural history and epidemiology of different isolates (species?); a better understanding of the importance of *Cryptosporidium* spp. as agents of diseases (both gastrointestinal and respiratory) that contribute to the morbidity and mortality of man and his domesticated animals; the development of in vitro cultivation and animal models; identification of the mechanisms of acquired immunity; identification of parasite antigens that are responsible for eliciting protective immunity; elucidation of the mechanisms by which this parasite and its metabolites or toxins may alter normal intestinal function; and the identification and development of an effective treatment.

REFERENCES

Alpert G, Bell L M, Kirkpatrick C E, Budnick L D, Campos J M, Friedman H M, Poltkin S A 1984 Cryptosporidiosis in a day care center. N Engl J Med 311: 860–861
Anderson B C 1985 Moist heat inactivation of *Cryptosporidium* sp. Am J Publ Hlth 75: 1433–1434
Anderson B C, Donndelinger T, Wilkins R M, Smith J 1982 Cryptosporidiosis in a veterinary student. J Am Vet Med Ass 180: 408–409
Angus K W 1983 Cryptosporidiosis in man, domestic animals, and birds: a review. J R Soc Med 76: 62–70
Anonymous 1984 Cryptosporidiosis among children attending day care centers – Georgia, Pennsylvania, Michigan, California, New Mexico. Morb Mort Weekly Rep 33: 599–601
Blagburn B L, Current W L 1983 Accidental infection of a researcher with human *Cryptosporidium*. J Infect Dis 148: 772–773

Blagburn B L, Lindsay D S, Giambrone J J, Sundermann C A, Hoerr F J 1987 Experimental cryptosporidiosis in broiler chickens. Poultry Sci 66: 442–449

Bogaerts J, Lepage P, Rouvonoy D, Vandepitte J 1984 *Cryptosporidium* spp., a frequent cause of diarrhea in Central Africa. J Clin Microbiol 20: 874–876

Campbell P N, Current W L 1983 Demonstration of serum antibodies to *Cryptosporidium* sp. in normal and immunodeficient humans with confirmed infections. J Clin Microbiol 18: 165–169

Casemore D P 1987 The antibody response to *Cryptosporidium*: development of a serological test and its use in a study of immunologically normal persons. J Infect 14: 125–134

Clarke J J 1895 A study of coccidia met with in mice. J Microsc Sci 37: 277–302

Crawford F G, Vermund S H 1988 Human cryptosporidiosis. CRC Crit Rev Microbiol 16: 113–159

Current W L 1983 Human cryptosporidiosis. N Engl J Med 309: 614–615

Current W L 1986 *Cryptosporidium*: its biology and potential for environmental transmission. CRC Crit Rev Envir Control 17: 21–31

Current W L 1989 *Cryptosporidium* spp. In: Walzer P D, Genta R M (eds) Parasitic infections in the compromised host. Marcel Dekker Inc., New York pp 281–341

Current W L, Bick P W 1989 The immunobiology of *Cryptosporidium* spp. Path Immunopath Res 8: (in press)

Current W L, Haynes T B 1984 Complete development of *Cryptosporidium* in cell culture. Science 224: 603–605

Current W L, Long P L 1983 Development of human and calf *Cryptosporidium* in chicken embryos. J Infect Dis 148: 1108–1113

Current W L, Reese N C 1986 A comparison of endogenous development of three isolates of *Cryptosporidium* in suckling mice. J Protozool 33: 98–108

Current W L, Snyder D B 1988 Development of and serologic evaluation of acquired immunity to *Cryptosporidium baileyi* by broiler chickens. Poultry Sci 67: 720–729

Current W L, Reese N C, Ernst J V, Bailey W S, Heyman M B, Weinstein W M 1983 Human cryptosporidiosis in immunocompetent and immunodeficient persons: studies of an outbreak and experimental transmission. N Engl J Med 308: 1252–1257

Current W L, Upton S J, Haynes T B 1986 The life cycle of *Cryptosporidium baileyi* n. sp. (Apicomplexa, Cryptosporidiidae) infecting chickens. J Protozool 33: 289–296

D'Antonio R G, Winn R E, Taylor J P, Gustafson T L, Current W L, Rhodes M M, Gary G W, Zajac R A 1985 A waterborne outbreak of cryptosporidiosis in normal hosts. Ann Intern Med 103: 886–888

Driscoll M S, Thomas V L, Sanford B A 1988 *Cryptosporidium* infection in day care centers. Drug Intell Clin Pharm 22: 636

Fayer R, Ungar B L P 1986 *Cryptosporidium* spp and cryptosporidiosis. Microbiol Rev 50: 458–483

Fayer R, Perryman L E, Riggs M W 1989 Hyperimmune bovine colostrum neutralizes *Cryptosporidium* sporozoites and protects mice against oocyst challenge. J Parasitol 75: 151–153

Fayer R, Anderson C, Ungar B L P, Blagburn B L 1989 Efficacy of hyperimmune bovine colostrum for prophylaxis of cryptosporidiosis in calves. J Parasitol 75: (in press)

Forgacs P, Tarshis A, Ma P, Federman M, Mele L, Silverman M L, Shea J A 1983 Intestinal and bronchial cryptosporidiosis in an immunodeficient homosexual man. Ann Intern Med 99: 793–794

Garcia L S, Current W L 1989 Cryptosporidiosis: clinical features and diagnosis. CRC Crit Rev Clin Microbiol (in press)

Garcia L S, Bruckner D A, Brewer T C, Shimzu R Y 1983 Techniques for the recovery and identification of *Cryptosporidium* oocysts from stool specimens. J Clin Microbiol 18: 185–190

Garcia L S, Brewer T C, Bruckner D A 1987 Fluorescent detection of *Cryptosporidium* oocysts in human fecal specimens by using monoclonal antibodies. J Clin Microbiol 25: 119–121

Hart A, Baxby D 1985 Management of cryptosporidiosis. J Antimicrob Chemother 15: 3–4

Heine J, Pholenz J F L, Moon H W, Woode G N 1984 Enteric lesions and diarrhea in gnotobiotic calves monoinfected with *Cryptosporidium* species. J Infect Dis 150: 768–775

Jokipii L, Pohjola S, Jokipii A M M 1983 *Cryptosporidium*: a frequent finding in patients with gastrointestinal symptoms. Lancet i: 358–361

Koch K L, Phillips D L, Current W L 1985 Cryptosporidiosis in hospital personnel: evidence for person-to-person transmission. Ann Intern Med 102: 593–596

Levine N D 1984 Taxonomy and review of the coccidian genus *Cryptosporidium* (Protozoa, Apicomplexa). J Protozool 31: 94–98

Lewis I J, Hart C A, Baxby D 1985 Diarrhoea due to *Cryptosporidium* in acute lymphoblastic leukemia. Arch Dis Child 60: 60–62

Louie E, Borkowsky W, Klesius P H, Haynes T B, Gordon S, Bonk S, Lawrence H S 1987 Treatment of cryptosporidiosis with oral bovine transfer factor. Clin Immunol Immunopath 44: 329–334

Ma P, Soave R 1983 Three step stool examination for cryptosporidiosis in ten homosexual men with protracted watery diarrhea. J Infect Dis 147: 824–828

Madore M S, Rose J B, Gerba C P, Arrowood M J, Sterling C R 1987 Occurrence of *Cryptosporidium* oocysts in sewage effluents and selected surface waters. J Parasitol 73: 702–705

Mata L, Bolanos H, Pizarro D, Vives M 1984 Cryptosporidiosis en ninos de Costa Rica: estudio transversal y longitudinal. Rev Biol Trop 32: 129–135

Miesel J L, Perera D R, Meligro C, Rubin C E 1976 Overwhelming watery diarrhea associated with *Cryptosporidium* in an immunosuppressed patient. Gastroenterology 70: 1156–1160

Miller R A, Holmberg R E, Clausen C R 1983 Life-threatening diarrhea caused by *Cryptosporidium* in a child undergoing therapy for acute lymphocytic leukemia. J Pediatr 103: 256–259

Moon H W, Woodmansee D B, Harp J A, Abel S, Ungar B L P 1988 Lacteal immunity to enteric cryptosporidiosis in mice: immune dams do not protect their suckling pups. Infect Immun 56: 649–653

Navin T R 1985 Cryptosporidiosis in humans: a review of recent epidemiologic studies. Eur J Epidemiol 1: 77–83

Nime F A, Burek J D, Page D L, Holscher M A, Yardley J H 1976 Acute enterocolitis in a human being infected with the protozoan *Cryptosporidium*. Gastroenterology 70: 592–598

Panciera R J, Thomassen R W, Garner F M 1971 Cryptosporidial infection in a calf. Vet Pathol 8: 479–484

Pitlik S, Fainstein V, Rios A, Guarda L, Mansell P W A, Hersh E M 1983 Cryptosporidial cholecystitis. N Engl J Med 308: 976

Reese N C, Current W L, Ernst J V, Bailey W S 1982 Cryptosporidiosis of man and calf: a case report and results of experimental infections in mice and rats. Am J Trop Med Hyg 31: 226–229

Rose M E 1987 Immunity to *Eimeria* infections. Vet Immunol Immunopath 17: 333–343

Sallon S, Deckelabum R J, Schmid I I, Harlap S, Baras M, Spira D T 1988 Cryptosporidium, malnutrition, and chronic diarrhea in children. Am J Dis Child 142: 312–315

Saxon A, Weinstein W 1987 Oral administration of bovine colostrum anticryptosporidia antibody fails to alter the course of human cryptosporidiosis. J Parasitol 73: 413–415

Soave R 1985 Diagnosis, management, and prognosis of human cryptosporidiosis. Annual Meeting of the American Society of Tropical Medicine and Hygiene, Miami, FL, abstract No. 135

Soave R, Ma P 1985 Cryptosporidiosis: travelers' diarrhea in 2 families. Arch Intern Med 145: 70–72

Stibbs H H, Ongereth J 1985 Detection of *Cryptosporidium* oocysts in fecal smears and river water. Proc. 60th Annual Meeting of the American Society of Parasitology, Athens, GA, abstract No. 100

Sundermann C A, Lindsay D S, Blagburn B L 1987 Evaluation of disinfectants for ability to kill avian *Cryptosporidium* oocysts. Companion Animal Practice, November: 36–39

Tyzzer E E 1907 A sporozoan found in the peptic glands of the common mouse. Proc Soc Exp Biol 5: 12–13

Tyzzer E E 1910 An extracellular coccidium, *Cryptosporidium muris* (gen et sp nov.) of the gastric glands of the common mouse. J Med Res 23: 487–516

Tyzzer E E 1912 *Cryptosporidium parvum* (sp. nov.), a coccidium found in the small intestine of the common mouse. Arch Protistenkd 26: 394–412

Tzipori S 1983 Cryptosporidiosis in animals and humans. Microbiol Rev 47: 84–96

Tzipori S, Angus K W, Campbell I, Gray E W 1980 Cryptosporidium: evidence for a single species genus. Infect Immun 30: 884–886

Tzipori S, Campbell I 1981 Prevalence of *Cryptosporidium* antibodies in 10 animal species. J Clin Microbiol 14: 455–456

Tzipori S, Robertson D, Chapman C 1986 Remission of diarrhea due to cryptosporidiosis in an immunodeficient child treated with hyperimmune bovine colostrum. Br Med J 293: 1276–1277

Ungar B L P, Soave R, Fayer R, Nash T E 1986 Enzyme immunoassay detection of immunoglobulin M and G antibodies to *Cryptosporidium* in immunocompetent and immunocompromised persons. J Infect Dis 153: 570–578

Ungar B L P, Gilman R H, Lanata C F, Perez-Schael I 1988 Seroepidemiology of *Cryptosporidium* infection in two Latin American populations. J Infect Dis 157: 551–556

Upton S J, Current W L 1985 The species of *Cryptosporidium* (Apicomplexa: Cryptosporidiidae) infecting mammals. J Parasitol 71: 625–629

Walsh J A, Warren K S 1979 Selective primary care. An interim strategy for disease control in developing countries. N Engl J Med 301: 967–974

K

Discussion of paper presented by W. L. Current

Discussed by T. A. Hart
Reported by H. C. Neu

Current's presentation provided a major review of the small amount of knowledge we have about *Crytosporidium*. During the discussion a number of important facts were emphasized. Specific species of *Cryptosporidium* will infect only certain species. *C. parvum* will infect only mammals and *C. baileyi* only turkeys and chickens. Life cycles are different, and the organisms have different karyotypes. It is probable that *Cryptosporidium* has been around for years, but had not been recognized because of the small size of the parasite, and the dismissal of it as a yeast when seen in animal diarrhoea. However serological testing of stored blood for antibody has not been done.

There are marked differences in human or calf isolates since some produce minimal disease and others produce fulminant diarrhoea. The reasons for the differences among the isolates are unknown.

Unfortunately diarrhoea is not produced in the suckling mouse model, and in the guinea pig the diarrhoea is compensated for by the ability of the large bowel to fill with fluid. Malabsorption is present in models, but villi between parasitized areas of the gut are maintained, and whether diarrhoea is a toxic, secretory process has not been established.

Albumin is lost via the intestine and diarrhoea occurs even on parenteral nutrition. Major factors in the disease in AIDS would appear to be in the auto-infection cycle and in the lack of acquired immunity that occurs in the animal models, making it difficult to study the AIDS related illness.

An individual can have more than one episode of disease. The disease is less severe after several episodes if the individual is immunologically normal. Administration of gammaglobulin from individuals with antibodies against the parasite to an infected hypogammaglobulinaemic individual did not alter disease. Whether colostrum from the cow has any effect is questionable, since calves born to cows which have antibodies develop diarrhoea. Colostrum from naturally infected cows does not protect AIDS patients. IgG, IgM, IgA antibodies have been found, but the amount of secretory IgA produced is unknown.

Cryptosporidium spp. are viable as long as they are kept moist and cool. Thus there remains a potential for nosocomial spread.

Hart stressed the importance of *Cryptosporidium* as a cause of diarrhoea in children, where it might be cause for 6–20% of diarrhoea in developing countries.

274

Table 14.3 Duration of diarrhoea

Organism	Mean duration (days)
Cryptosporidium	12.4
Aeromonas spp.	11.6
Adenovirus	8.6
Astrovirus	7.3
Calcivirus	8.4
Rotavirus	5.9
Campylobacter	7.7
Salmonella	6.5
Shigella	6.8

Unlike rotavirus and enterotoxigenic *E. coli*, it does not cause a rapid dehydration but the diarrhoea persists for a longer time (Table 14.3) and thereby produces malnutrition and further immunocompromise.

The problem of purification of water supplies has not been solved, and communities can suffer severe outbreaks. Recurrent attacks occur even in individuals with a good antibody response.

Finally, how often *Cryptosporidium* causes respiratory infections is unknown. Malnourished children with measles in Africa have had respiratory disease with *Cryptosporidium* and even immunocompetent children have had respiratory illness. Experimental animals readily develop respiratory illness since the organism will complete its life cycle on any mucosal surface.

Much needs to be learned about *Cryptosporidium* and the infections it produces. The pathogenesis of the diarrhoea and the mechanisms controlling immunity are inadequately known. Better understanding of the biochemistry of *Cryptosporidium* should make it possible to develop agents to inhibit or kill the parasite. Knowledge of secretory proteins may provide targets for vaccines.

15. *Pneumocystis carinii*: advances in biology, prophylaxis and treatment

W. T. Hughes

INTRODUCTION

During the first third of the twentieth century *Pneumocystis carinii* was discovered and thought to be an obscure protozoan in the lungs of rodents. During the next third of the century the organism was recognized as the cause of pneumonitis in humans, but only in debilitated infants and severely immunocompromised children and adults with cancer, organ transplants and other forms of immunosuppression. Cases were seen mainly in cancer hospitals and large tertiary care centres. During the last third of the century, the prevalence of *P. carinii* pneumonitis has skyrocketed. This rapid and profound escalation of cases has been due to the epidemic of acquired immunodeficiency syndrome (AIDS) which began in 1981.

Of the 90 000 cases of AIDS that have occurred in the United States, approximately 75% (67 500 cases) have had *P. carinii* pneumonitis at least once. Current estimates are that without any prophylaxis 40 000 cases of the pneumonitis will occur in human immunodeficiency virus (HIV)-infected patients during 1989 and that more than 60 000 cases will occur during the year 1992. Already, *P. carinii* pneumonitis is the most frequent cause of death due to a reportable infectious disease in the United States.

This precipitous impact on human health has made vivid the dearth of information on the biological characteristics of *P. carinii* and has created the need for new modalities of treatment and prevention.

Within the last few years, many excellent comprehensive reviews of *P. carinii* pneumonitis have been published. Therefore, this commentary will deal only with the very recent advances reported predominantly within the last 2–3 years. Even here all of the reported studies cannot be considered. Since the major advances have occurred in studies of the organism and of treatment and prophylaxis, these topics will be addressed.

ORGANISM

Taxonomy

P. carinii has challenged taxonomists for over seven decades. Most have agreed that it must be categorized as either fungus or protozoon. Morphological and tinctorial characteristics, host–parasite interactions, biochemical and histochemical determinations and susceptibility to antimicrobial drugs have not provided a sufficient pattern for phylogenetic placement. Recently, application of techniques of molecular biology has given further insight into the nature of the organism.

Edman et al (1988), obtained 16s-like rRNA from *P. carinii* washed from infected rat lungs. The sequences of the RNA were compared with published sequences of 16s rRNA of *Trypanosoma brucei*, *Dictystelium discoidem*, *Neurospora crassa*, *Zea mays*, *Rattus norvegicus* and *Saccharomyces cerevisiae*. A close evolutionary link between *P. carinii*, *S. cerevisiae* and *N. crassa* was observed using a 'distance matrix' method devised on the structural distance of organisms determined on the average number of base changes per position. These investigators were of the opinion that this feature qualified *P. carinii* as a fungus.

Studies were carried out by Stringer et al (1988), and Cushion et al (1988a), on 18s rRNA from *P. carinii* derived from infected rat lung. The sequence of 386 nucleotides was compared with sequences from eight other taxa. Greatest homology was noted with *S. cerevisiae* and *N. crassa*. Greater divergence was noted from sequences of *Toxoplasma gondii*, *Plasmodium berghei* and *Apicomplexa*. They interpreted these observations as evidence for the fungus nature of *P. carinii*.

Studies in Japan (Watanabe et al 1988) suggested that a 5s rRNA from *P. carinii* was phylogenetically related to the 'Rhizopoda/Myxomycota/Zygomycota'.

Other studies reported in 1988 provide some evidence to support a protozoal classification for *P. carinii*. Gradus et al (1988) isolated DNA from *P. carinii* and calculated the quantity contained in a single organism, since the DNA content of cells has been used in taxonomy. They found the DNA per cell to range from 0.22 to 0.34 pg. When this value was compared with the DNA content of other protozoa and the yeast *Saccharomyces*, the quantity was closer to that of protozoa than to the fungus (Table 15.1). The DNA of *Saccharomyces* (0.02 pg/cell) was 10–15 times less than that of *P. carinii*, whereas there was only the difference of 0.12–0.13 pg/cell between *Toxoplasma gondii* and *P. carinii*. To place these measurements in greater perspective, the DNA content of viruses is in the range of 0.0005 pg/cell, the content of bacteria is about 0.007 pg/cell and that of some plant cells is around 100.0 pg/cell. The percentage of guanine-plus-cytosine $(G + C)$

Table 15.1 Comparison of DNA content of *P. carinii* to that of protozoa and fungi

Organism	DNA content (pg/cell)
Eimeria tenella	0.73
Trichomonas vaginalis	0.53
Entamoeba histolytica	0.45
Trichomonas gallinae	0.40
Pneumocystis carinii	0.22–0.34
Toxoplasma gondii	0.10
Trypanosoma cruzi	0.077
Trypanosoma gambiense	0.077
Trypanosoma equipiderum	0.077
Plasmodium berghei	0.05
Saccharomyces	0.02

(Modified from Gradus et al 1988)

comprising DNA has been used as an indicator of genetic relatedness among microbes. The assumption has been that the more closely related organisms, such as bacteria, have similar proportions of G + C. The G + C content of *P. carinii* DNA was found to be 33 mol/dl by Worley et al (1988). On comparison of G + C percentage of *P. carinii* to that of established protozoa and fungi no pattern is discernible (Table 15.2).

The ribosomal RNA of *P. carinii* has been investigated by Fishman et al (1988). They found the 18s and 26s RNAs of *P. carinii* to resemble the size of those of *Toxoplasma gondii*.

Other studies describing protozoal features of *P. carinii* include those of Yoneda & Walzer (1983). These investigators demonstrated, by the use of freeze-fracture electron microscopy techniques, circular structures about 60 nm diameter on the outer surface of the organisms which were believed to be evidence of membrane fusion, a phenomenon limited to protozoa. Also, the ultrastructural investigations of Vossen et al (1976) revealed a microtubular system of the intracystic sporozoite of *P. carinii* that was similar to that found in sporozoa. Tubules about 20–26 nm in diameter were found just below the pellicle. These tubular units had an electron-transparent central core of about 10 nm and an outer osmiophilic layer.

The susceptibility of *P. carinii* to antimicrobial agents is clearly that of a protozoon rather than a fungus (Table 15.3).

The problem of taxonomic placement of *P. carinii* may not be easily solved. Taxonomy is not based on a single determinant. It is dependent on an organism's morphology, physiology, metabolic functions, DNA–RNA sequences, phylogenetic position and other known features of uniqueness. Thus, well-defined criteria for categorization of fungi and protozoa are lacking. The point is clearly made by

Table 15.2 Comparison of guanine + cytosine (G + C) component of *P. carinii* DNA to that of known protozoa and fungi

Organism	Fungus or protozoon	% DNA as G + C
Trypanosoma cruzi	P	50.2
Plasmodium berghei	P	40.7
Candida parapsilosis	F	40.4
Saccharomyces cerevisae	F	40.0
Candida albicans	F	35.1
Pneumocystis carinii	?	33.0
Trichomonas vaginalis	P	29.0
Tetrahymena paluta	P	25.0

Table 15.3 Comparison of susceptibility of *P. carinii* to antifungal and antiprotozoan drugs

Antimicrobial agents	Examples of susceptible organisms	Susceptibility of *P. carinii*
Trimethoprim–sulphamethoxazole	*Isospora*	+
Pyrimethamine–sulphadiazine	*Toxoplasma, Plasmodia*	+
Pentamidine isethionate	*Trypanosoma, Leishmania*	+
Dapsone	*Plasmodium*	+
Amphotericin B	*Candida, Cryptococcus*	−
Ketoconazole	*Candida, Cryptococcus*	−

Sogin et al (1989) who after analysis of the 16s rRNA of the protozoon *Giardia lamblia* proposed a new perspective on the evolution of nucleated cells. They described extensive differences of *G. lamblia* and other eukaryotes including diverse protozoa. Thus, if comparisons of gene sequences become the basis for taxonomic placement, *P. carinii* may eventually receive its proper title. Currently it is more urgent to learn the biological characteristics of *P. carinii* than to argue the family tree.

Cloning of DNA from *P. carinii*

During 1988, three groups of investigators reported studies of *P. carinii* DNA. Gradus et al (1988) in Oklahoma City isolated DNA from rat-derived *P. carinii* and determined the content per cell to be from 0.22 to 0.34 pg.

Tanabe et al (1988) isolated *P. carinii* DNA from infected rat lungs and cloned the genomic DNA fragments into a plasmid and used them as probes in the DNA (Southern) hybridization analysis of both *P. carinii* of rat and human sources.

Wakefield et al (1988) in Oxford succeeded in extracting *P. carinii* DNA from infected rat lungs. They were able to clone the fraction and identify recombinants of non-rat origin through the use of negative colony hybridization probing with genomic rat DNA. In further studies the British investigators tested recombinants in an in situ hybridization assay using specimens from *P. carinii*-infected and uninfected human and rat lungs.

These developments provide important steps in the further study of the biology, genetics and taxonomy of *P. carinii*. Furthermore, the use of cloned sequences of *P. carinii* DNA and hybridization techniques offer great potential for clinical applications.

Carbohydrates in *P. carinii*

Yoshikawa et al (1988) utilized colloidal gold labelled concanavalin A (con-A) and *Macura pomifera* (MPA) lectins to elucidate the carbohydrate receptors on the trophozoite and cyst forms of *P. carinii*. Their findings showed that binding sites for these lectins were found on the pellicle and on the cell surface of the developmental stages. The electron-dense outer layer contained the respective carbohydrates for these lectins, but the electron-lucent middle layer did not contain MPA-specific carbohydrates.

A panel of fluorescein isothiocyanate conjugated lectins was used by Cushion et al (1988b) to study respective carbohydrates in *P. carinii*. These experiments indicated that both the cyst and trophozoite forms have mannose, *N*-acetylglucosamine and *N*-acetylgalactosamine as the predominant surface carbohydrates. No evidence for the presence of sialic acid and β-galactose was found.

Pesanti & Shanley (1988), using biotin-conjugated lectins and avidin–peroxidase reactions detected receptors to con-A and wheat germ agglutinin on *P. carinii*. They also found gold-labelled con-A on tubular extensions of *P. carinii* examined by electron microscopy.

Monoclonal antibodies to *P. carinii*

Recently, monoclonal antibodies specific for *P. carinii* have been developed in several laboratories (Graves et al 1986, Lee et al 1986, Gigliotti et al 1986,

Linder et al 1987, Matsumoto et al 1987, Beckers 1988, Kovacs et al 1989). Antigens of 25, 35, 65, 90, 110, 116 and 120 kD were identified in rat *P. carinii* isolates and an antigen of 82 kD has been identified in human organisms. Gigliotti et al (1986), found monoclonal antibodies that reacted with *P. carinii* from diverse species including human, rat, rabbit and ferret. They also described antibodies unique to certain species-derived *P. carinii*. Kovacs et al (1989), identified antigen of rat *P. carinii* with molecular weights of 40–100 kD and of human *P. carinii* with molecular weights of 22–95 kD. These studies, even when technical variations are considered, indicate a variety of antigeneic sites on *P. carinii* with differences in organisms derived from man and lower animals. Gigliotti et al (1988), have purified and characterized a surface glycoprotein of ferret *P. carinii*. This acidic glycoprotein (isoelectric point 5.0–5.7) contains both mannose and/or glucose and *N*-acetyl glucosamine residues. The passive administration of monoclonal antibody for this antigen to infected ferrets and rats effectively reduced the severity of *P. carinii* infection (Gigliotti & Hughes 1988).

Current concept of developmental stages of *P. carinii* in vitro
Several suggestions for the life cycle and stages of development of *P. carinii* have been put forth in the past. These have been based primarily on 'still life' studies by light microscopy and transmitted electron microscopy of infected lungs from man and lower animals. Pifer et al (1977), observed the developmental stages of *P. carinii* in vitro by following an organism in culture by phase contrast microscopy. This technique did not provide sufficient visualization to determine the method of replication. Recently Cushion et al (1988c), have utilized a similar approach to study *P. carinii* derived from rat cultured in A549 cell monolayers. From these studies they propose the life cycle depicted in Figure 15.1.

TREATMENT AND PREVENTION

Anti-*P. carinii* activity has been demonstrated for several drugs. However, only two trimethoprim–sulphamethoxazole (TMP–SM) and pentamidine isethionate, are in general use. These are equally effective for the treatment for *P. carinii* pneumonitis but the oral as well as intravenous routes of administration and lower adverse reaction rates make TMP–SM the drug of choice in most instances. Pentamidine must be given intravenously or intramuscularly. Some patients fail to respond to either drug and those with AIDS have a remarkably high rate of side-effects from both drugs. Thus, a more effective and safe drug would be desirable.

   P. carinii pneumonitis can be prevented by the administration of TMP–SM. However, patients with AIDS are often deprived of this prophylaxis because of adverse effects.

   Consideration will be given here to the development of new approaches to this treatment and preventions of *P. carinii* pneumonia.

Treatment
Promising results have been obtained for additional drugs in the treatment of *P. carinii* pneumonitis. Those that have reached clinical trials will be reviewed.

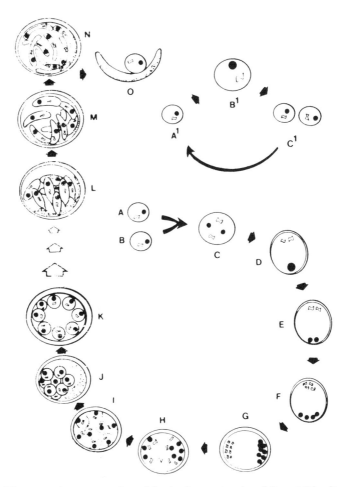

Figure 15.1 Diagrammatic representation of the development cycles of *P. carinii* in vitro. *The Asexual Cycle.* (A^1), trophic form; (B^1) mitotic replication of trophic form; (C^1) trophic forms, products of binary fission. *The Sexual Cycle.* A and B, isogametic forms; C, karyogamy; D, early precyst, diploid zygote; E, intermediate precyst, beginning of mitotic replication of nuclei; F, intermediate precyst, 4 nuclei; G, intermediate precyst, completion of nuclear replication, 8 nuclei; H, late precyst, migration of nuclei to periphery; I, late precyst, initiation of compartmentalization of daughter forms; J, early cyst, completed separation of daughter forms; K, mature cyst, 8 rounded daughter forms within a thick wall; L, cyst containing ellipsoidal daughter forms; M, cyst containing elongated daughter forms; N, cyst containing thin, very elongated daughter forms; O, collapsed, excysted cyst with trophic form. The progressive elongation of the daughter forms within the cyst stages L to N, may present the process required for excystation. These forms have been seen repeatedly in culture and in infected rat lung homogenates, although the actual process of excystment was not observed. (Reproduced with permission, from Cushion et al 1988a)

Pentamidine by the aerosol route

As early as 1973 Waldman et al showed that in rats pentamidine administered in an aerosol permitted the delivery of the drug into the lung without systemic concentrations that might adversely affect other organs. Later Bernard et al (1985) reported a systematic study of the use of aerosolized pentamidine in rats and showed that this route of administration for long-term use was not associated with significant toxicity. Debs et al (1987) showed that the administration of a dose of 5.0 mg/kg per day for a 2-week period resulted in a 75% cure rate for *P. carinii* pneumonitis in infected rats. Girard et al (1987) used three times this dose over a 3-week period and obtained similar cure rates. In 1987, Conte et al treated 13 AIDS patients with mild *P. carinii* pneumonitis using 4.0 mg/kg per day of aerosolized pentamidine for 14 days. Nine (69%) patients had a satisfactory response but 3 (33%) of these had early relapses. Also, in 1987, Montgomery et al treated 15 episodes of *P. carinii* pneumonia in AIDS patients using a total dose of 600 mg pentamidine by aerosol given daily for 21 days. Thirteen (87%) of the 15 patients responded to this therapy. The only local adverse reaction was cough in 12 (69%) of the patients.

In contrast to the reports of Conte and Montgomery, Godfrey-Faussett et al (1988) had success in 2 (15%) of 13 patients treated with 8.0 mg/kg per day of aerosolized pentamidine for 15–17 days. The reason for these differences is not apparent. However, the particle size delivered by nebulizers differs from one type of unit to another and nebulizers of different types were used in these studies. Armstrong (1988) mentions his experience of therapeutic failures with aerosolized pentamidine at Memorial Sloan-Kettering Cancer Center and urges that this mode of therapy not be used alone for treatment for *P. carinii* pneumonia.

Difluoromethylornithine (Eflornithine)
Difluoromethylornithine (DFMO), an ornithine decarboxylase inhibitor, was found to be ineffective against *P. carinii* in the rat model by Hughes & Smith (1984) and effective by Clarkson et al (1988). Reports of clinical trials of DFMO in the treatment of *P. carinii* pneumonitis have been limited to patients who have failed other forms of treatment and the studies have been uncontrolled (Golden et al 1984, McLees et al 1987). These investigators described favourable responses in some patients. Unfortunately, conclusive data are lacking on the efficacy of this drug. However, Pesanti et al (1988) were surprisingly unable to detect ornithine decarboxylase activity in *P. carinii*.

Trimetrexate
A clever approach to the development of anti-*P. carinii* drugs has been taken by investigators at the National Institutes of Health in Washington. Allegra et al 1987a, assayed antifolate compounds in vitro with *P. carinii* dihydrofolate reductase and found that trimetrexate, the quinazoline analogue of methotrexate, had activity some 1500 times greater than pyrimidines. Kovacs et al (1988) showed efficacy in the steroid-treated rat model for *P. carinii*, protecting the mammalian folate metabolism with calcium leucovorin. The design of this therapeutic approach is based upon the fact that *P. carinii*, presumably, must synthesize folates while mammalian cells can utilize preformed exogenous folates.

Trimetrexate has now been studied clinically. Allegra et al (1987b) demonstrated favourable response rates in AIDS patients with *P. carinii* pneumonia treated with intravenous trimetrexate plus leucovorin. In 16 patients treated initially with the drugs, 63% responded with improvement. A similar response was found in another group of 16 patients who had failed conventional therapy. A third group received trimetrexate and leucovorin plus sulphadiazine and 71% of these 17 patients responded favourably. Relapse of the pneumonitis occurred at the rates of 60% for those in the first group to only 6.0% for those in the group treated also with sulphadiazine. Although adverse reactions occurred in 34% of the 49 episodes treated, only one patient required withdrawal of the drug.

Diaminodiphenysulphone (dapsone)
In 1984, Hughes & Smith found dapsone to be highly effective in the treatment of murine *P. carinii* pneumonitis. They also demonstrated a synergistic effect when trimethoprim was combined with dapsone. Leoung et al (1986) treated 15 patients with *P. carinii* pneumonitis and AIDS with dapsone–trimethoprim for 21 days. All of the patients responded to therapy. Adverse reactions were common and 2 of the patients eventually required withdrawal of the drugs. When dapsone was used therapeutically without trimethoprim, the results were less impressive, although 61% of 18 cases responded favourably (Mills et al 1988).

A randomized double-blind controlled study by Medina et al (1987), compared trimethoprim–dapsone with TMP–SM in the treatment of 58 AIDS patients with *P. carinii* pneumonitis. Both regimens were administered over 21 days. The treatments were successful in 27 (93%) of the 29 patients in each group. However, neutropenia was encountered in 5 of 29 patients in the sulphamethoxazole group but only 1 of 29 in the dapsone group. Also, elevation of serum transaminases was encountered more frequently in the sulphamethoxazole group.

Prevention
Although TMP–SM has been highly effective and safe for the prevention of *P. carinii* pneumonitis in non-AIDS patients, for unknown reasons AIDS patients have a high rate of adverse reactions. Thus, an alternative approach is needed for those who cannot take this regimen.

Studies in cancer patients at high risk for *P. carinii* pneumonitis have shown that TMP-SM administered on only 3 consecutive days per week is as effective as continuous daily doses (Hughes et al 1977, Hughes et al 1984). An advantage of the intermittent scheme is a significant reduction in the cases of systemic opportunistic mycoses when compared with daily doses of TMP–SM.

Only one study has been published to evaluate in a controlled manner prophylaxis for *P. carinii* pneumonitis in AIDS patients. Fischl et al (1988) compared daily TMP–SM given to one group to an untreated control group in closely matched patients with AIDS and Kaposi's sarcoma. Of the 30 patients taking TMP–SM, no cases of the pneumonitis occurred, whereas 16 (53%) of the 30 untreated control developed *P. carinii* pneumonitis. The mean survival for the TMP–SM group was 22.6 months and the mean survival of the untreated group was 12.6 months (Fig. 15.2). Adverse reactions occurred in 50% of the patients but only 5 (17%) required discontinuation of the drug. A similar rate of reactions occurred in the untreated group. This study indicates that TMP–SM is as effective in AIDS patients as in non-AIDS patients, that at least some of the adverse reactions attributed to TMP–SM may not be related to the drugs and that some patients may be able to tolerate the drugs despite rashes and transient neutropenia.

For patients who cannot take TMP–SM prophylaxis two alternative experimental approaches look promising.

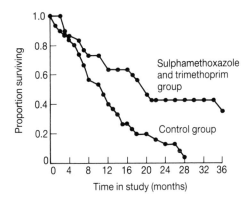

Figure 15.2 Proportion of surviving patients with acquired immunodeficiency syndrome-associated Kaposi's sarcoma receiving sulphamethoxazole and trimethoprim chemoprophylaxis vs no prophylaxis, using Kaplan-Meier product-limit method. Closed circles represent patients receiving sulphamethoxazole and trimethoprim suppressive therapy; open circles represent patients receiving no suppressive therapy. (Reproduced with permission, from Fischl et al 1988)

Aerosolized pentamidine prophylaxis

Bernard et al (1987, 1988a, 1988b) administered aerosolized pentamidine at 60 mg per dose weekly for 4 weeks and then biweekly thereafter to patients with AIDS. In an historical control group the rate of *P. carinii* pneumonitis was 6.7 per 100 patient months. The rate of the pneumonitis in the pentamidine-treated patients was 0.52 per 100 patient months for all of the 191 patients studied. For those who had previously had *P. carinii* pneumonitis the recurrence rate on pentamidine was 1.7 per 100 patient months.

Conte et al (1988) administered 300 ng aerosolized pentamidine once monthly to 103 patients with AIDS or AIDS-related complex (ARC). Two-thirds of these patients also received azidothymidine (AZT). After 6 months of prophylaxis 82% of patients had remained free of *P. carinii* pneumonitis.

Feigal et al (1988) administered approximately 36 mg aerosolized pentamidine every 2 weeks to 211 human immunodeficient virus (HIV)-infected patients. Overall, by 5 months 9.9% of the patients had experienced *P. carinii* pneumonitis.

The true efficacy of aerosolized pentamidine is unknown since controlled studies have not been done.

Dapsone prophylaxis

Animal studies showed dapsone to be highly effective as prophylaxis for *P. carinii* infection (Hughes & Smith 1984). An open clinical trial of prophylactic dapsone was reported in 1987 (Metroka et al) in which 156 patients with AIDS or ARC with less than 200 T_4 lymphocytes/mm^3 were given 100 mg of dapsone daily by mouth. *P. carinii* pneumonitis occurred in only 1 (0.6%) of the patients. In contrast, 14 (74%) of 19 case-matched control patients receiving no prophylaxis developed the pneumonitis. Anaemia was a significant adverse effect and 39 (25%) of the 156 patients required blood transfusion. Rash, methaemoglobinaemia, nausea and increase in serum lactic dehydrogenase values were also noted but were not deleterious.

Recently, an animal study has suggested that dapsone may have prolonged prophylactic effects and that widely spaced doses might be effective. Hughes (1988) showed that while 11 (73%) of 15 untreated control rats had *P. carinii* pneumonia after 10 weeks of immunosuppression, none of the animals given dapsone, 125 mg/kg daily, weekly, biweekly or monthly had evidence of infection. This study suggests that such widely spaced doses might reduce the toxicity encountered with daily usage. No such studies have been reported in man.

CONCLUSION

Within the past 3 years important developments have occurred with *P. carinii*. It has continued to escalate as a cause of human disease because of the AIDS epidemic. Some knowledge has been gained of the organism's biology. Cloning of the *P. carinii* DNA has provided an important step towards further understanding of the nature of the organism and the development of diagnostic techniques. Also, new modalities of prevention and treatment have advanced to clinical use.

It seems reasonable to predict that *P. carinii* will soon gain a position as one of the major infectious diseases of man.

ACKNOWLEDGEMENTS

This work was supported in part by the National Cancer Institute Cancer Center Support (CORE) Grant P30 CA21765, Grant R01-AI 20673–06 from the National Institute of Allergy and Infectious Diseases, and the American Lebanese Syrian Associated Charities (ALSAC).

REFERENCES

Allegra C J, Kovacs J A, Drake J C et al 1987a Activity of antifolates against *Pneumocystis carinii* dihydrofolate reductase and identification of a potent new agent. J Exp Med 165: 926
Allegra C J, Chabner B A, Tuazon C U et al 1987b Trimetrexate for the treatment of *Pneumocystis carinii* pneumonia in patients with the acquired immunodeficiency syndrome. N Engl J Med 317: 978–985
Armstrong D 1988 Aerosol pentamidine. Ann Intern Med 109: 852–854
Beckers P J A 1988 Recent developments in the immunobiology of pneumocystis. Parasitology 28: 117–121
Bernard E M, Donnelly H J, Koo H P et al 1985 Aerosol administration improved delivery of pentamidine to the lungs (Abstract). In: Program and Abstracts of the 25th Interscience Conference of Antimicrobial Agents and Chemotherapy Washington DC American Society for Microbiology, p 193
Bernard E, Schmitt H, Pagel L, Seltzer M, Armstrong D 1987 Safety and effectiveness of aerosol pentamidine for prevention of PCP in patients with AIDS. Interscience Conference on Antimicrobial Agents and Chemotherapy, Minneapolis, American Society of Microbiology, Abstract 944
Bernard E M, Schmitt H J, Lifton A et al 1988a Prevention of *Pneumocystis carinii* pneumonia with aerosol pentamidine (Abstract). IV International Conference on AIDS, Stockholm, Sweden, June 12–16
Bernard E M, Schmitt H J, Lifton A M, Dickmeyer M, Seltzer M, Armstrong D 1988b Aerosol pentamidine prevents PCP among patients with AIDS. Interscience Conference on Antimicrobial Agents and Chemotherapy, Los Angeles, Abstract 1118

Clarkson A B Jr, William D E, Rosenberg C 1988 Efficacy of DL-alpha-difluoromethylornithine in a rat model of *Pneumocystis carinii* pneumonia. Antimicrob Agents Chemother 32: 1158–1163

Conte J E, Hollander H, Golden J A 1987 Inhaled or reduced-dose intravenous pentamidine for *Pneumocystis carinii* pneumonia. Ann Intern Med 107: 495–498

Conte J E, Chernoff D, Feigal D, Hollander H, Golden J 1988 Once monthly inhaled pentamidine for the prevention of *Pneumocystis carinii* pneumonia. Interscience Conference on Antimicrobial Agents and Chemotherapy, Los Angeles, Abstract 1111

Cushion M T, Ruffolo J J, Walzer P D 1988a Analysis of the development stages of *Pneumocystis carinii in vitro*. Lab Invest 58: 324–331

Cushion M T, Blase M A, Walzer P D 1988b Isolation of RNA from *Pneumocystis carinii*. Proceedings 41st Annual Meeting Society of Protozoologists. Bristol, England, July 18–22

Cushion M T, DeStafano J A, Walzer P D 1988c *Pneumocystis carinii*: surface reactive carbohydrates detected by lectin probes. Exp Parasitol 67: 137–147

Debs R J, Blumenfeld W, Brunette E N et al 1987 Successful treatment with aerosolized pentamidine of *Pneumocystis carinii* pneumonia. Antimicrob Agents Chemother 31: 37–41

Edman J C, Kovacs J A, Masur H, Santi D V, Elwood H J, Sogin M L 1988 Ribosomal RNA sequence shows *Pneumocystis carinii* to be a member of the fungi. Nature 334: 519–522

Feigal D W, Kandall K, Fallat R 1988 Pentamidine aerosol prophylaxis for *Pneumocystis carinii* pneumonia: efficacy in 211 AIDS and ARC patients. Interscience Conference on Antimicrobial Agents and Chemotherapy, Los Angeles, Abstract 1113

Fischl M A, Dickinson G M, La Voie L 1988 Safety and efficacy of sulfamethoxazole and trimethoprim chemoprophylaxis for *Pneumocystis carinii* pneumonia in AIDS. J Am Med Ass 259: 1185–1189

Fishman J A, Ullu E, Armstrong M, Richards F F 1988 Organization of DNA and RNA from rat *Pneumocystis carinii*. Proceedings 41st Annual Meeting Society of Protozoologists, Bristol, England, July 18–22

Gigliotti F, Hughes W T 1988 Passive immunoprophylaxis with specific monoclonal antibody confers partial protection against *Pneumocystis carinii* pneumonitis in animal models. J Clin Invest 81: 1666–1668

Gigliotti F, Stokes D C, Cheatham A B, Davis D S, Hughes W T 1986 Development of murine monoclonal antibodies to *Pneumocystis carinii*. J Infect Dis 154: 315–322

Gigliotti F, Ballou L R, Hughes W T, Mosley B D 1988 Purification and initial characterization of a ferret *Pneumocystis carinii* surface antigen. J Infect Dis 158: 848–854

Girard P M, Brun-Pascand M, Farinotti R, Tamister S, Kernbaum S 1987 Pentamidine aerosol in prophylaxis and treatment of murine *Pneumocystis carinii* pneumonia. Antimicrob Agents Chemother 31: 978–981

Godfrey-Faussett P, Miller R F, Semple S J 1988 Nebulized pentamidine. Lancet i: 645–646

Golden J A, Sjoerdsma A, Santi D V 1984 *Pneumocystis carinii* pneumonia treated with a-difluoromethylornithine: A prospective study among patients with the acquired immunodeficiency syndrome. West J Med 141: 613

Gradus M S, Gilmore M, Lerner M 1988 An isolation method of DNA from *Pneumocystis carinii*: a quantitative comparison to known parasitic protozoan DNA. Comp Biochem Physiol 89B: 75–77

Graves D C, McNabb S J N, Ivey M H, Worley M A 1986 Development and characterization of monoclonal antibodies to *Pneumocystis carinii*. Infect Immun 51: 125–133

Hughes W T 1988 Comparisons of dosages, intervals and drugs in the prevention of *Pneumocystis carinii* pneumonia. Antimicrob Agents Chemother 32: 623–625

Hughes W T, Smith B L 1984 Efficacy of diaminodiphenylsulfone and other drugs in murine *Pneumocystis carinii* pneumonitis. Antimicrob Agents Chemother 26: 436–440

Hughes W T, Rivera G K, Schell M J et al 1984 Successful intermittent chemoprophylaxis for *Pneumocystis carinii* pneumonitis. New Engl J Med 316: 1627

Hughes W T, Kuhn S, Chaudhary S et al 1977 Successful chemoprophylaxis for *Pneumocystis carinii* pneumonia. New Engl J Med 297: 1419

Kovacs J A, Allegra C J, Kennedy S, Swan J C, Drake J, Parrillo J E, Chabner B, Masur H 1988 Efficacy of trimetrexate, a potent lipid-soluble antifolate in the treatment of rodent *Pneumocystis carinii* pneumonia. Am J Trop Med Hyg 39: 491–498

Kovacs J A, Helpern J L, Lundgren B, Swan J C, Parrillo J E, Masur H 1989 Monoclonal antibodies to *Pneumocystis carinii*: identification of specific antigens and characterization of antigenic differences between rat and human isolates. J Infect Dis 159: 60–70

Lee C H, Bolinger C D, Bartlett M S, Kohler R B, Wilde C E, Smith J W 1986 Production of monoclonal antibody against *Pneumocystis carinii* by using a hybrid of rat spleen and mouse myeloma cells. J Clin Microbiol 23: 505–508

Leoung G S, Mills J, Hopewell P C, Hughes W, Wofsy C 1986 Dapsone-trimethoprim for *Pneumocystis carinii* pneumonia in the acquired immunodeficiency syndrome. Ann Intern Med 105: 45–48

Linder E, Lundin L, Vorma H 1987 Detection of *Pneumocystis carinii* in lung-derived samples using monoclonal antibodies to an 82 kDa parasite component. J Immunol Meth 98: 57–62

McLees B D, Barlow J L R, Kuzma R J et al 1987 Successful eflornithine (DFMO) treatment of *Pneumocystis carinii* pneumonia (PCP) in AIDS patients failing conventional therapy. Am Rev Resp Dis 135: A167

Matsumoto Y, Amogai T, Yamada M, Imanishi J, Yoshida Y 1987a Production of a monoclonal antibody with specificity for the pellicle of *Pneumocystis carinii* by hybridoma. Parasitol Res 73: 228–233

Matsumoto Y, Amogai T, Yamada M, Imanishi J, Yoshida Y 1987b Production of a monoclonal antibody with specificity for the pellicle of *Pneumocystis carinii* by using a hybrid of rat spleen and mouse myeloma cells. J Clin Microbiol 23: 505–508

Medina F, Leoung G, Mills J et al 1987 Oral therapy for *Pneumocystis carinii* pneumonia in AIDS. A randomized double-blind trial of trimethoprim sulfamethoxazole versus dapsone trimethoprim for first episode *Pneumocystis carinii* pneumonia in AIDS. Third International Conference on AIDS, Washington DC, Abstract F3.3

Metroka C E, Lange R, Braun N, O'Sullivan M, Josefberg H, Jacobus D 1987 Successful chemoprophylaxis for *P. carinii* pneumonia with dapsone in patients with AIDS and ARC. Third International Conference on AIDS, Washington DC, Abstract THP231

Mills J, Leoung G, Medina I, Hopewell P C, Hughes W T, Wofsy C 1988 Dapsone treatment of *Pneumocystis carinii* pneumonia in the acquired immunodeficiency syndrome. Antimicrob Agents Chemother 32: 1057–1060

Montgomery A B, Debs R J, Luce J M, et al 1987 Aerosolized pentamidine as sole therapy for *Pneumocystis carinii* pneumonia in patients with acquired immunodeficiency syndrome. Lancet ii: 480–483

Pesanti E L, Shanley J D 1988 Glycoproteins of *Pneumocystis carinii*: characterization by electrophoresis and microscopy. J Infect Dis 158: 1353–1359

Pesanti E L, Bartlett M S, Smith J W 1988 Lack of detectable activity of ornithine decarboxylase in *Pneumocystis carinii*. J Infect Dis 158: 1137–1138

Pifer L, Hughes W T, Murphy M J 1977 Propagation of *Pneumocystis carinii* in vitro. Pediat Res 11: 305–311

Sogin M L, Gunderson J H, Elwood H J, Alonso R A, Peattie D A 1989 Phylogenetic meaning of the kingdom concept: an unusual ribosomal RNA from *Giardia lamblia*. Science 243: 75–77

Stringer S L, Cushion M, Blase M, Walzer P D, Stronger J R 1988 Partial sequence of 18s ribosomal RNA from *Pneumocystis carinii*. Proceedings 41st Annual Meeting Society of Protozoologists, Bristol, England, July 18–22

Tanabe K, Fuchimoto M, Egawa K, Nakamura Y 1988 Use of *Pneumocystis carinii* genomic DNA clones for DNA hybridization analysis of infected human lungs. J Infect Dis 157: 593–596

Vossen M E M H, Beckers P J A, Meuwissen J H E Th, Stadhouders A M 1976 Microtubules in *Pneumocystis carinii*. Z Parasitenk 49: 291–292

Wakefield A E, Hopkin JM, Burns J, Hipkiss J B, Stewart T J, Moxon E R 1988 Cloning of DNA from *Pneumocystis carinii*. J Infect Dis 158: 859–862

Waldman R H, Pearace D E, Martin R A 1973 Pentamidine isethionate levels in lungs, livers and kidneys of rats after aerosol or intramuscular administration. Am Rev Resp Dis 108: 1004–1009

Watanbe J I, Nakamura Y, Tanabe K, Hori H 1988 5s ribosomal RNA sequence of *Pneumocystis carinii* and its phylogenetic association with 'Rhizopoda/Myxomycota/Zygomycota group'. Proceedings 41st Annual Meeting Society of Protozoologists, Bristol, England, July 18–22

Worley M A, Ivey M H, Graves D C 1988 Establishment of a genomic library for *Pneumocystis carinii*. Proceedings 41st Annual Meeting Society of Protozoologists, Bristol, England, July 18–22

Yoneda K, Walzer P D 1983 Attachment of *Pneumocystis carinii* to type 1 alveolar cells studied by freeze-fracture electron microscopy. Infect Immun 40: 812–816

Yoshikawa H, Morioka H, Yoshida Y 1988 Ultrastructural detection of carbohydrates in the pellicle of *Pneumocystis carinii*. Parasitol Res 74: 537–543

Discussion of paper presented by W. T. Hughes

Discussed by J. A. Kovacs
Reported by H. C. Neu

Pneumocystis carinii is worldwide in distribution. Ninety percent of rodents are infected, and most dogs, rabbits, cats, monkeys and chimpanzees are infected as well. Pneumocystis is transmitted by the aerosol route as shown by experiments with germ-free rats placed in isolator cages downwind from infected rats. If rats are immunosuppressed, immunosuppression stopped, and they are treated with trimethoprim–sulphamethoxazole and placed in a germ-free environment, the animals will, even in a germ-free isolator, develop pneumocystis again after a number of months if they are treated with steroids.

Pneumocystis has been isolated from ear fluid and occasionally from the spleen, liver and kidney. Why there is little dissemination in the immunocompromised host remains an unsolved problem. But it is possible that, as time goes by, more disseminated cases will appear. Since pentamidine will not reach some areas of the lung there may be atypical pulmonary presentations such as cystic lesions, lobar involvement and other atypical features.

Kovacs reported that, in addition to the ribosomal RNA homology with fungi, other studies suggest that *P. carinii* is a fungus. All protozoa have a bifunctional dihydrofolate reductase (DHFR)-thymidilate synthase (TS) enzyme that exist on a single, large molecular weight molecule ($> 100\,000$). In contrast, bacteria, fungi and mammalian cells possess these enzymatic activities on separate, smaller molecules. Kovacs et al have characterized the DHFR of both *P. carinii* and *T. gondii* (Kovacs et al submitted), and have found that while *T. gondii* does have a large molecular weight protein with both activities, *P. carinii* possesses a small molecular weight ($25\,000$) enzyme, and that TS and DHFR activities of *P. carinii* can be separated by affinity column chromatography. Recently both the DHFR (J Edman et al submitted) and TS (U Edman et al submitted) genes of *P. carinii* have been cloned and have been documented by Southern blotting to *P. carinii* chromosomes which can be separated by pulse-field electrophoresis showing that the genes for the enzymes reside on separate chromosomes. These studies document that *P. carinii* DHFR and TS are separate proteins; which is characteristic of fungi and not protozoa. Monoclonal cross-reactivity studies as well as staining studies also suggest that *P. carinii* is a fungus since it stains with mucicarmine.

Immunoblot studies using polyclonal sera directed against rat and human *P. carinii* have shown that the antigenic patterns of the two isolates are different.

In looking at human sera Kovacs and others have found that by immunoblot the majority of healthy and immunosuppressed humans have antibodies to *P. carinii* documenting prior exposure and suggesting that disease results from reactivation of latent infection.

Kovacs also commented on diagnosis of *P. carinii* pneumonia (PCP). Recent studies have found that induced sputum can be used to diagnosis PCP in about 55% of cases. To see if an indirect immunofluorescent assay using monoclonal antibodies could be utilized in detecting *P. carinii* in sputum, they undertook a collaborative study with the San Francisco General Hospital. In that study *P. carinii* could be detected in sputum by any stain in 94% of AIDS patients ultimately found to have PCP. Although both toluidine blue-O and a differential staining method were able to detect *P. carinii* in 75–80% of cases, the best results were seen with the immunofluorescent stain, which detected *P. carinii* in 92% of cases. Currently at the NIH more than 90% of cases of *P. carinii* are detected by examination of induced sputum.

There is still much work to be done with pneumocystis. The use of dapsone, pentamidine aerosol and other treatment modalities have offered alternative forms of therapy. Diagnosis is now rapid in AIDS patients. Unfortunately the disease is never eradicated, but only suppressed, so further work on lifelong suppression is necessary.

Plenary Lecture IV

Chairman: J. Verhoef

16. Rationally modulating the immune response: the importance of MHC–peptide interactions

J. B. Rothbard   R. Busch

INTRODUCTION

In the past few years, our understanding of the recognition of protein antigens by T lymphocytes has greatly expanded. Although some important details are still to be elucidated, an extraordinary mechanism of recognition has been defined, which requires antigen-specific receptors on the surface of two separate cells to come in contact.

The T lymphocytes appear to be essential components of a large percentage of the effector functions involved in the immune response, and their capacity to be stimulated by antigens is the basis of genetic differences in responsiveness between individuals. Consequently, understanding the molecular basis of the clonal expansion of this cell population provides an unprecedented opportunity to modulate the response rationally, either by selectively expanding certain cells, as is required in vaccine immunizations, or by specifically decreasing a deleterious population of T cells, as in the case of treating allergies or autoimmune syndromes. In this paper we attempt to describe our current understanding of T-cell recognition of peptide–major histocompatibility complex (MHC) complexes, with particular emphasis on the experimental strategies employed by our laboratory.

A fundamental characteristic of the vertebrate immune system is its capacity to recognize and respond to a wide spectrum of antigens. At the present time three different classes of molecules have been shown to bind antigen: (1) the immunoglobulins, (2) the antigen receptor of T cells, and (3) the class I and II major histocompatibility proteins. Each set of proteins has evolved a separate mechanism to allow them to interact with a diversity of ligands.

The best understood are the antibodies, which generate the greatest diversity of antigen-combining sites by a combination of genetic rearrangement of the exons encoding the variable, joining, diversity and constant regions during B-cell development (Honjo 1983) and subsequent somatic mutation of the rearranged immunoglobulin gene (Moller 1987). The antigen receptors of T cells are closely related to the immunoglobulins, both in their primary structure and genetic organization. Their diverse antigen-combining sites appear to arise from similar

This paper was prepared for the meeting but unfortunately could not be presented.

genetic rearrangements as for antibodies, however subsequent somatic mutation has never been detected (Davis & Bjorkman 1988). The third group of antigen-binding molecules, the class I and II major histocompatibility proteins, has evolved separately. Even though they both contain domains which resemble immunoglobulins in their tertiary structure, the antigen-combining site is folded in a distinctly different manner (Bjorkman et al 1987a). The proposed site is composed of an 8-stranded β-pleated sheet supporting two helical segments (Bjorkman et al 1987b). The most extraordinary feature of these molecules is that even though the proteins encoded for by the MHC represent one of the most polymorphic family of molecules known, the residues forming the binding site of any single allele are invariable. Nevertheless, each allele can bind a very large number of diverse peptide sequences.

The capacity of MHC class II molecules to bind peptide antigens initially was demonstrated using equilibrium dialysis (Babbitt et al 1985). The peptide–MHC class II complex subsequently was shown to be sufficiently stable to be isolated using gel filtration (Buus et al 1986). Even though an individual MHC allele was shown to interact with a variety of T-cell determinants, binding was selective; not all sequences were capable of binding, nor did all bind with equal affinity (Buus et al 1987).

These studies also revealed that the kinetics of the formation and dissociation of the complex were unusual. Both rates were extremely slow, requiring hours, rather than seconds or minutes to be detected. These extraordinary kinetics were not simply characteristic of detergent-solubilized class II molecules, because similar rates have been shown for class II molecules embedded in lipid monolayers (Watts & McConnell 1986) and recently using intact cells (Busch et al submitted, Ceppellini et al submitted). Recent detailed investigation of the formation of the peptide–MHC class II complex has identified an intermediate, present in the initial minutes of the reaction that precedes the formation of the more stable complex (Sadegh-Nasseri & McConnell 1989).

The solution of the crystal structure of HLA A2 has provided a framework on which these experiments can be interpreted. In addition to providing information on the folded polypeptide backbone, the initial X-ray diffraction data also contained data which allowed the putative antigen-combining site to be localized, which surprisingly appeared constitutively occupied with a mixture of ligands (Bjorkman et al 1987b). The presence of a diverse spectrum of bound ligands has been confirmed recently by isolating material, ranging in molecular weight between 2 and 20 kD, that was susceptible to proteolysis, from preparations of purified MHC class II molecules (Buus et al 1988). Consequently, the complex kinetics might be explained, partially by the need to displace a resident ligand.

Our laboratory has concentrated on trying to understand the capacity of MHC molecules to bind a range of ligands by attempting to identify common features among immunogenic peptides and to determine whether high-affinity interactions correlated with increased immunogenicity. We reasoned that for the initial T-cell determinants to have been identified, they must have bound the MHC proteins with sufficient affinity to be highly represented in a polyclonal response. Consequently, any structural similarity in their primary sequence might be a logical beginning to an investigation of peptide–MHC interactions. This assumption was based on the ability of proteolytic enzymes to bind a variety of substrates, many in a similar location in the enzymatic site, by contacting a small number of critical moieties in the ligand.

Because of their small number, we initially did not distinguish between helper and cytotoxic determinants, nor did we segregate ones recognized by murine, rat, or guinea-pig T cells from those capable of stimulating human lymphocytes. An empirical analysis revealed a linear pattern composed of a charged amino acid or a glycine followed by 2 or 3 hydrophobic amino acids and ending with a polar residue that was present in a surprisingly high percentage of the sequences (Rothbard & Taylor 1988). Support for the importance of this loose pattern was that in the few cases where the critical amino acids in recognition were defined, none of the residues, composing these motifs, could be deleted and the peptide still be recognized by a T cell.

As the list of T-cell determinants grew, they could be segregated by the H-2 or HLA allele with which they were originally defined. When analysed in this fashion, additional similarities were apparent. When the peptides were aligned based on a pair of hydrophobic amino acids, homologous residues were present at relative positions 1, 4, 5 and 8, with the hydrophobic residues being at positions 4 and 5. If the homologous residues constituted important, common contacts with the MHC molecule, then they represented evidence that many of our assumptions had validity and partially explained why these and more detailed patterns had predictive value. In addition, the spacing of the homologous residues in the peptide sequences provided additional information on the conformation of the bound peptide. For example, residues at positions 1, 4, 5, and 8 form a common surface of a helix when a peptide adopts this conformation. This conformation of the determinant also was postulated by DeLisi & Berzofsky (1985) in a separate analysis.

These ideas were tested in two separate series of experiments following a common strategy. The experimental design was based on the premise that if the patterns were valid, then their presence implied that many peptides not only adopted a similar conformation when bound, but they also must interact with the same MHC residues in the combining site and consequently there must be a preferred location for the bound ligand. Furthermore, clonal specificity would be dictated in this model by only some, and not all, of the amino acids composing the determinants, and they should be able to be identified by exchanging amino acids between determinants. Those residues that form critical contacts exclusively with the MHC molecules should be exchangeable, whereas those interacting with the T-cell receptor would not be able to be replaced, and recognition by the T-cell clone should be retained.

Two DR1 restricted T-cell clones, one specific for an influenza matrix peptide and the other stimulated by a sequence from the haemagglutinin were used in the initial set of experiments (Rothbard et al 1988). Two sets of hybrid peptides were synthesized based on an alignment of the sequences that had structural similarities at relative positions 1, 4, 5, and 8. One was composed of residues from the influenza haemagglutinin peptide substituted for the corresponding residues in the matrix sequence, while the other contained amino acids of the matrix peptide replacing those in the haemagglutinin sequence. When the hybrid peptides were tested, only those peptides that contained 6 substitutions, which were spaced in the sequence to constitute a facade of a putative helix, were recognized by the clones. However, the stimulatory capacity of each was significantly less than either of the natural sequences. In addition, a proline had to be replaced in the hybrid peptide formed by substituting the matrix residues into the haemagglutinin background to generate a response. This was rationalized to be due to the problem proline posed in the conformational flexibility of the peptide, but it was not unequivocally demonstrated.

Even though these experiments supported the model, the experimental design had two shortcomings; (1) the only experimental readout was the proliferation of T-cell clone; MHC binding was not examined, and (2) not all possible hybrid peptides were synthesized and the proposed amino acids necessary for T-cell recognition could have been fortuitously identified, particularly because the amino acids that were not exchanged were quite homologous. These criticisms were addressed in a study using cytotoxic T cells (Rothbard et al 1989). In this case residues from an influenza nucleoprotein-peptide were substituted for corresponding amino acids in an HLA CW3 peptide also seen by K^d-restricted cells. This series of experiments was more exhaustive, because (1) a number of different alignments of the two peptides were used as the basis for exchange of amino acids, (2) the ability of the hybrid molecules to bind the restriction element was examined indirectly by competitively interfering with T cell recognition, and (3) once a hybrid peptide was recognized successfully by the T-cell clone, the importance of each substituted amino acid was tested by individually reverting it to the original residue of the other determinant.

Only one of the four possible alignments of the two peptides tested resulted in hybrid peptides which could stimulate the clone or compete for binding of the natural sequence consistently throughout the set. As with the class II system, substitution of 6 amino acids resulted in partial recognition, however, the presence of a seventh improved the potency of the peptide. Five of the 6 residues were required for recognition and the spacing of the 6 essential amino acids was consistent with the peptide adopting a helical conformation when bound. Substitution of less than 5 of these amino acids in the sequence did not interfere with the peptide's capacity to compete with the natural sequence for recognition, but did eliminate all recognition by the T cell, proving that these modifications affected the interaction with the T-cell receptor of the clone, but not the restriction element. These data were combined with additional information on the effects of point substitutions on both binding and recognition by the T-cell clone to generate a tentative model of the peptide–class I complex.

As informative of the postulated interactions between the peptides and the MHC proteins as these experiments were, they did not involve an assay that directly measured MHC binding. Two groups have attempted to define the orientation of peptide determinants when part of the complex, by correlating the inability of natural determinants containing point substitutions to stimulate the T-cell clone with their capacity to bind the restriction element. Their logic was that if a substitution of an amino acid eliminated T-cell recognition, but not its capacity to bind the restriction element, then that residue must be oriented so that it does not contact the MHC protein. If the substitution eliminated the T-cell response and also its ability to bind the class II protein, then that residue makes an important contact with the restriction element. Allen and his colleagues used this strategy to explore the interactions between $1-A^k$ and a lysozyme peptide (Allen et al 1987). Individual substitution of every position in the peptide sequence with alanine generated a family of analogues whose ability to bind the purified class II molecule and/or stimulate a T-cell clone provided sufficient information to allow a helical conformation of the bound peptide to be postulated. However, the results of a more extensive study using a similar strategy to dissect a helper determinant in ovalbumin failed to identify residues unequivocally interacting with either macromolecule (Sette et al 1987). Consequently, a regular conformation could not be identified, primarily because the majority of peptides containing single substitutions were still able to bind the class II protein.

Even though Grey and his colleagues interpreted their data as proof that the peptide did not bind as a helix (Sette et al 1987), we reasoned that if, as previously emphasized, the structure of the antigen-combining site of the MHC molecule has evolved to bind multiple, unrelated peptides, then the ability to tolerate many point substitutions in a peptide with only slight effects on the apparent affinity of binding might not be surprising. Consequently, an unnaturally large side-chain might cause greater steric interference with binding than substitution with any natural amino acid, thereby allowing us to observe a greater reduction in binding upon altering a critical residue.

In the model of the complex we proposed (Rothbard et al 1988), the side-chains of the amino acids composing the upper face of a helical peptide extend out of the antigen-combining site and the residues which form the opposite facade and the sides of the helix make important contacts with complementary residues of the HLA molecule. Substitution of individual residues of the peptide by a bulky amino acid should differentially affect the stability of the complex depending on the steric requirements of each contact and the relative importance of each amino acid in binding.

To test this hypothesis, a set of peptides containing a derivative of biotinylated lysine with an additional hydrocarbon spacer, long-chain biotin (LCB) (Hofmann et al 1982), substituted for each residue of the haemagglutinin peptide was synthesized. This modification was chosen not only for usefulness for this application, but also for the development of an assay to detect immunogenic peptides binding to MHC class II molecules on the surface of intact cells. The latter assay is integral to this discussion and needs to be explained.

The initial experiments used a T-cell determinant from influenza haemagglutinin (HA; residues 307–319) (Rothbard et al 1988), which was recognized by a HLA-DR1 restricted T-cell clone. The peptide was biotinylated on the alpha amino group and assayed for its ability to bind Epstein–Barr virus transformed human B lymphocytes (B-LCL) homozygous for HLA-DR1. These cells were chosen because they were homozygous, well-characterized cell lines that express unusually high levels of HLA class II proteins. Because of concerns of high background fluorescence and a low specific signal, the peptide was not directly fluoresceinated. Instead, it was conjugated to a biotinyl group to take advantage of the amplification that can be obtained by using multiply fluoresceinated streptavidin.

When the DR1-homozygous B-LCL, MAJA, was incubated with the peptide, stained with fluoresceinated streptavidin, and analysed for green fluorescence by flow cytometry, the cell surface fluorescence was approximately five times higher than in the absence of peptide (Fig. 16.1a). The signal was two orders of magnitude less intense than that obtained by indirect immunofluorescence with a monoclonal antibody specific for a determinant present on many human class II molecules.

All detectable fluorescence was shown to be specific by using RJ 2.2.5 cells (Accolla 1983). These cells, like the MAJA line, are human B-lymphoblastoid cells transformed by Epstein–Barr virus, except that they do not express class II proteins because of a mutation in a regulatory protein required for class II expression (Hume et al 1987). Consequently, they provide an excellent control for the specificity of the fluorescent signal, because they should display an identical cell surface except for the absence of MHC class II proteins. When RJ 2.2.5 cells were used in the assay, the fluorescence in the presence of peptide was indistinguishable from background (Fig. 16.1b). This demonstrated that the fluorescent signal on the cells expressing DR1 was entirely specific and strongly suggested that the peptide bound to class II MHC proteins or other proteins whose expression was co-regulated.

L cells transfected with genes encoding α and β chains of human class II molecules (Lechler et al 1988) were used to demonstrate that the peptide binds to HLA-DR. A distinct fluorescent signal was observed when the HA peptide was incubated with cells transfected with DR1, but absent on normal L cells (Fig. 16.1c). In contrast, the fluorescence on L cells expressing DQw1 was indistinguishable from that of untransfected cells (data not shown). However, because the level of DQ expression on these transfectants was low, the possibility that the peptide can weakly interact with DQ cannot be ruled out.

Further evidence that the peptide directly interacted with HLA-DR on the surface of B-LCL was that the fluorescent signal could be modulated by co-incubating the B-LCL with peptide and an anti-DR monoclonal antibody (Shackelford et al 1983). Increasing amounts of antibody progressively reduced the fluorescent signal (Fig. 16.2a). The reduction of the fluorescent signal closely paralleled the saturation of cell surface DR1 by the antibody (Fig. 16.2b), supporting the conclusion that the fluorescent signal is due exclusively to a peptide–MHC class II complex.

The natural determinant also was shown to compete with the biotinylated peptide, demonstrating that both occupy the same site on DR1. Half inhibition could be obtained at a seven-fold molar excess of the competitor over the biotinylated peptide (Fig. 16.2c). As the concentration of the competitor was increased, the fluorescence decreased, reaching 80% inhibition at a molar ratio of 110. A higher excess of competitor could not be obtained because of the limited solubility of the natural determinant and the need for relatively large μmol/l amounts of biotinylated peptide in order to observe a distinct fluorescent signal.

The ease of the assay and the availability of the homozygous B-LCL allowed us to examine the ability of the biotinylated HA peptide to bind to 22 cell lines expressing different DR types (Fig. 16.3). Remarkably, even though the fluorescent signal (Fig. 16.3a) significantly varied between cell lines, detectable fluorescence distinct from background was present in each case with the exception of the

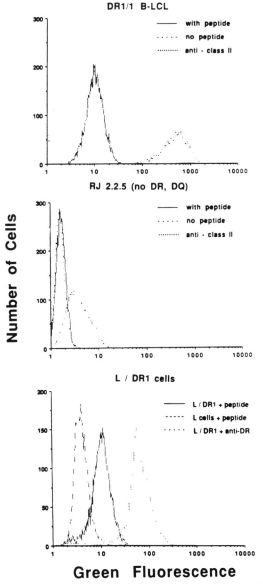

Green Fluorescence

Figure 16.1 Binding of a biotinylated analogue of HA 307–319 to surfaces of B cells transformed by Epstein–Barr virus. (a) The DR-homozygous B-LCL, MAJA (HLA-A2,3, B35, C4, Bw6, DR1 Dw1, DQw1, DP4) was incubated with HA 307–319 containing long chain biotin at the amino terminus and stained with FITC-streptavidin (———). Surface expression of class II MHC proteins was shown by indirect immunofluorescence using the anti HLA-D mAb. 31.1 (DeKretser et al 1982) (......). Background fluorescence in the absence of biotinylated peptide was determined by incubation only with streptavidin (. . . . .). (b) Binding of the HA analogue (—) and 31.1 mAb (.....) to the class II-deficient B-cell line, RJ 2.2.5 (Accolla 1983) HLA-A3, 19; B51, 35; C3,4; Bw4, 6; DR, DQ-negative; DP-low). Fluorescence in the absence of peptide (. . . . .) is indistinguishable from fluorescence with peptide. (c) Binding of the biotinylated HA peptide to L cells transfected with HLA-DR1. Transfectants (clone 5–3.1, Lechler et al 1988) (———) or untransfected L cells (- - - - -) were incubated with 100 µmol/l peptide overnight. The levels of DR expression (.....) on the transfected L cells were measured by indirect immunofluorescence using the anti-DR monoclonal antibody, L243 (Shackelford et al 1983)

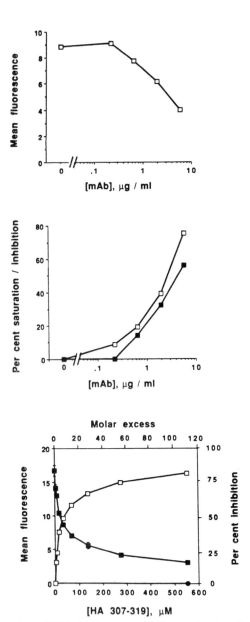

Figure 16.2 Inhibition of peptide binding by an anti-DR monoclonal antibody and the natural HA determinant. (a) MAJA cells were grown in heat-treated serum, incubated with the peptide (50 μmol/l). In the presence of varying amounts of purified L243 anti-DR antibody, stained, and analysed as in Figure 16.1. Results are displayed as mean fluorescence per cell minus background (approx. 2 at all concentrations of L243). At concentrations above 10 μg/ml, the antibody agglutinated the cells. (b) Comparison of the reduction in fluorescent signal by L243 (■) and the fraction of DR molecules bound by antibody (□) as determined by indirect immunofluorescence using varying amounts of L243 as in (a), followed by fluoresceinated rabbit anti-mouse Ig. (c) MAJA cells were co-incubated with the biotinylated HA analogue and varying amounts of HA 307–319 (shown as molarity and molar excess on bottom and top axes, respectively). Both the fluorescence (■; scale on left) and the fractional reduction in fluorescent signal (□; scale on right) are shown. The unbiotinylated peptide had no effect on background fluorescence, which was subtracted. RJ 2.2.5 cells incubated with biotinylated peptide and competitor gave no signal (●)

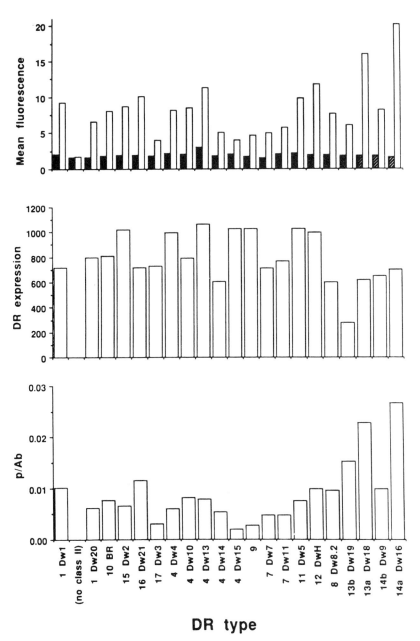

Figure 16.3 Binding of the HA peptide to B-LCL homozygous for different DR alleles. (a) Mean fluorescence on cell lines homozygous for the DR types indicated, when incubated with peptide (□) and without peptide (■). The cell lines used (haplotypes in brackets) were MAJA (DR1 Dw1), LWAGS (DR1 Dw20), EFI-ND (10BR), PGF (DR15 Dw2), WT18 (DR16 Dw21), WT20 (DR17 Dw3), PRIESS (DR4 Dw4), AL10 (DR4 Dw10), JHF (DR4 Dw13), PE117 (DR4 Dw14), HIN-ND (DR4 Dw15), KOZ (DR9), MANN (DR7 Dw7), DBB (DR7 Dw11), IDF (DR11 Dw5), HERLUF (DR12 Dw H), OLL (DR8 Dw8.2), DAUDI (DR13b Dw19), ARNT (DR13a Dw18), WT52 (DR14b Dw9), and AZL (DR14a Dw16). (b) Mean fluorescence on the same cells stained with directly fluoresceinated L243 anti-DR monoclonal antibody (Becton-Dickinson). (c) Relative peptide binding (from panel a) divided by relative antibody binding (from panel b)

class II-deficient cell line. The variation in fluorescence could not be explained by differences in DR expression between cell lines (shown in Fig. 16.3b). When peptide binding was corrected for these variations by dividing the fluorescence obtained with peptide by that obtained with the anti-DR monoclonal antibody (Fig. 16.3c), significant differences between cell lines remained, which allowed classification of the cells into groups having haplotypes with high (DR14a Dw16, DR13a Dw18, DR13b Dw19, DR16 Dw21) low (DR17 Dw3, DR9, DR4 Dw15), or intermediate (all others) capacity to associate with the HA peptide.

Even the lowest levels of cell surface fluorescence measured in this assay are relevant to T-cell responsiveness: DR4 Dw15 expressing cells, which bound the biotinylated HA analogue most weakly, presented the natural HA determinant to an HA-specific T lymphocyte clone equally well over a range of concentrations as the autologous restriction element, DR1 Dw1, which binds the biotinylated peptide at intermediate levels. (J. Rothbard et al 1989). This does not imply that, either in a natural infection or in the presence of a spectrum of competitive peptides, the quantitative differences in peptide binding to the DR alleles might not be an important factor determining immune responsiveness.

We do not believe that the broad specificity of binding reported here is unique to the HA peptide. Four other T-cell determinants also bind the 22 B-LCL, but the high-binding alleles are not identical for each peptide (Busch et al submitted). If generally true, these results indicate that a major factor in MHC restriction of T-cell recognition must arise from MHC–T-cell receptor interactions (Davis & Bjorkman 1988) and not simply from different capacities to bind peptide (Guillet et al 1987).

The assay also can be used to explore the conformation of the peptide when part of the MHC complex. When peptides containing lysine–LCB at each position were incubated with the cells, marked differences were seen in the resultant fluorescent signal (Fig. 16.4a). Strong fluorescence was present when lysine-LCB was placed either at the amino terminus or substituted for proline 307, lysine 308, valine 310, asparagine 313, lysine 316, and alanine 318. In contrast, no detectable fluorescence was observed when peptides containing lysine–LCB at residues 311 and 312 were used, while substitution at 309, 314, 315, or 317 resulted in reduced fluorescence.

A loss of the fluorescent signal upon biotinylating any residue might occur because the ability of the peptide to bind to DR1 is reduced by the modification, or because the peptide still binds but with the biotinyl group sterically unavailable to streptavidin. In the latter case, no fluorescent signal should be apparent at any concentration, because steric inaccessibility should not depend on the amount of peptide in the assay. The appearance of a fluorescent signal when analogues containing lysine–LCB at 309, 311, and 312 were used at concentrations well above 50 µmol/l (data not shown) indicated that biotinylation affected the apparent affinity of the analogues for DR1.

The ability of the analogues to bind to the restriction element on cell surfaces could have been affected by the biotinylation in a number of ways: (1) by interfering with a critical contact between the peptide and the class II proteins; (2) by altering the propensity of the peptide to adopt the conformation in which it bound to DR1; or (3) by changing the susceptibility of the analogue to proteolytic

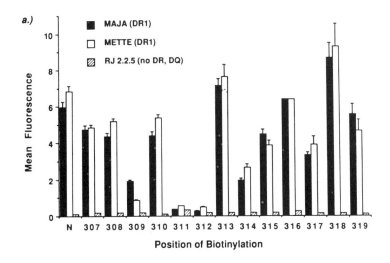

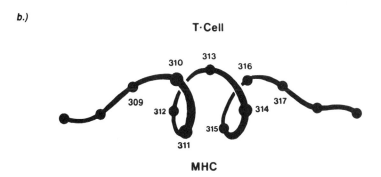

Figure 16.4 Differential binding of analogues of HA 307–319, biotinylated at each position, to DR1-homozygous, EBV-transformed B cells. (a) Each peptide (50 mmol/l was incubated with transformed B cells homozygous for DR1 Dw1 (MAJA [■] and METTE [□]) or the DR-negative B-cell line, RJ2.2.5 [■], stained, and analysed by flow cytometry. The relative amount of peptide bound to cells was judged by the intensity of green fluorescence per cell, averaged over all viable cells. Background as determined by control incubations in the absence of biotinylated peptide was subtracted. The results shown are the average of three assays with the standard deviation displayed with error bars. (b) Model of the conformation adopted by the peptide when bound to DR1, deduced from the binding results shown in (a). Residues 309–317 are folded into an a-helix, with an orientation that permits residues 310, 313, and 316 to point away from, while 309, 311, 312, 314, 315, and 317 would be directed towards the antigen-combining site. The amino-acids at both termini, which tolerate biotinylation, are not drawn as part of the helix because of their apparent conformational flexibility

degradation. The second possibility was unlikely because each of the 14 peptide analogues had indistinguishable circular dichroism spectra (data not shown) in trifluoroethanol (TFE)/water mixtures containing TFE concentrations at which the helical propensities of closely related, unbiotinylated HA analogues were significantly different (see below). The third possible explanation for the different fluorescent signals generated by each analogue, differential proteolysis, was more difficult to disprove. However, none of the low fluorescent signals was increased in the presence of a cocktail of protease inhibitors (TPCK, PMSF, leupeptin, aprotinin, and soybean trypsin inhibitor). Therefore, the differences in fluorescence appear to arise from the varying capacity of the class II molecule to bind the analogues, reflecting the differential effect of biotinylation at each position on the affinity of the interaction.

If this interpretation is true, then the assay provides a quantitative measure of the involvement of each amino acid of the peptide in the formation of the complex: the lower the signal, the more important the amino acid is. Therefore we can conclude that tyrosine 309, lysine 311, glutamine 312, and, to a lesser extent threonine 314, leucine 315, and leucine 317 contribute to the formation of the complex.

The peptide might bind to DR1 in a variety of ways. However, the distinct variations in fluorescence observed when the different analogues were assayed implied that the number of conformations and orientations of the bound peptide was limited. In all possible modes of binding, residues 311 and 312 form critical contacts with the restriction element, because biotinylation at these positions eliminated the fluorescent signal at the peptide concentration used. A further constraint on the possible conformations of the bound peptide was that the fluorescent profile peaked at every third residue (310, 313 and 316) within the central portion of the peptide, with significantly less fluorescence in between. The periodicity suggested that the central core adopted a helical conformation. However, the results were not consistent with the peptide being helical over its entire length because analogues containing lysine-LCB at 308 and 318 resulted in a strong signal. If the peptide adopted a perfect helix with 310, 313, and 316 pointing up, these residues should point down. The ability to tolerate substitution with biotinylated lysine at both ends of the peptide might be explained by an increased accessibility of the termini of the helix or by deviations from an ideal a-helix. A model based on this interpretation of the pattern of fluorescence is shown in Figure 16. 3b, consisting of a helical core (residues 309–317), with the two amino acids at each end of the peptide exhibiting greater conformational freedom and not modelled as part of the repeating structure.

Obviously we are examining whether the set of biotinylated peptides binds purified HLA DR1 in a similar manner as found on the surface of cells. Even though we believe that based on preliminary experiments, they shall, this is clearly a necessary part of the investigation. Whether the haemagglutinin peptide adopts this conformation when bound by other DR alleles is also being examined. In addition, similar analyses of other defined T-cell determinants can easily be performed and will reveal whether the behaviour of this peptide represents a general mode of binding or just one of many variations of a peptide–MHC complex. Regardless of the results, the described assays in this report appear to have tremendous potential to identify quickly the peptide residues most critical in binding MHC proteins and represents a new strategy, which when combined with other described methods, should allow investigators to generate working models of MHC–peptide interactions. These in turn can be used rationally to design peptides and isosteric chemical analogues which should be capable of specifically binding individual HLA alleles. Such compounds represent the next generation of immune modulators and might be important therapeutics for both allergies and autoimmune syndromes.

Our collective understanding of this extraordinary system of molecular recognition has transformed this section of immunology from confusing phenomenological observations to one of the best-defined ligand receptor interactions yet known.

REFERENCES

Accolla R 1983 Human B cell variants immunoselected against a single Ia antigen subset have lost expression of several Ia antigen subsets. J Exp Med 157: 1053–1060

Allen P, Matsueda G, Evans R, Dunbar J, Marshall G, Unanue E 1987 Identification of the T cell and Ia contact residues of a T cell antigenic epitope. Nature 327: 713–716

Babbitt B, Allen P, Matsueda G, Haber E, Unanue E 1985 The binding of immunogenic peptides to Ia histocompatibility molecules. Nature 317: 359–362

Bjorkman P, Saper M, Samraoul B, Bennett W, Strominger J, Wiley D 1987a Structure of the human class I histocompatibility antigen, HLA-A2. Nature 329: 506–511

Bjorkman P, Saper M, Samraoul B, Bennett W, Strominger J, Wiley D 1987b The foreign antigen binding site and T cell recognition regions of class I histocompatibility antigens. Nature 329: 512–517

Busch R, Howland K, Fenton C, Rothbard J Binding of peptides to MHC class II proteins on B cell surfaces. (submitted)

Buus S, Sette A, Colon S, Miles C, Grey H 1986 Isolation and characterisation of antigen-Ia complexes in T cell recognition. Cell 47: 1071–1076

Buus S, Sette A, Colon S, Miles C, Grey H 1987 The relation between major histocompability complex (MHC) restriction and the capacity of Ia to bind immunogenic peptides. Science 235: 1353–1357

Buus S, Setta A, Colon S, Miles C, Grey H 1988 Autologous peptides constitutively occupy the antigen binding site on Ia. Science 242: 1045–1046

Ceppellini R, Frumento G, Ferrara G, Tosi R, Chersi A, Pernis B Binding of labeled influenza matrix peptide 17–29 to HLA-DR in living B lymphoid cells. (submitted)

Davis M, Bjorkman P 1988 T cell antigen receptor genes and T cell recognition. Nature 334: 395–400

DeKretser T et al 1982 Demonstration of two distinct light chains in HLA-DR associated antigens by two-dimensional gel electrophoresis. Eur J Immunol 12: 214–221

DeLisi C, Berzofsky J 1985 T cell antigenic sites tend to be amphipathic structures. Proc Natl Acad Sci USA 82: 7048–7052

Guillet J, Lai M, Briner J, Buus S, Sette A, Grey H, Smith J, Gefter M 1987 Immunological self, non-self. Science 235: 865–870

Hofmann K, Titus G, Montibeller J, Finn F 1982 Avidin binding of carboxyl substituted biotin and analogues. Biochemistry 21: 978–982

Honjo T 1983 Immunoglobulin genes. Annu Rev Immunol 1: 499–528

Hume C, Accolla R, Lee J 1987 Defective HLA class II expression in a regulatory mutant is partially complemented by activated ras oncogenes. Proc Natl Acad Sci USA 84: 8603–8607

Lechler R, Bal V, Rothbard J, Germain R, Sekaly R, Long E, Lamb J 1988 HLA-DR restricted antigen induced activation of human helper T lymphocyte clone using transfected murine cell lines. J Immunol 141: 3003–3007

Moller O (ed) 1987 Role of somatic mutation in the generation of lymphocyte diversity. Immunol Rev 96: 1–162

Rothbard J, Taylor W 1988 A sequence pattern common to T cell epitopes. EMBO J 7: 93–98

Rothbard J, Lechler R, Howland K, Fenton C, Rothbard J 1988 Structural model of HLA-DR1 restricted T cell antigen recognition. Cell 52: 515–523

Rothbard J, Pemberton R, Bodmer H, Askonas B, Taylor W 1989 Identification of residues necessary for clonally specific recognition of a cytotoxic T cell determinant. EMBO J (in press)

Sadegh-Nasseri S, McConnell H 1989 A kinetic intermediate in the reaction of an antigenic peptide and I-E^k. Nature 337: 274–275

Sette A, Buus S, Colon S, Smith J, Miles C, Grey H 1987 Structural characteristics of an antigen required for its interaction with Ia and recognition by T cells. Nature 28: 395–399

Shackelford D, Lampson L, Strominger J 1983 Separation of three class II antigens from a homozygous human B cell line. J Immunol 130: 289–294

Watts T, McConnell H 1986 High affinity fluorescent peptide binding to I-A^d in lipid membranes. Proc Natl Acad Sci USA 83: 9660–9664

Index

United Nations Children's Fund (UNICEF) 222
Uracil 245–52
Uracil phosphoribosyltransferase 247, 248

Variant surface glycoproteins (VSG) 25, 102–10
anatomy of molecule 122–5
antigen expression by metacyclic stage 108–10
as macromolecular diffusion barrier 121–2
discussion 141–3
gene conversion 106
gene expression sites 106–8
gene repertoire 105–6
genes for 104–5
GPI anchor 126–9
M-VSGs 108–10

membrane attachment of *T. brucei* 121–40
N-glycosylation 124
primary amino-acid sequence 122–3
sequence diversity 117
subgroups 123–4
three-dimensional structure 124–5
Veterinary parasitology 3–16
Veterinary vaccines 15

Walsh/Warren test criteria of morbidity and mortality 233
World Health Organization 217, 218
Wuchereria 228

Yellow fever 229

Zea mays 277